Analysis of Drugs and Metabolites by Gas Chromatography – Mass Spectrometry

ANALYSIS OF DRUGS AND METABOLITIES
BY GAS CHROMATOGRAPHY-MASS SPECTROMETRY

VOLUME 1: Respiratory Gases, Volatile Anesthetics, Ethyl Alcohol, and Related Toxicological Materials

VOLUME 2: Hypnotics, Anticonvulsants, and Sedatives

VOLUME 3: Antipsychotic, Antiemetic, and Antidepressant Drugs

VOLUME 4: Central Nervous System Stimulants

VOLUME 5: Analgesics, Local Anesthetics, and Antibiotics

VOLUME 6: Cardiovascular, Antihypertensive, Hypoglycemic, and Thyroid-Related Agents

IN PREPARATION

VOLUME 7: Natural, Pyrolytic, and Metabolic Products of Tobacco and Marijuana

OTHER VOLUMES IN PREPARATION

ANALYSIS OF DRUGS AND METABOLITES BY GAS CHROMATOGRAPHY–MASS SPECTROMETRY

VOLUME 6
Cardiovascular, Antihypertensive, Hypoglycemic, and Thyroid-Related Agents

Benjamin J. Gudzinowicz
*Department of Pathology
Rhode Island Hospital
Providence, Rhode Island*

Michael J. Gudzinowicz
*Center in Toxicology
Department of Biochemistry
School of Medicine
Vanderbilt University
Nashville, Tennessee*

With the Assistance of

Horace F. Martin

*Department of Pathology, Rhode Island Hospital
Providence, Rhode Island
and
Division of Biological and Medical Sciences
Brown University, Providence, Rhode Island*

and

James L. Driscoll
Joanne Hologgitas

*Department of Pathology, Rhode Island Hospital
Providence, Rhode Island*

MARCEL DEKKER, INC.,   New York and Basel

Library of Congress Cataloging in Publication Data (Revised)

Gudzinowicz, Benjamin J.
  Analysis of drugs and metabolites by gas
chromatography--mass spectrometry.

  Includes bibliographical references and indexes.
  CONTENTS: v. 1. Respiratory gases, volatile
anesthetics, ethyl alcohol, and related toxicological
materials.--v. 2. Hypnotics, anticonvulsants, and
sedatives.--v. 3. Antipsychotic, antiemetic, and
antidepressant drugs. [etc.]
  1. Drugs--Analysis. 2. Gas chromatography,
3. Mass spectrometry. 4. Drug metabolism.
I. Gudzinowicz, Michael J., joint author. II. Title. [DNLM: 1. Drugs--Analysis. 2. Chromatography, Gas. 3. Spectrum analysis, Mass.
QV25.G923a]
RS189.G83   615'.1901   76-56481
ISBN 0-8247-6757-8(V.6)

COPYRIGHT © 1979 by MARCEL DEKKER, INC. ALL RIGHTS RESERVED

Neither this book nor any part may be reproduced or transmitted in any form or by any means, electronic or mechanical, including photocopying, microfilming, and recording, or by any information storage and retrieval system, without permission in writing from the publisher.

MARCEL DEKKER, INC.
270 Madison Avenue, New York, New York 10016

Current printing (last digit):
10 9 8 7 6 5 4 3 2 1

PRINTED IN THE UNITED STATES OF AMERICA

Dedicated to

HELEN L. GUDZINOWICZ
a devoted and understanding wife and mother

PREFACE

In the past two decades, remarkable progress has been made in the analysis of drugs, pharmaceuticals, and related toxicological materials. In great measure, these notable advances can be attributed to technological advancements in two specific types or areas of analytical instrumentation; namely, gas chromatography and integrated gas chromatography-mass spectrometry.

Since James and Martin revealed to the scientific community their gas chromatographic technique which permitted the separation of fatty acid mixtures into their individual components, the rapid growth of gas chromatography has been very evident. This remarkable progress can be directly correlated with the improvements that we have witnessed over the years in gas chromatographic stationary phase, carrier gas, column, and temperature- and pressure-controlling technology. Furthermore, it has assumed a position of even greater analytical significance since the advent of highly specific, rapid, sensitive detection systems.

On the other hand, the integrated GC-MS analytical system is rather unique and exceptional in that it combines the mass spectrometer's unexcelled identification potential with the gas chromatograph's separation capabilities. Although the integration of GC and MS was first reported in 1957 by Holmes and Morrell, it nevertheless remained a dormant, costly, and seemingly unappreciated technique until 1970. Since then, with improved instrumentation at a more reasonable price and newly developed operating techniques, numerous publications have appeared in the literature showing its applicability to a wide variety of difficult analytical problems, thus opening up new horizons for analytical research in toxicology, biochemistry, pharmacology, forensics, medicine, etc. To be able to monitor a drug, its persistence and metabolic fate in biological fluids of man via mass fragmentography at picogram concentration levels provides the researcher with a tool of immeasurable significance.

PREFACE

Because much has been written over the years about the analysis of drugs and their metabolites by either or both techniques, the objectives of these volumes are several-fold: (1) to compile from existing literature in a chronological manner the various GC and/or GC-MS procedures available for the analysis of specific drugs and their metabolites, (2) to describe with as much detail as possible all procedures (qualitative and quantitative) in order that they might be reproduced faithfully in one's laboratory, and (3) to indicate, wherever possible, not only the results, precision, accuracy, and limits of detection achieved by a given procedure, but also its applicability to pharmacokinetic studies. For this reason, in addition to the text, which is well referenced in each section, many illustrations of actual applications and tables of data for each instrumental technique are included as aids to the analyst for his greater appreciation and understanding of the limitations as well as potentials ascribed to each method. As stated in the past, from an analytical chemist's point of view, it is hoped that this deliberately combined visual and factual approach will find acceptance by the reader who would otherwise rely only on his interpretation of the written word relative to some published procedure.

Without wishing to be repetitious, in retrospect it must be again stated that this volume really represents the end result of many tedious and arduous investigations by numerous eminent scientists whose research efforts have appeared in the literature throughout the world. We are indeed humbly indebted to them, and to those journals, publishers, and organizations that granted special copyright permission to the authors.

Benjamin J. Gudzinowicz
Michael J. Gudzinowicz

CONTENTS

Preface v

Contents of Other Volumes ix

Chapter 1. CARDIOVASCULAR DRUGS 1

    I. Digitalis-Type Glycosides 1
    II. Antiarrhythmic Agents 32
    III. Coronary Vasodilators 137
    IV. Coumarin-Type Anticoagulants 165
    V. Diuretics 194
    VI. Antisclerosis (Antihyperlipidemia) Drugs 218
    References 238

Chapter 2. ANTIHYPERTENSIVE, HYPOGLYCEMIC, AND THYROID-RELATED DRUGS 255

    I. Antihypertensive Drugs 255
    II. Hypoglycemic Agents 288
    III. Thyroid Hormones and Drugs 343
    References 384

Author Index 389

Subject Index 409

CONTENTS OF OTHER VOLUMES

Volume 1 RESPIRATORY GASES, VOLATILE ANESTHETICS, ETHYL ALCOHOL, AND RELATED TOXICOLOGICAL MATERIALS

    Chapter 1. Respiratory Gases, Volatile Anesthetics, and Related Toxicological Materials

    Chapter 2. Ethyl Alcohol and Volatile Trace Components in Breath, Body Fluids, and Body Tissues

Volume 2 HYPNOTICS, ANTICONVULSANTS, AND SEDATIVES

    Chapter 1. Hypnotics, Anticonvulsants, and Sedatives: Barbiturate Compounds

    Chapter 2. Hypnotics, Anticonvulsants, and Sedatives: Nonbaributate Compounds

    Chapter 3. Hypnotics, Anticonvulsants, and Sedatives: Nonbarbiturate Compounds (Continued)

Volume 3 ANTIPSYCHOTIC, ANTIEMETIC, AND ANTIDEPRESSANT DRUGS

    Chapter 1. Antipsychotic and Antiemetic Drugs: Phenothiazine, Butyrophenone, and Thioxanthene Derivatives

    Chapter 2. Antidepressant Drugs: Monoamine Oxidase Inhibitors, Tricyclic Antidepressants, and Several Related Compounds

Volume 4 CENTRAL NERVOUS SYSTEM STIMULANTS

Chapter 1. Amphetamines, Xanthines, and Related Compounds

Chapter 2. Phenylethylamine-, Tryptamine-, and Propranolol-Related Compounds

Volume 5 ANALGESICS, LOCAL ANESTHETICS, AND ANTIBIOTICS

Chapter 1. Narcotics, Narcotic Antagonists, and Synthetic Opiate-like Drugs

Chapter 2. Antipyretic, Antiinflammatory, and Antihyperurlcemic Agents; Local Anesthetics; and Antibiotics

Volume 7 NATURAL, PYROLYTIC, AND METABOLIC PRODUCTS OF TOBACCO AND MARIJUANA

Chapter 1. Natural, Pyrolytic, and Carcinogenic Products of Tobacco

Chapter 2. Natural, Pyrolytic, and Metabolic Products of Marijuana

OTHER VOLUMES IN PREPARATION

Analysis of Drugs and Metabolites by Gas Chromatography–Mass Spectrometry

Chapter 1

CARDIOVASCULAR DRUGS

In this chapter, drugs with the ability to alter cardiovascular function will be considered: digitalis-type glycosides, antiarrhythmic, antianginal, anticoagulant, and diuretic drugs, as well as pharmacological approaches to atherosclerosis using agents aimed at altering hyperlipidemia.

I. DIGITALIS-TYPE GLYCOSIDES

As noted by Goth [1]:

> Certain steroids and their glycosides have characteristic effects on the contractility and electrophysiology of the heart. Most of these glycosides are obtained from the leaves of the foxglove, Digitalis purpurea or Digitalis lanata, or from the seeds of Strophanthus gratus. These cardioactive steroids [Fig. 1.1] are widely used in the treatment of heart failure and in the management of certain arrhythmias. They are collectively referred to as digitalis.
> Although catecholamines, methylxanthines, and glucagon also increase the contractility of the myocardium, digitalis must accomplish its effect by a unique mechanism and is by far the most important drug in the treatment of heart failure.

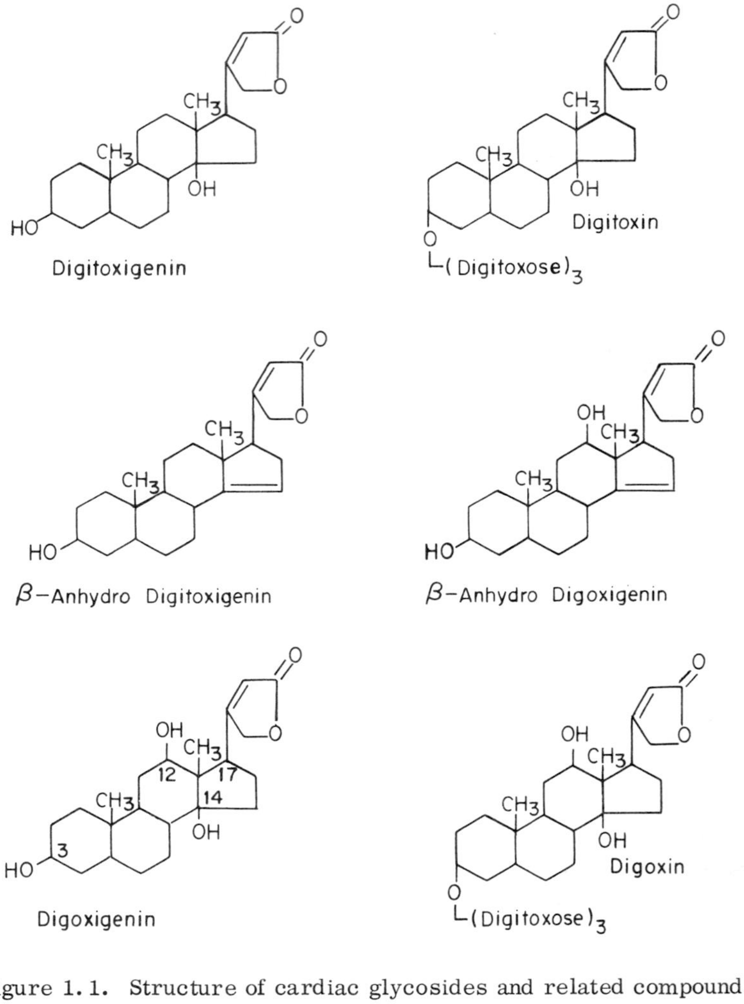

Figure 1.1. Structure of cardiac glycosides and related compounds.

In recent years various aspects of the pharmacokinetics of drugs have appeared in the literature and, in this regard, Chow and Ronfeld [2] compiled data for antibiotics and antiarrhythmics which included percent of drug absorbed intact, time of peak concentration, volume of distribution, elimination half-life (β phase), percent of drug excreted unchanged, renal clearance, and plasma binding. Such information for digitoxin and digoxin are as shown in Table 1.1.

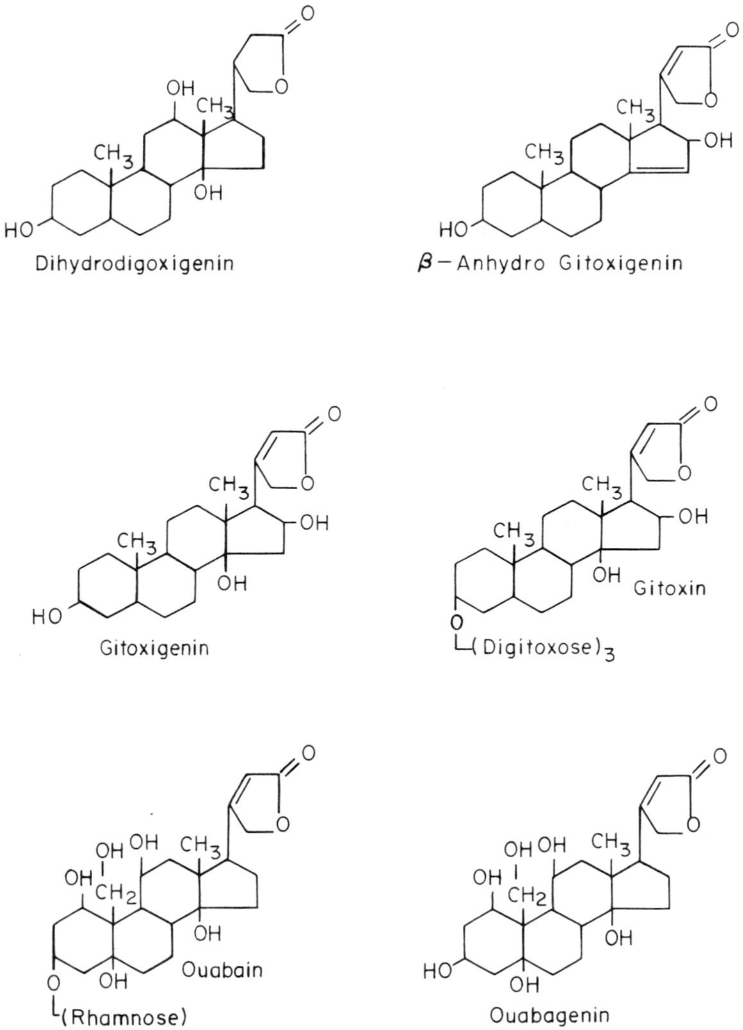

DIGITALIS-TYPE GLYCOSIDES

Figure 1.1. (continued)

Of the most commonly used glycosides, the structure of digitoxin is characterized by a steroid nucleus with an unsaturated lactone attached in the C-17 position. The three sugars attached to the C-3 position are unusual 20-deoxyhexoses. The molecule without the sugars is called an aglycone or genin. The steroidal structure and the unsaturated lactone are

TABLE 1.1

Pharmacokinetic Data for Digitoxin and Digoxin[a]

	Digitoxin	Digoxin
Percent absorbed intact	90-100 [3]	45-56 Lanoxin tablet [9,10] 67 Lanoxin elixir [9] 80-83 (IM) Lanoxin
Time of peak conc. (hr)	1 [4,5]	0.5-0.75 [9] 1-2 (IM) [9,11]
Volume of distribution V_d	35 liters[b] [6]	580 liters [12]
$t_{1/2}\ \beta$ phase (hr)	6 days [3,7]	36 [13]
Percent excreted unchanged	8 [6]	76 [9]
Renal clearance (ml/min)	Negligible	140[b]
Percent plasma protein binding	96 (bound to albumin) [8]	23 [8]
Therapeutic conc. (ng/ml)	15-20 [7]	0.76-1.60 [3]

[a]Adapted from Chow and Ronfeld [2].
[b]Calculated value.

essential for the characteristic cardioactive effect. On the other hand, as noted by Goth, digoxin differs from digitoxin in that its structure contains an OH group at the C-12 position whereas ouabain differs from both in its steroid portion; its aglycone is known as G-strophanthidin, and the sugar to which it is attached in the glycoside is rhamnose.

These and structurally related compounds were examined by gas chromatography as early as 1961, when Vanden Heuvel and Horning [14] undertook an investigation to determine the chromatographic behavior of the sapogenins, which are naturally occurring steroids that, in addition to a spiroketal system, have a varying degree of substitution with keto and hydroxyl groups.

With an argon ionization detector and a 6-ft by 5-mm column packed with 0.75% SE-30 on 100-140 mesh Gas Chrom P and operated isothermally at 225°C, the relative retention times of the compounds investigated all yielded single, well-defined peaks. The times are listed in Table 1.2.

Several correlations between structure and relative retention times

TABLE 1.2
Relative Retention Times of Various Sapogenins[a,b]

Compound	C_{25}[c]	C_5[d]	Substituents	Time[e]
Sarsasapogenin	Neo	β	3β-OH	2.57
Smilagenin	Iso	β	3β-OH	2.47
Yamogenin	Neo	Δ^5	3β-OH	2.66
Diosgenin	Iso	Δ^5	3β-OH	2.64
Tigogenin	Iso	α	3β-OH	2.71
Yuccagenin	Iso	Δ^5	$2\alpha, 3\beta\text{-}(OH)_2$	4.68
Gitogenin	Iso	α	$2\alpha, 3\beta\text{-}(OH)_2$	4.81
Chlorogenin	Iso	α	$3\beta, 6\alpha\text{-}(OH)_2$	5.40
Hecogenin	Iso	α	3β-OH 12-Keto	4.96
Mexogenin	Iso	β	$2\beta, 3\beta\text{-}(OH)_2$ 12-Keto	7.82
Manogenin	Iso	α	$2\alpha, 3\beta\text{-}(OH)_2$ 12-Keto	8.76
Kammogenin	Iso	Δ^5	$2\alpha, 3\beta\text{-}(OH)_2$ 12-Keto	8.33
Cholestane				1.00[f]

[a]From Vanden Heuvel and Horning [14], courtesy of the Journal of Organic Chemistry.
[b]Conditions: Column, 6 ft x 5 mm; 0.75% SE-30 polymer on 100/140 mesh Gas Chrom P; 225°C; 14 psi; argon ionization detector.
[c]The configurations are 25L or neo and 25D or iso.
[d]The notation refers to 5-H.
[e]Relative to cholestane.
[f]Time, 7.0 min.

were reported by Vanden Heuvel and Horning, based on the chromatographic retention time data. For example, they noted that:

1. An additional hydroxyl or carbonyl incorporated into the structure led to a very large increase in retention time.

2. Compounds with differing ring A/B relationship could be resolved (tigogenin and smilagenin).
3. Compounds with a Δ^5 structure gave retention times which differed from those noted for their corresponding saturated compounds.
4. A relatively small effect due to a change in configuration of the methyl group at C-25 was noted; this effect paralleled their observations on the behavior of C-25 epimers in the steroidal amine series.

Since a number of stereoid hormones are synthesized from sapogenins, the investigators postulated that these steroid transformation reactions could be monitored by gas chromatography.

Since the determination of the urinary excretion of digitalis compounds can improve dose control of digitalis in difficult clinical situations [15] and the aglycone moieties of digitalis compounds are steroids as evidenced by the structures of digitoxigenin and digoxigenin, Jelliffe and Blankenhorn [16] investigated their gas chromatographic behavior with a Barber Colman model 10 gas chromatograph equipped with an argon ionization detector and a 12-ft by 4-mm-i.d. glass column packed with 0.75% SE-30 coated onto 100-140 mesh, silanized Gas Chrom P. Whereas the free hydroxy compounds could not be chromatographed directly, trimethylsilyl (TMSi) ether derivatives of digitoxin, digoxin, digitoxigenin, and digoxigenin were prepared with hexamethyldisilazane and trimethylchlorosilane added to catalyze the reaction

$$2ROH + (CH_3)_3SiNHSi(CH_3)_3 \rightarrow 2ROSi(CH_3)_3 + NH_3 \qquad (1.1)$$

The digitoxigenin-TMSi and digoxigenin-TMSi derivatives (shown below) yielded single, reproducible, symmetrical peaks with the following operating parameters: column temperature, 228°C; detector temperature, 220°C; flash heater temperature, 348°C; detector voltage, 1000 V; argon carrier-gas flow rate, 104 ml/min; electrometer gain, 10^{-9} A. The retention times for cholestane (reference marker), digitoxigenin-TMSi, and digoxigenin-TMSi were 6.2, 37.5, and 47.5 min, respectively. However, no useful peaks were obtained for digitoxin, digoxin, and digoxigenin.

In 1967, Wilson, Johnson, Perkins, and Ripley [17] chromatographed on a single column the TMSi ether derivatives of digoxigenin, digoxigenin monodigitoxoside, digoxigenin bisdidigitoxoside, and digoxin as well as the free sterols digoxigenin, digitoxigenin, and gitoxigenin.

The aglycones of digoxin and digitoxin were determined quantitatively by hydrolyzing the glycosides in a dilute hydrochloric acid-dioxane solution followed by GC analysis of the TMSi derivatives of the resulting sterols. In their procedure, the TMSi derivatives were prepared by adding 1 ml of silanizing mixture (hexamethyldisilazane-trimethylchlorosilane-pyridine,

10:1:10 volume ratios) to the dry alcohol. The mixture was shaken intermittently for 30 min, transferred to a 2-ml septum-capped tube, and finally centrifuged at 2000 X g for 30 min, which sedimented the suspended particles. An aliquot of the clear solution was then injected into a Barber-Colman 5000 series gas chromatograph equipped with hydrogen flame detectors and three U-shaped columns: column A, 6 ft by 6 mm i.d., packed with 1% SE-30 coated on 80-100 mesh Gas Chrom Q; column B, 6 ft by 6 mm i.d., packed with 1.6% SE-30 on 80-100 mesh Gas Chrom Q; and column C, 1 ft by 4 mm i.d., packed with 1.6% SE-30 on 80-100 mesh Gas Chrom Q. Whereas the injection block temperature was maintained at column temperature, the detector temperature was 320°C for all runs except when temperature-programming was used; in this case the temperature was held at 340°C. The retention times of the various compounds on the different columns used are given in Table 1.3, which also includes the nitrogen carrier-gas flow rate, the type of column used, and its operating temperature.

Using temperature programming with column C (programming commenced 1 min after sample injection and proceeded at 6°C/min from 230 to 330°C) and a nitrogen carrier-gas flow rate of 60 ml/min, the retention times of digoxigenin TMSi ether, digoxigenin monodigitoxoside TMSi ether, digoxigenin bisdigitoxoside TMSi ether, and digoxin TMSi ether were 5.18, 11.80, 18.75, and 24.10 min, respectively.

TABLE 1.3

Retention Times of Sterol and Sterol-TMSi Derivatives[a]

Compound	Retention times (min)				
	Column A[b]	Column B[c]	Column B[d]	Column C[e]	Column C[f]
Digoxigenin		30.20			
Digitoxigenin		19.85			
Gitoxigenin		16.35			
Digoxigenin TMSi ether	1.89		20.60		
Digoxigenin monodigitoxoside TMSi ether	9.58			2.3	1.30
Digoxigenin bisdigitoxoside TMSi ether				10.30	5.08
Digoxin TMSi ether					18.70
Digitoxigenin TMSi ether			16.40		
Gitoxigenin TMSi ether			20.60		
Ouabain TMSi ether	15.67				

[a]Adapted from Wilson et al. [17].
[b]Column temperature, 285°C; nitrogen carrier-gas flow rate, 100 ml/min.
[c]Column temperature, 250°C; nitrogen carrier-gas flow rate, 100 ml/min.
[d]Column temperature, 250°C; nitrogen carrier-gas flow rate, 100 ml/min.
[e]Column temperature, 285°C; nitrogen carrier-gas flow rate, 100 ml/min.
[f]Column temperature, 300°C; nitrogen carrier-gas flow rate, 125 ml/min.

TABLE 1.4

Analysis of Sterol TMSi Ether Concentration[a]

Sterol TMSi ether chromatographed	Sample no.	Mμmoles of sample injected	Average peak area[b]	Relative standard deviation
Digoxigenin	1	3.12	46.1	±8.04
	2	6.66	131.4	±4.20
	3	9.07	194.9	±6.18
	4	12.93	286.2	±1.90
Digoxigenin (hydrolyzed)	1	1.91	15.1	±4.74
	2	12.35	271.3	±2.14
Digoxigenin (from hydrolyzed digoxin)	1	1.93	21.3	±3.54
	2	3.20	51.9	±5.57
	3	8.05	157.0	±6.82
	4	11.25	244.3	±6.23
Digitoxigenin	1	2.74	32.4	±5.72
	2	6.36	126.2	±7.68
	3	13.15	290.9	±2.45
Digitoxigenin (from hydrolyzed digitoxin)	1	3.96	62.0	±8.62
	2	6.94	139.1	±3.01
	3	11.92	262.2	±3.78

[a]From Wilson et al. [17], courtesy of <u>Analytical Chemistry</u>.
[b]Numbers representing peak areas derived from electronic counter in integrator used with gas chromatograph.

As reported by Wilson et al.:

In Table [1.4] are listed the results obtained from chromatographing varying quantities of digoxigenin TMSi ether. For each determination ten injections of 1 μl of sample and ten injections of only the corresponding syringe needle contents were performed. Peak areas were corrected for needle content, which accounted for approximately 6% of the total uncorrected peak areas.

Linearity of detector response and quantitative recovery of hydrolyzed glycoside aglycone TMSi ether are shown in Figure [1.2]. Quantitation of peak areas for unhydrolyzed digoxigenin TMSi ether involved measurement of only one peak, whereas hydrolyzed

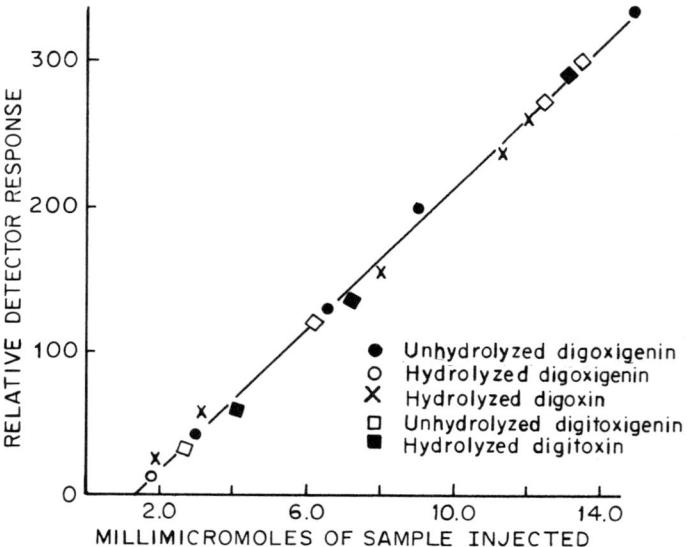

Figure 1.2. Linearity of detector response to TMSi ethers. From Wilson et al. [17], courtesy of <u>Analytical Chemistry</u>.

digoxigenin or hydrolyzed digoxin always yielded two peaks. When more than one peak occurred, the sum of the areas of both peaks was ascertained in computing the points presented in Figure [1.2].

From the four different concentrations of unhydrolyzed digoxigenin TMSi ether [Table 1.4] a standard reference line (best-fit line using the method of least squares) was found to conform to the equation: $y = -30.6 + 24.6x$. The equation for the line which includes all of the points determined for hydrolyzed digoxigenin and hydrolyzed digoxin was $y = -29.0 + 24.5x$. The correlation coefficient for these two sets of data was 0.99, which is indicative of a very high degree of dependability in their direct interrelationship.

The equation for a best-fit standard reference line which includes all points determined for digitoxigenin and hydrolyzed digitoxin was $y = -29.7 + 24.5x$.

The observation that the intercept of the best-fit straight line in Figure [1.2] occurs on the abscissa rather than at the origin indicates that some irreversible adsorption occurred on the column [18]. This, however, does not indicate incomplete conversion of the sterol to the TMSi ether, as has recently been reported for estrogens by Lau [19].

In 1968, Maume, Wilson, and Horning [20] also noted that cardenolides may be converted to volatile derivatives by silylation; the level of silylation being reagent dependent. For example, the use of hexamethyldisilazane-trimethylchlorosilane leads to TMSi ether formation for all relatively unhindered hydroxyl groups (3β, 12β, 16β). When bis(trimethylsilyl)acetamide-trimethylchlorosilane is employed, the unsaturated lactone ring is converted to an enol form, with subsequent formation of a TMSi enol ether. All hydroxyl groups, including the tertiary 14β-hydroxyl group and the enol derived from the lactone side chain, are converted to TMSi ethers with trimethylsilylimidazole-bis-(trimethylsilyl)acetamide-trimethylchlorosilane at 60°C.

The separation of the silyl derivatives were carried out with a Barber-Colman series 5000 gas chromatograph equipped with flame ionization detectors and 12-ft by 4-mm-i.d. W-shaped glass columns packed with either 1% SE-30 or 1% OV-17 coated on 100-120 mesh Gas Chrom P. Separations and determinations of methylene unit (MU) values listed in Table 1.5 were carried out by temperature programming at a rate of 1°C/min from 200 to 260°C (SE-30) or 230 to 290°C (OV-17). For their GC studies, the other operating parameters were injector temperature, 260°C; detector temperature, 300°C; nitrogen carrier-gas flow rate, 55 ml/min. Spectral investigations were performed with a LKB model 9000 integrated GC-MS instrument equipped with a 9-ft glass coiled column packed with 1% SE-30. The accelerating voltage was maintained at 70 eV to obtain mass spectra with the current and ion source temperature set at 60 μA and 250°C, respectively.

The use of HMDS-TMCS reagent led to the formation of a single major reaction product for digitoxigenin (D-2), digoxigenin (D-3) and gitoxigenin (G-3). The mass spectra indicated that this product was a mono-TMSi ether for digitoxigenin; di-TMSi ethers were formed for digoxigenin and gitoxigenin. The mass spectra (illustrated in Fig. 1.3 for digitoxigenin) contained in each instance an ion fragment corresponding to loss of 18 amu [M-18 and M-90-18 for digitoxigenin, and also M-90-90-18 for digoxigenin, gitoxigenin, and dihydrodigoxigenin (DHD-3)]. They noted that the conclusion to be drawn from these data is that the reaction occurred under these conditions for 3β-, 12β-, and 16β-hydroxyl groups, but not for the 14β-hydroxyl group or for the lactone group. This method for derivative formation is not recommended because the derivatives of digoxigenin and gitoxigenin are not separated with SE-30 or OV-17 columns (see Table 1.5 and Fig. 1.4).

The products obtained with the noncatalyzed BSA reagent were similar to those obtained when TMCS was added as catalyst. In each instance a single major reaction product was formed. The mass spectra indicated that the derivative from digitoxigenin contained two TMSi groups, and that the derivatives from digoxigenin and gitoxigenin contained three TMSi groups. Dihydrodigoxigenin, however, gave a derivative containing only two TMSi groups. The mass spectrum of the ether from D-2 (Fig. 1.5)

TABLE 1.5

MU Values of Silyl Derivatives of Cardenolides[a]

Compound	MU value[b]	
	SE-30	OV-17
Digitoxigenin (D-2)		
3β,14-Dihydroxy-5β-card-20(22)-enolide	34.45	
3β-trimethylsilyloxy	34.46	39.71
3β,23-di-(trimethylsilyloxy) (enol ether)	32.00	34.55
3β,14β,23-tri-(trimethylsilyloxy) (enol ether)	32.23	33.42
Digoxigenin (D-3)		
3β,12β,14-Trihydroxy-5β-card-20(22)-enolide	36.00	
3β,12β-di-(trimethylsilyloxy)	35.41	38.95
3β,12β,23-tri-(trimethylsilyloxy) (enol ether)	32.64	34.22
3β,12β,14β,23-tetra-(trimethylsilyloxy) (enol ether)	32.83	33.20
Gitoxigenin (G-3)		
3β,14,16β-Trihydroxy-5β-card-20(22)-enolide	33.91	
3β,16β-di-(trimethylsilyloxy)	35.41	39.07
3β,16β,23-tri-(trimethylsilyloxy) (enol ether)	32.93	34.47
3β,14β,16β,23-tetra-(trimethylsilyloxy) (enol ether)	32.85	33.23
Dihydrodigoxigenin (DHD-3)		
3β,12β,14-Trihydroxy-5β-cardenolide		
3β,12β-di-(trimethylsilyloxy)	34.33	37.87
3β,12β,14β-tri-(trimethylsilyloxy)	33.84	35.33

[a]From Maume et al. [20], courtesy of Marcel Dekker, Inc.
[b]Determined with 1% SE-30 and 1% OV-17 columns by temperature programming at a rate of 1°C/min.

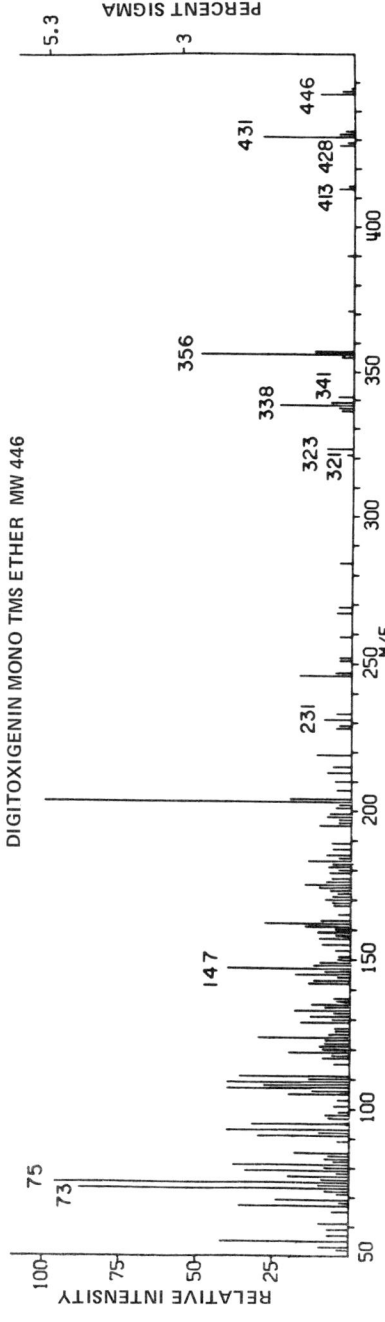

Figure 1.3. Mass spectrum for the mono TMSi ether of digitoxigenin (3-TMSi ether). Peaks providing structural information include those at the following amu values: 446 (M), 431 (M-15), 428 (M-18), 413 (M-18-15), 356 (M-90), 341 (M-90-15), 338 (M-90-18), 323 (M-90-18-15), 321 (M-side chain-D ring-H) and 231 (M-90-side chain-D ring-H). Peaks at 73, 75, and 147 amu are usually found in spectra for TMSi ethers of alicyclic and aliphatic alcohols. From Maume et al. [20], courtesy of Marcel Dekker, Inc.

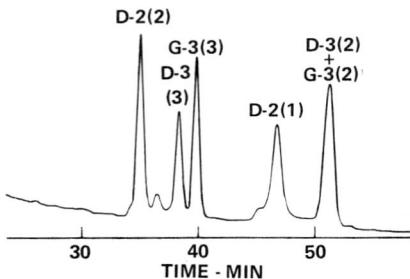

Figure 1.4. GLC separation of TMSi ethers resulting from the reaction of digitoxigenin, digoxigenin, and gitoxigenin with BSA-TMCS in pyridine. The TMSi ethers of the enol form of the lactone side chain are not stable under these conditions. The initial products of the reaction are the TMSi ethers shown in Figure 1.7 (D-2, D-3, G-3); these are gradually converted to simpler ethers with TMSi groups at positions 3, 12, and 16 only. The latter ethers are those of digitoxigenin (3-TMSi ether) [D-2 (1)], digoxigenin (3,12-di-TMSi ether) [D-3(2)], and gitoxigenin (3,16-di-TMSi ether) [G-3(2)]. The conditions were the same as those for the separation in Figure 1.7. From Maume et al. [20], courtesy of Marcel Dekker, Inc.

showed a peak at M-18, and a metastable ion peak at 483 amu (calculated for 518 $\xrightarrow{-18}$ 500, m* = 482.6). The derivatives from D-3 and G-3 showed peaks at M-18, M-90-18, and M-90-90-18, and a metastable ion peak at 571 amu (calculated for 606 $\xrightarrow{-18}$ 588, m* = 570.5). Peaks were also observed at M-72 for each derivative.

Finally, when TSIM-BSA-TMCS was used at 60°C as silylating reagent, reaction occurred for all hydroxyl groups and for the lactone ring, and a single reaction product was obtained for all cardenolides. The mass spectra (illustrated for D-2 in Fig. 1.6) showed no evidence of loss of 18 amu at any stage (the loss of 72 amu for enol ether cleavage was observed). These data indicate that the 14β-hydroxyl group, although a tertiary group, formed a TMSi ether under these conditions.

From the data in Table 1.5, it can be seen that the best GC separations of the TMSi derivatives were obtained using a SE-30 column and BSA-TMCS reagent; this separation is illustrated in Figure 1.7. As noted by the authors, the retention behavior of the derivatives observed with an OV-17

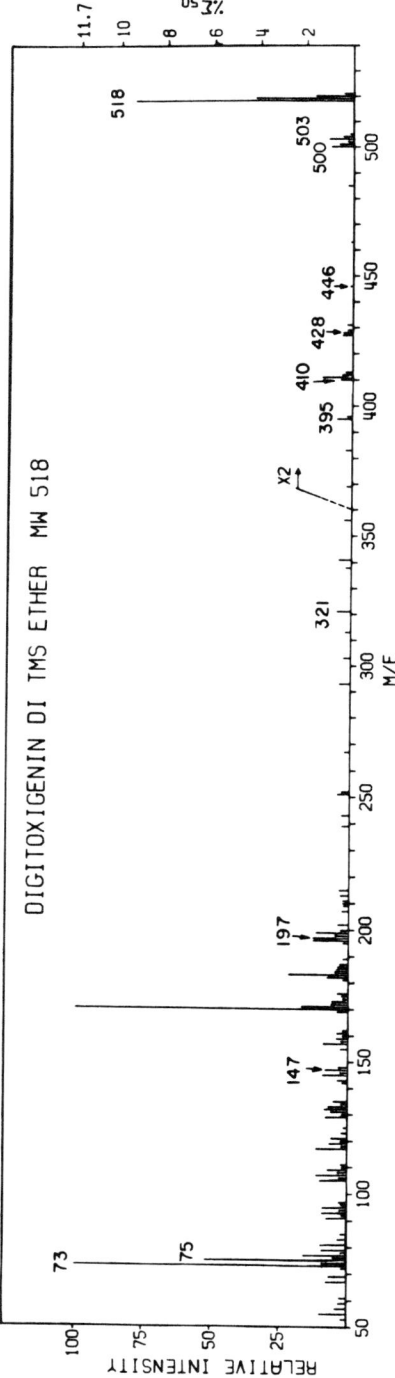

Figure 1.5. Mass spectrum for the di-TMSi ether of digitoxigenin (3,23-di-TMSi ether). Peaks providing structural information include those at the following amu values: 518 (M), 503 (M-15), 500 (M-18), 446 (M-72), 428 (M-72-18 and M-90), and 395 (M-90-18-15). From Maume et al. [20], courtesy of Marcel Dekker, Inc.

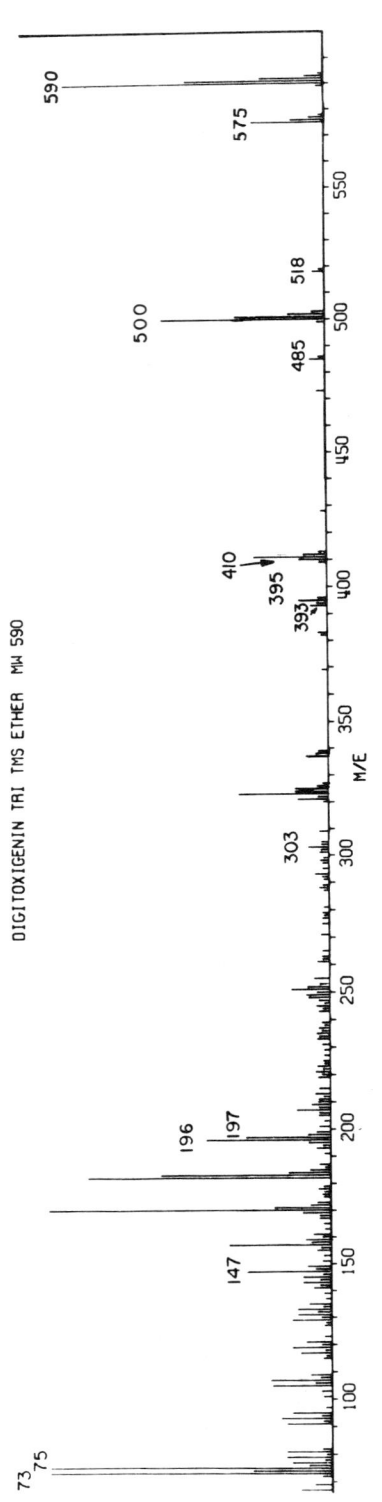

Figure 1.6. Mass spectrum for the tri-TMSi ether of digitoxigenin (3,14,23-tri-TMSi ether). Peaks providing structural information include those at the following amu values: 590 (M), 575 (M-15), 518 (M-72), 500 (M-90), and 485 (M-90-15). From Maume et al. [20], courtesy of Marcel Dekker, Inc.

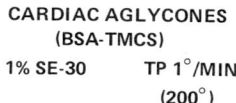

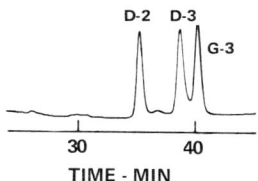

Figure 1.7. GLC separation of TMSi ethers of digitoxigenin, (3,23-di-TMSi ether) (D-2), digoxigenin (3,12,23-tri-TMSi ether) (D-3), and gitoxigenin (3,16,23-tri-TMSi ether) (G-3) prepared by silylation with BSA-TMCS in the presence of a minimum amount of pyridine. The 14β-hydroxyl group does not undergo reaction under these conditions, but a TMSi ether is formed for the enol form of the lactone side chain. Conditions: column, 1% SE-30 on 100-120 mesh acid-washed and silanized Gas Chrom P, 12 ft by 4 mm; temperature programmed at 1°C/min from 200°C. From Maume et al. [20], courtesy of Marcel Dekker, Inc.

column follows an expected pattern. As the functional groups are converted to ethers, the MU values decrease, but it is not always possible to separate all three cardenolides. The separation of the free steroids is possible with the SE-30 column (see Table 1.5), but this is not advisable because multiple products (presumably due to dehydration) are observed. The reactions observed with DHD-3 were normal; the lactone structure did not enolize.

In 1969, Tan [21] developed a simple and efficient method for the identification of digitalis steroid cardenolides as their "β"-anhydro derivatives, resulting in greatly reduced retention times and enhanced resolution. In this investigation, two series of compounds were studied (cardenolides and cardadienolides) which were converted to either TMSi or acetate derivatives as shown in Figure 1.8. The silyl derivatives were prepared using either N,O-bis-(trimethylsilyl)-acetamide (BSA) or hexamethyldisilazane as reagent with trimethylchlorosilane added as catalyst. The acetylated products were formed by reacting the parent compound overnight with equal (0.2-ml) volumes of anhydrous pyridine and acetic anhydride at 35°C.

The general procedure for the preparation of "β"-anhydro derivatives (compounds B1 through B9) was as follows:

Basic Structures

Series A   Series B

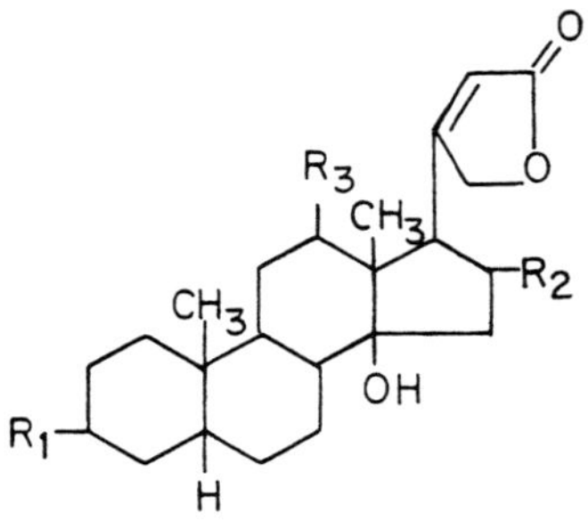

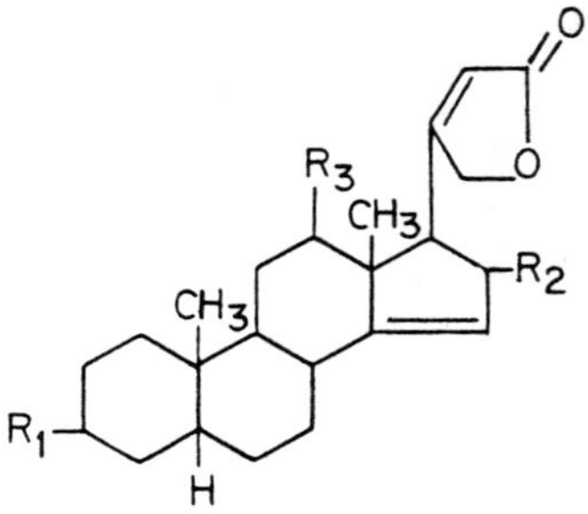

Series	Identification number	Substituents		
		R_1	R_2	R_3
A, B	1	-OH	H	H
A, B	2	-OH	-OH	H
A, B	3	-OH	H	-OH
A, B	4	-OTMSi	H	H
A, B	5	-OTMSi	-OTMSi	H
A, B	6	-OTMSi	H	-OTMSi
A, B	7	-OAc	H	H
A, B	8	-OAc	-OAc	H
A, B	9	-OAc	H	-OAc

Figure 1.8. Structures of cardenolides/cardadienolides studied and their derivatives. Adapted from Tan [21].

For GC analysis, compounds B4-B9 were prepared in situ directly from the corresponding 14β-hydroxylated parent cardenolides A4-A9, by addition of the thionyl chloride-benzene-pyridine reagent [22] at 4°C. Dehydration occurred within 15 min.

The cardadienolides B1-B3 were prepared from compounds A1-A3, respectively, via their TMSi derivatives, followed by dehydration with thionyl chloride-benzene-pyridine reagent in the cold and subsequent hydrolysis of the TMSi group by treatment with 90% methanol at room temperature. However, it should be noted that the tertiary 14β-hydroxy group is neither affected by esterification nor etherification, this conclusion supported by IR spectral evidence. As pointed out by Tan, "the so-called cardioactive steroids are distinguished by the presence of a tertiary hydroxy group at the C-14 ring junction. The pseudoaxial configuration of the alcohol group makes this class of naturally occurring compounds unique among the steroids. Together with the conjugated five-membered lactone ring in the case of the cardenolides, or the doubly conjugated six-membered pyrone ring in the case of the bufadienolides, this oxygenated substituent defines the strong biological activity of the cardiotonic steroids." Hence, use was made of the inherent instability, offered by the unique combination of a tertiary C-14 hydroxy group and a C-17 lactone ring, present in a 1,3-pseudodiaxial steric relationship. Capable of selectively acetylating or silylating only the secondary hydroxy groups at positions 3β, 12β, or 16β, while leaving the 14β-OH group intact, an easy method was provided for the preparation in situ of $\Delta^{14(15)}$-cardadienolides B1-B9 that were suitable for GC analysis. The mechanism for cardadienolide formation is indicated below, where N is a nucleophilic species:

The GC separation of these compounds was performed with a Hewlett-Packard model 402 gas chromatograph equipped with flame ionization detectors and three glass column systems: column A, 90 cm by 0.4 cm, packed with 3% SE-30 coated on 100-120 mesh Gas Chrom Q; column B, 180 cm by 0.3 cm, packed with 3% OV-1 coated on 100-120 mesh Gas Chrom Q; and column C, 180 cm by 0.3 cm, packed with 3% QF-1 coated on 100-120 mesh Gas Chrom Q. The other operating parameters were as follows: column temperature, 250°C; injector temperature, 275°C; detector temperature, 285°C; helium carrier-gas flow rate, 23 ml/min for column A and 33 ml/min for columns B and C. As indicated above, more polar liquid stationary phases were investigated since previous reports on the GC analysis of cardenolides and bufadienolides on a nonselective phase provided separations with varying degrees of success [16,17,23].

Using the designated columns and operating conditions, the retention times of the compounds illustrated in Figure 1.8 are listed in Table 1.6.

Wilson and Ripley [24] demonstrated in 1969 that TMSi ether derivatives of digoxigenin, digitoxin, and gitoxin could be resolved on a GC column packed with OV-17 as liquid stationary phase. At 340°C, separation of the glycoside derivatives was effected by permitting differing degrees of

TABLE 1.6

Retention Times of Cardenolides/Cardadienolides and Their Derivatives[a]

Compound[b]	Retention times (min)		
	Column A	Column B	Column C
A1	12.90	22.70	53.30
A2	11.68	21.60	67.00
A3	22.45	29.70	51.75
A4	12.85	22.60	43.00
A5	14.95	24.80	49.25
A6	15.67	29.10	46.00
A7	16.37	28.80	110.03
A8	15.44	27.20	92.50
A9	23.62	39.20	150.00
B1	8.00	13.85	20.10
B2	4.92	8.80	13.03
B3	6.43	11.58	10.43
B4	8.05	14.30	17.93
B5	9.37	16.30	21.60
B6	11.10	19.35	23.05
B7	10.33	17.90	44.90
B8	12.50	22.00	54.30
B9	15.85	28.10	39.60

[a]Adapted from Tan [21].
[b]Compounds identified in Figure 1.8.

dipole-induced dipole interaction between solute and liquid phase. In the case of digoxin TMSi ether, the sphere of influence of the dipole of the lactone ring in the aglycone was sterically hindered, resulting in varying effectiveness of induction of electron delocalization in the π electron system of the aromatic groups of the liquid phase.

DIGITALIS-TYPE GLYCOSIDES

The derivatives of the sterols were prepared as follows:

1. Acetates were prepared by heating 1 mg of sterol and 0.5 ml of pyridine-acetic anhydride solution (10:3, v/v) in a 16/125-mm culture tube lined with Teflon at 75°C for 1.5 hr.

2. Trimethylsilylation was accomplished by dissolving 1 to 6 mg of sterol in 1 ml of "silanizing mixture" which contained hexamethyldisilazane, pyridine, and trimethylchlorosilane in a volume ratio of 10:10:1. Reaction was permitted to occur at room temperature for at least 60 min.

The aglycones digitoxigenin (D-2), digoxigenin (D-3), and gitoxigenin (G-3), the sterol acetates, and the sterol TMSi derivatives were resolved chromatographically using a Barber-Colman 5000 series gas chromatograph equipped with hydrogen flame detectors and five different U-shaped column systems: column A, 6 ft by 5 mm i.d., packed with 2.5% OV-1 on 80-100 mesh Chromosorb W-HP; column B, 6 ft by 5 mm i.d., packed with 1% OV-1 on 80-100 mesh Chromosorb W-HP; column C, 6 ft by 5 mm i.d., packed with 2.5% OV-17 on 80-100 mesh Chromosorb W-HP; column D, 1 ft by 4 mm i.d., packed with 2.5% OV-1 on 80-100 mesh Chromosorb W-HP; and column E, 1 ft by 4 mm i.d., packed with 2.5% OV-17 on 80-100 mesh Chromosorb W-HP. With the nitrogen carrier-gas flow rate and detector temperature maintained at 100 ml/min and 340°C, respectively, the injector and column temperatures were identical during isothermal operation, but in the cases of temperature programming, the injector temperature was set at the lower (starting) temperature of the column.

For the determination of molecular weights and, thus, the extent of substitution of the sterol derivatives eluted from the GC columns, mass spectral data were obtained using LKB 9000 integrated GC-MS instrument equipped with a 9-ft by 6-mm glass column packed with 1% SE-30 coated on Gas Chrom P. The operating conditions selected for the GC-MS unit were accelerating voltage, 70 eV; filament current, 60 μA; ion source temperature, 250°C; column temperature, temperature programmed from 230°C at 1°C/min after sample injection.

The data obtained by Wilson and Ripley using columns A, B, and C, as shown in Table 1.7, were essentially identical, with the following observations noted:

1. Relative retention orders of the sterol acetates were similar to those of the free sterols on both OV-1 and OV-17.

2. Retention times of the sterol acetate were 5.5 times greater on column C (OV-17) than on column A (OV-1).

3. Relative affinities for OV-17, as compared to OV-1, were consistent with the postulate that the more extensive π-electron system of

TABLE 1.7

Gas Chromotographic Retention Time Relationships of Aglycones and Their Various Derivatives[a]

Aglycones and derivatives	1.0% OV-1 (column B) Isothermal: 260°C		2.5% OV-1 (column A) Isothermal: 290°C		2.5% OV-17 (column C) Isothermal: 290°C	
	Retention time (min)	Retention relative to derivatives of D-3 (%)	Retention time (min)	Retention relative to derivatives of D-3 (%)	Retention time (min)	Retention relative to derivatives of D-3 (%)
Digitoxigenin (D-2)	7.6		6.0		18.5	
Gitoxigenin (G-3)	7.0		5.6		16.9	
Digoxigenin (D-3)	13.1		9.8		39.8	
Dihydrodigoxigenin (DHD-3)	11.5		8.6		24.0	
D-2-Ac	9.4	74	7.1	78	38.4	76
G-3-Ac	8.6	68	6.5	71	35.1	70
D-3-Ac	12.7	100	9.1	100	50.4	100
DHD-3-Ac	10.4	82	7.9	87	39.3	78
D-2-TMSi ether	7.5	88	5.7	90	20.9	121
G-3-TMSi ether	8.5	100	6.3	100	17.7	103
D-3-TMSi ether	8.5	100	6.3	100	17.1	100
DHD-3-TMSi ether	7.5	88	5.2	82	14.0	82

[a]From Wilson and Ripley[24], courtesy of Analytical Chemistry

those aglycones possessing conjugated lactone rings permits a stronger interaction with the aromatic groups of the liquid phase than one could predict from consideration of group dipole moments alone.

4. Relative retention times of the aglycones and the acetates on columns A and C were correlated with (a) assumed molecular weight differences, (b) assumed vapor pressure differences, and (c) the frequency of occurrence of various groups with an appreciable dipole moment.

5. The retention order of the aglycone-TMSi ethers on OV-17 was obviously related to molecular characteristics other than vapor pressure differences.

6. Relative affinities on OV-17 are generally consistent with the hypothesis that steric hindrance of the lactone greatly influences the degree of separation of the aglycone TMSi ethers. For example, a CPK model of the 17α-epimer of the $3\beta, 12\beta, 14, 16\beta$-aglycone tetraol as illustrated in Figure 1.9 indicates that the TMSi ether of the 12β-ol would provide more pronounced shielding of the lactone ring than would the same derivative of the 16β-ol.

With the shorter columns D and E subjected to temperature programming, GC retention time relationships of glycoside TMSi ether derivatives are shown in Table 1.8.

Wilson and Ripley summarized these findings in the following manner:

The separations achieved for trisaccharide glycoside TMSi ethers demonstrated clearly that the affinity of gitoxin TMSi ether for OV-17 is significantly greater than that of digoxin TMSi ether and is less than that of digitoxin TMSi ether. If we assume (a) that dipole-dipole interactions between the aromatic liquid phase and the 14β-OH (as well as the lactone ring) were significant during gas chromatography of the aglycone TMSi ethers and that they became much less significant during GC of the trisaccharide TMSi ethers and (b) that vapor pressure differences provide an immeasurably small contribution to retention time differences in the cases of the trisaccharide TMSi ethers, the relative retention time relationships observed for the trisaccharide TMSi ethers correlate with results expected from gas chromatography of the aglycone TMSi ethers. The importance of dipole-induced dipole interactions in determining relative affinity of the various glycoside TMSi ether derivatives for OV-17 is more clearly demonstrated than was the case for the aglycone TMSi ethers at the lower temperatures.

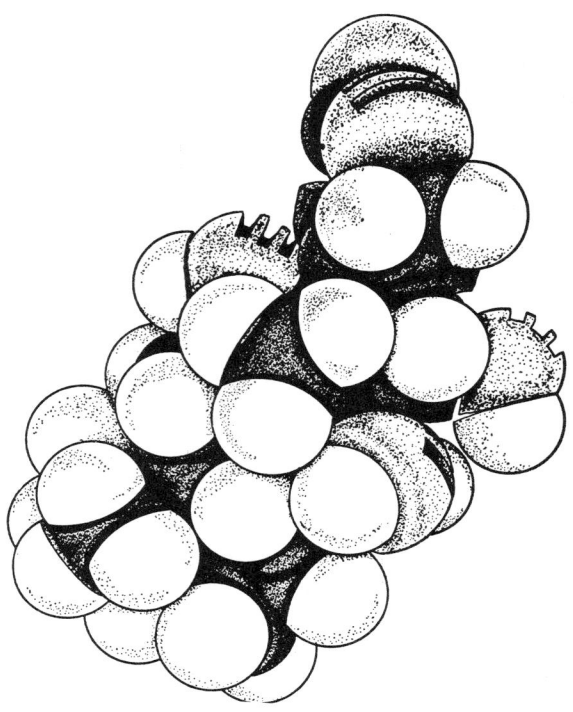

Figure 1.9. A CPK model demonstrating the van der Waals radii of the 17α-epimer of diginatigenin, 3β, 12β, 14, 16β tetrahydroxy-5β, -card-20(22)-enolide, in which the 3β hydroxyl group is hidden. From Wilson and Ripley [24], courtesy of Analytical Chemistry.

Using an approach previously suggested by Jelliffe [25], Watson and Kalman [26] described a method for the determination of digoxin in human plasma using electron-capture detection. The procedure involved addition of a labeled internal standard, ^{3}H-digoxin, extraction with methylene chloride, and preliminary purification on a Florisil column followed by thin-layer chromatography on silica gel. The spot attributed to digoxin [R_f = 0.23 using benzene-methanol (5:1) as eluant] was removed from the TLC plate by suction into a Pasteur pipette, the narrow ends of which were packed with a small plug of silanized glass wool, and eluted with three 0.5-ml volumes of acetone into a 3-ml glass tube. Following centrifugation, the acetone was transferred to another 3-ml silanized glass tube and evaporated under nitrogen by placing the tip of the tube in a sand bath maintained at 50°C. Heptafluorobutyric anhydride was added to the residue

TABLE 1.8

Gas Chromatographic Retention Time Relationships of
Glycoside TMSi Ether Derivatives[a]

	2.5% OV-1 (column D)	2.5% OV-17 (column E)
	Temperature programmed from 240 to 340°C at 7.5°C/min	Temperature programmed from 240 to 340°C at 7.5°C/min
Glycoside trimethylsilyl ether derivatives	Retention time (min)	Retention time (min)
Gitoxigenin	2.2	3.6
Gitoxin	15.8	20.7
Dihydrodigoxigenin	2.0	3.0
Digitoxigenin (D-2)	2.0	4.0
Digitoxigenin monodigitoxoside (D-2-MD)	7.0	10.0
Digitoxigenin bisdigitoxoside (D-2-BD)	11.7	14.5
Digitoxin	15.8	21.6
Digoxigenin (D-3)	2.2	3.6
Digoxigenin monodigitoxoside (D-3-MD)	7.1	9.3
Digoxigenin bisdigitoxoside (D-3-BD)	11.7	13.7
Digoxin	15.8	19.5
TMSi ether mixtures		
D-2 and D-3	2.0; 2.2	4.0; 3.6
D-2-MD and D-3-MD	7.0; 7.0	10.0; 9.3
D-2-BD and D-3-BD	11.8; 11.8	14.5; 13.7
Digitoxin and digoxin	15.9; 15.9	21.6; 19.5

[a]From Wilson and Ripley [24], courtesy of Analytical Chemistry.

to form the heptafluorobutyrate derivative by placing the stoppered tube and its contents to a depth of 2 cm into the holes of a heating block maintained at 90°C. The HFB derivative was again chromatographed on a 5-cm by 20-cm silica plate using benzene-ethyl acetate (7:3). In this system the R_f of the HFB derivative was 0.35. After TLC separation, the HFB derivative was removed from the plate and then extracted into acetone which was subsequently evaporated as previously described. Following the addition to the residue of 12 to 50 µl of benzene solution containing 0.72 ng/µl of digitoxigenin heptafluorobutyrate as internal standard, a 2-µl aliquot was withdrawn and injected into the gas chromatograph.

In this investigation, a Tracor MT 220 gas chromatograph equipped with a ^{63}Ni (14.5 mCi) electron-capture detector and a 4-ft by 3.5-mm-i.d. glass column packed with 3% OV-1 on Gas Chrom Q was used; the other GC conditions employed were carrier-gas (10% methane: 90% argon) flow rate, 100 ml/min; detector temperature, 350°C; column temperature, 240°C; ECD operation, 55-V pulse of 10 usec duration every 300 usec. With these GC conditions, the retention times of the HFB derivatives of digoxigenin and digitoxigenin were about 9.00 and 11.37 min, respectively.

Relative to the above procedure, Watson and Kalman noted that:

1. The overall recovery as determined by tritium counting averaged 25%.

2. Formation of the digoxigenin HFB derivative from digoxin by the direct action of heptafluorobutyric anhydride was about 80%.

3. The minimum detectable quantity of pure standard digoxigenin HFB was about 0.5 ng. The minimum detectable concentration from plasma extract was about 0.10 ng.

Quantitative data were obtained via a standard curve prepared by chromatographing varying amounts of digoxigenin HFB from 0.30 to 1.6 ng with 1.44 ng of digitoxigenin HFB; the peak height ratios were then plotted versus the weight ratios. After the determination of the ratio of the peak heights of digoxigenin HFB and the internal standard from the chromatogram of a given plasma sample, the amount of digoxin in the aliquot could be obtained by referring this ratio to the standard curve.

In 1972, Watson, Tramell, and Kalman [27] extended their previous studies to the identification of submicrogram amounts of digoxin, digitoxin, and their metabolites which were separated by paper chromatography and then by thin-layer chromatography. Appropriate spots were identified by their R_f values in comparison with known markers (internal standards) and then further characterized by gas chromatography after making volatile derivatives with heptafluorobutyric anhydride. In this present study, they described the extension of the reaction with heptafluorobutyric anhydride to bis- and monodigoxigenin digitoxosides as well as digitoxin and its corresponding metabolic products. Since the reaction of HFBA with digoxin and its metabolites (its bis- and monoglycosides and its aglycone) yielded digitoxigenin HFB, it was necessary to separate these glycosides prior to derivative formation.

The GC conditions and instrument employed were essentially those previously reported [26] with several slight modifications: a 4-ft by 2-mm-i.d. U-shaped column packed with 3% OV-1 on Gas Chrom Q; and a helium carrier-gas flow rate of 50 ml/min. With these slight changes, the retention times of digoxigenin HFB and digitoxigenin HFB were 9.0 and 11.3 min, respectively.

Finkle, Cherry, and Taylor [28] developed a simple GC system utilizing four columns and three liquid phases, complemented by a direct solvent-extraction scheme designed to detect common poisons, drugs, and human metabolites encountered in forensic toxicology to a sensitivity limit of 2 μg/ml in blood, urine, or tissue specimens. Relative retention data for almost 600 different substances were tabulated in two indices, one providing reference GC information for any of the substances prior to an analysis and the other allowing tentative identification of unknown GC peaks (see Chapter 1 of Volume 2 for column, GC operating, extraction, and coding details). In their tabulated data, the relative retention times and the column system used for digitalin and digitoxin were as follows: digitalin, RRT = 1.92, column system I; digitoxin, RRT = 1.92, column system I.

Kibbe and Araujo [29] also proposed a rapid quantitative GC method for assaying digoxin in both tablet and powder form. The TMSi derivative of digoxin was prepared using a mixed silylating reagent, hexamethyldisilazane:trimethylchlorosilane:pyridine in a 10:1:10 volume ratio, after it had been converted to digoxigenin. Sample preparation for GC analysis consisted of the following:

> A sample of either 0.1 mg of powdered digoxin or the equivalent amount in tablet form was dissolved in 2 ml of a pyridine-water (50%, v/v) solution. A volume of 0.1 ml of 0.1 N sodium hydroxide was added, and the mixture was heated on a steam bath for 30 min to convert completely the digoxin to digoxigenin. The solution was then evaporated to dryness and redissolved in 100 μl of dry pyridine. An aliquot of 10 μl of a stock solution containing 2 μg/μl of cholesterol in pyridine was added. From this solution, a 1-μl sample was injected into the chromatograph and the areas under the curves were calculated by means of a disk integrator.

If silyl derivatives were needed, the sample to be silylated was made to react with 1 ml of the reagent at room temperature before injecting into the gas chromatograph.

In this study, Kibbe and Araujo used a Varian model 2100 GC system equipped with flame ionization detectors and three column types: column A, 2-m by 2-mm-i.d. U-shaped glass, packed with 2.5% OV-1 on 80-100 mesh Chromosorb A; column B, 0.5-m by 4-mm-i.d. U-shaped copper, packed with 2.5% OV-1 on 80-100 mesh Chromosorb A; column C, 0.5-m by 4-mm-i.d. U-shaped copper, packed with 3% OV-17 on 80-100 mesh Chromosorb A. To obtain the retention time data shown in Table 1.9, the following GC conditions were employed: injector temperature, 330°C; column temperature, 285°C; detector temperature, 330°C; nitrogen carrier-gas flow rate, 50 to 100 ml/min; hydrogen flow rate, 35 ml/min; air flow rate, 300 ml/min.

They noted that the results indicated that both silylated and nonsilylated compounds exhibited similar retention times using all three columns and, from this standpoint, there appeared to be no advantage in silylating the compound.

For quantitative studies, the standard curve was generated by plotting A_D/A_C against W_D/W_C, where A_D and A_C are the areas under the curve for digoxigenin and cholesterol, respectively, and W_D and W_C are the respective weights for digoxigenin and cholesterol. The results along with the analysis of variance are shown in Table 1.10.

In 1976, Anbar and St. John [30] developed a field ionization and desorption source, comprising a rough metal surface at the end of a short, thin metal rod, and a heatable structure which allows its reproducible placement within 50 μm from a counterelectrode. The field desorbing rod is extremely simple to prepare, and a new one may be used for each sample. Successfully operated at ambient temperature to 350°C, among the number of examples of field ionization and field desorption spectra of inorganic and organic compounds obtained by this source was the field ionization spectrum of adsorbed digitoxigenin as shown in Figure 1.10. As noted by

TABLE 1.9

Retention Time (min)[a]

	Column A	Column B	Column C
Cholesterol (unsilylated)	2.0	0.67	0.5
Cholesterol (silylated)	2.0	0.67	0.5
Digoxigenin (unsilylated)	15.0	5.33	3.67
Digoxigenin (silylated)	15.0	5.00	3.67

[a]From Kibbe and Araujo [29], courtesy of Journal of Pharmaceutical Sciences.

TABLE 1.10

Standard Curve Data for Digoxigenin-Cholesterol[a]

$\dfrac{A_D}{A_C}$ [b]	$\dfrac{W_D}{W_C}$ [c]
3.48	16.47
2.08	10.83
2.50	8.95
1.51	7.58
0.89	6.55

Analysis of Variance

Source	df	Sum of squares	Mean square	F ratio
Regression	1	22.68	22.67	29.66
Residual	4	3.06	0.76	
Total	5	25.72		

Variables in Equation

Coefficient	0.20
Standard error	0.0013
Intercept	0.057

[a]From Kibbe and Aranjo [29], courtesy of Journal of Pharmaceutical Sciences.
[b]Area ratio (digoxin-cholesterol).
[c]Weight ratio (digoxin-cholesterol).

Anbar and St. John, there is substantial dehydration during this ionization process, and only about 35% molecular ions are observed. Somewhat lower, but still very significant, dehydration has been observed for this compound using Beckey's dendrite source [31].

Knight [32] described a GC method for the analysis of Fenugreek sapogenins whose structures are illustrated below:

	R₁	R₂	R₃			R₁	R₂	R₃	
I	H	CH₃	H	Diosgenin	III	H	CH₃	H	Tigogenin
II	CH₃	H	H	Yamogenin	IV	CH₃	H	H	Neotigogenin
V	H	CH₃	OH	Yuccagenin	VII	H	CH₃	OH	Gitogenin
VI	CH₃	H	OH	Lilagenin	VIII	CH₃	H	OH	Neogitogenin

As noted by Knight:

The seed of the Fenugreeek plant (<u>Trigonella foenum-graecum</u>) is a potentially useful source of diosgenin (I), a widely used raw material for steroid manufacture.

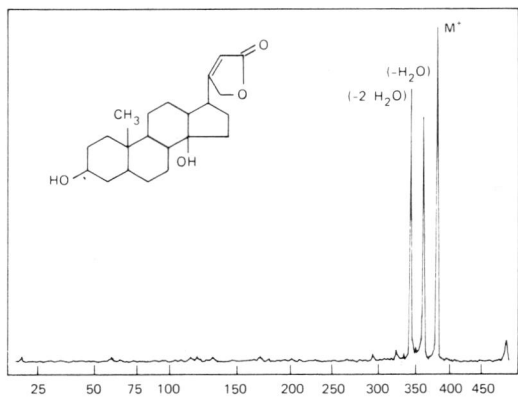

Figure 1.10. Field ionization spectrum of adsorbed digitoxigenin, mol. wt. 374.5, 150°C. From Anbar and St. John [30], courtesy of <u>Analytical Chemistry</u>.

Assay of the crude steroidal sapogenins obtained by acid hydrolysis of the plant material presents some problems, however, because together with diosgenin a considerable amount of the C_{25}-epimer yamogenin (II) is found, from which it can only be separated with some difficulty. In addition, there is usually some of a 5α-dihydro analog tigogenin (III) present plus the polar sapogenins gitogenin (VII) and yuccagenin (V).

A gas-liquid chromatographic assay for diosgenin in dioscorea root has been described [33] in which the acid hydrolysis products are chromatographed without derivatization. This works well when diosgenin is substantially the only sapogenin present, but it fails to separate the C_{25}-epimers from each other or from the 5α-dihydro analogs, and the more polar 2α,3β-dihydroxy steroids (V-VIII) are decomposed on the column.

Because of the many shortcomings cited above, Knight developed a method which would allow simultaneous determination of all these compounds without elaborate sample preparation. To accomplish this goal, derivatization was employed:

1. TMSi ethers were prepared by dissolving 10 mg of the sapogenin in a mixture of pyridine (0.5 ml) and bis-(trimethylsilyl)trifluoroacetamide (1 ml) and warming to 60°C until the reaction was complete.

2. Trifluoroacetate derivatives were prepared by dissolving the sapogenin in a mixture of chloroform (0.5 ml) and trifluoroacetic anhydride (0.5 ml). After 15 min at room temperature, the solution was evaporated to dryness in a stream of nitrogen at room temperature and the residue redissolved in chloroform prior to injection.

The TMSi- and TFA-sapogenin derivatives were analyzed with a Varian model 2440 gas chromatograph equipped with flame ionization detectors and three column systems: column A, 6-ft by 3-mm-i.d. glass, packed with 2% SE-30 on 100-120 mesh Chromosorb Q for free sapogenins; column B, 6-ft by 3-mm-i.d. glass, packed with 3% OV-17 on 100-120 mesh Chromosorb Q for TMSi ethers; and column C, 6-ft by 3-mm-i.d. glass, packed with 3% QF-1 on 100-120 mesh Chromosorb Q for trifluoroacetates.

The best separation was obtained when the TFA derivatives were chromatographed on QF-1, when eight compounds could be detected, which were arranged in four neo-iso pairs. Operating the QF-1 column in a temperature-programmed mode (following a 20-min preprogram hold, the temperature was programmed from 200 to 230°C at 2°C/min) (Note: No other GC conditions specified), the retention times of the TFA derivatives of diosgenin, yamogenin, tigogenin, neotigogenin, yuccagenin, lilagenin, gitogenin, and neogitogenin were approximately 31.80, 32.50, 33.60,

34.20, 39.60, 40.25, 42.40, and 43.10 min, respectively. It was also noted that, when refluxed in ethanolic HCl, the peaks ascribed to the neo-sapogenins were all greatly reduced because of conversion to the isoforms. When treated with ethanolic HCl, the dehydration of the 5-en-2-ol components to give 3,5-dienes was confirmed by GC; the 3,5-diene peak in the chromatogram having a retention time of nearly 13.75 min.

II. ANTIARRHYTHMIC AGENTS

In addition to digitalis, which is the principal drug of choice for certain types of arrhythmias (atrial fibrillation, atrial flutter, and paroxysmal atrial tachycardia), other prominent antiarrhythmic agents used today [34] are quinidine, procainamide, lidocaine, diphenylhydantoin, atropine, propranolol, and isoproterenol, as well as some more recently introduced — for example, disopyramide, α,α-dimethyl-4-$(\alpha,\alpha,\beta,\beta$-tetrafluorophenethyl) — benzylamine, aprindine, and mexiletine.

As in the case of digoxin and digitoxin, Chow and Ronfeld [2] compiled pharmacokinetic data for diphenylhydantoin, lidocaine, procainamide, quinidine, and propranolol which included percent of drug absorbed intact, time of peak concentration, volume of distribution, elimination half-life (β phase), percent of drug excreted unchanged, renal clearance, and plasma binding; this information is shown in Table 1.11.

Some of these drugs (for example, lidocaine, diphenylhydantoin, propranol, and isoproterenol) have been discussed in detail in other volumes of this series. Therefore, only more recent GC and/or GC-MS studies of these antiarrhythmics will be included in this chapter.

A. Quinidine

As early as 1965, Brochmann-Hanssen and Fontan [55] demonstrated that the diastereoisomers, quinidine and quinine, as well as cinchonine and cinchonidine, could be resolved using liquid stationary phases more polar than SE-30, as shown in Table 1.9 of Volume 5.

In their study of alkaloids using 3-ft by 0.07-in.-i.d. glass columns operated at temperatures ranging from 175 to 240°C, they noted that the polar alkaloid codeine, containing a hydroxyl group, exhibits greater interaction with the more polar phases, whereas the less polar lactone and ester moieties in atropine, homatropine, cocaine, hydrastine, and pilocarpine are less affected by the increase in the liquid-phase polarity.

Lactone alkaloids had greater relative retention times with the XE-60 liquid stationary phase than the HI-EFF-8B coating, and it was primarily

ANTIARRHYTHMIC AGENTS

due to these variances in polarity that pilocarpine was easily separated from codeine with XE-60, whereas no separation of this pair of alkaloids was possible with HI-EFF-8B. The relative retention times of the 11 alkaloids plotted against the stationary phases (SE-30, XE-60, EGSS-Y, and HI-EFF-8B) arranged in order of increasing polarity are shown in Figure 1.6 of Volume 5. From such a plot, one can determine the best phase necessary to perform gas chromatographic separations of mixtures. For example, atropine and scopolamine would require a very efficient column for separation on silicone rubber SE-30, but the same mixture is readily resolved on the more polar stationary phases, and this is also true for the principal opium alkaloids, such as morphine, codeine, and thebaine.

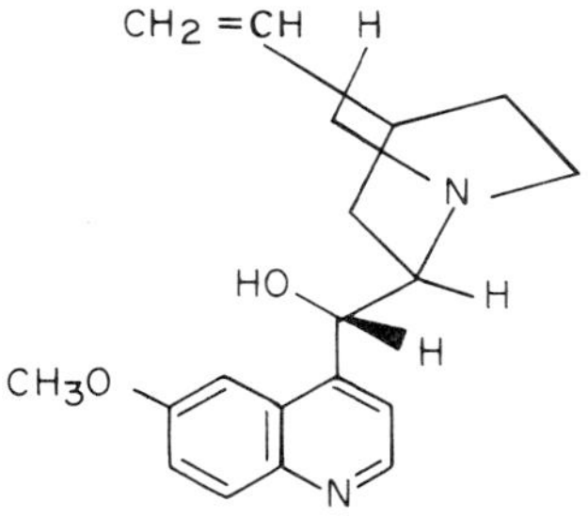

Quinidine

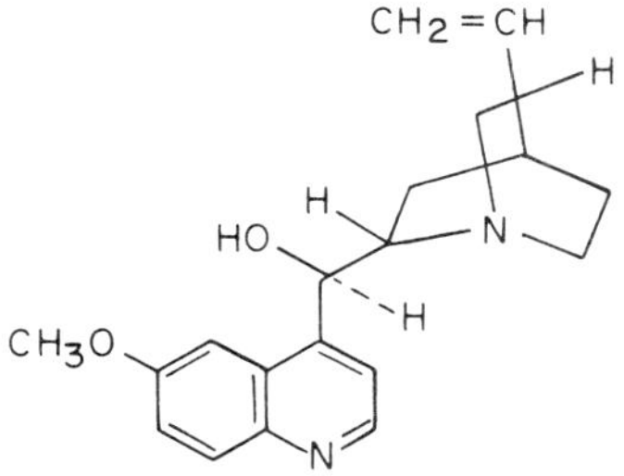

Quinine

Shortly thereafter, in 1969, Palmer, Martin, Baggett, and Wall [56] showed by mass spectrometry, GC-MS, and other analytical techniques (IR, UV, NMR, and TLC) that oral administration of quinidine preparations to humans yielded a wide range of urinary metabolites found as the free, or to a minor extent, as the β-glucosiduronate conjugates. The major metabolites isolated and characterized were two oxidative modifications of quinidine, and of 2'-quinolone and hydroxyquinuclidine derivatives. Also found were polyoxygenated quinidine derivatives.

As reported by Palmer et al.:

Gas chromatographic studies were made with a Varian Aerograph model 2100-2 instrument using a flame ionization detection system with 4-ft by 0.25-in. glass column with either a 3.8% SE-30 or 3.8% OV-17 silicone phase on 100-120 mesh Chromosorb HP-AWS. The trimethylsilyl (TMSi) derivatives for GC studies were made by heating a solution of the sample (100 to 200 μg) in a 1:2:9 mixture of trimethylchlorosilane:hexamethyldisilazane:anhydrous pyridine or bis-(trimethylsilyl)-acetamide or in bis-(trimethylsilyl)-trifluoroacetamide (Regisil) at 100°C for 10 to 15 min. After cooling, the solution

TABLE 11.1

Pharamacokinetic Data for Some Antiarrhythimic Drugs[a]

	A 98 (PO) [35]	B —
Percent adsorbed intact		
Time of peak conc. (hr)	4 [35]	0.50 (IM) [39] 0.25 (intercostal) [39]
Volume of distribution (V_d)	0.64 liter/kg [36]	1.7 liter/kg [40]
$t_{1/2}\ \beta$ phase (hr)	22 [37]	1.5 [40]
Percent excreted unchanged	<5 [35]	<10 [41]
Renal clearance (ml/min)	Negligible	192[c]
Percent plasma protein binding	88 [36]	66 [42]
Therapeutic	10-18 [38]	2-5 [43]

[a]Adapted from Chow and Ronfeld [2].
[b]A = diphenylhydantoin; B = lidocaine; C = procainamide; D = propranolol; E = quinidine.
[c]Calculated value.

(20 to 40 nl) was injected as such into the gas chromatograph. All evaporations were made under reduced pressure and all solvents used for recrystallization were freshly purified and distilled immediately before use. GC-MS on the LKB 9000 studies used a 5-ft chrom-chromatographic column with a 3.8% OV-17 packing as previously described. All separation and reaction procedures were routinely monitored by both TLC and GC, enabling immediate combination of like materials prior to bulk evaporation or the product work-up.

Based on mass spectral studies of the free and silylated metabolites, they postulated that "metabolite 5, therefore, can now be firmly assigned structure A, with B being its corresponding enolic form responsible for

Drug[b]		
C	D	E
95 (PO) [44]	0.4 (PO) [46]	90 (PO) [49]
<1 [45]	1.6 [46]	2.0-4.0 [50]
2 liters/kg [44]	2.6 liters/kg [47]	146 liters/kg [50,51]
3.5 [44]	3.1 (single dose) [46] 4.5 (multidose) [46]	7.2 [52]
48 [44]	Negligible	10-15 [50]
220[c]	Negligible	6.6[c]
	93 [47]	82 [53]
4-8 [44]	0.04-0.08 [48]	2-8 [54]

Metabolite 5 (Structure A)   ⇌ (pH>10 / H+)   Metabolite 5 (Structure B)

the observed base-induced bathochromic shift (UV spectrum)." As for metabolite 4, they concluded that the oxygen function in the quinuclidine part of its structure could be present as an N-oxide, a hydroxyl group or, more unlikely, in the ring following a rearrangement of the N-oxide. However, a comparison of the mass spectrum of its TMSi derivative to that of the parent compound showed that it formed a bis-TMSi derivative (M^+ = 484), in contrast to the mono-TMSi derivative (M^+ = 396) formed by quinidine. Also, the principal fragments of metabolite 4 each had one TMSi group (m/e 224 and 261) as opposed to the m/e 136 and 261 fragments found in quinidine. The formation of a bis-TMSi derivative by metabolite 4 is conclusive evidence that the oxygen is present as a hydroxyl group in the quinuclidine ring system.

The differences in mass spectral patterns among quinidine, metabolite 4, and metabolite 5 are shown in Figure 1.11.

More qualitative in nature, other GC and GC-MS investigations were performed by Finkle and co-workers [28,57,58] and Moffat [59]. In 1971, Finkle et al. [28] developed a GC system utilizing four columns and three liquid phases to detect common poisons, drugs, and human metabolites encountered in forensic toxicology (see Chapter 1 of Volume 2 for column, GC operating, extraction, and coding details). Included among their data were the relative retention times and the column system used for quinidine and quinine: quinidine, RRT = 0.46, column system VII; quinine, RRT = 0.50, column system VII. Other antiarrhythmic drugs chromatographed were procainamide, RRT = 0.72, column system II; lidocaine, RRT = 1.82, column system I; diphenylhydantoin, RRT = 1.43, column system II; diphenylhydantoin (methyl derivative), RRT = 0.55, column system II; atropine, RRT = 0.54, column system II; propranolol, RRT = 0.51, column system II; and isoproterenol, RRT = 0.98, column system I.

In 1972, Finkle et al. [57] generated reference mass spectral data for 133 drugs of abuse via a two-column GC-MS (quadrupole) system after each drug had been extracted and presented to the instrument in a form compatible with that encountered in human toxicological analysis.

Using an all-glass jet separator as a GC-MS interface, the data reported were obtained with a Finnigan GC-MS system, model 3000-003 gas chromatograph peak identifier capable of scanning with unit resolution to mass 500. In lieu of column effluent splitting, a total ion monitor was employed with a strip chart recorder. The GC system was based on that previously described by Finkle et al. [28] and used two columns, each packed with 2.5% SE-30 coated on 80-100 mesh Chromosorb G. The columns were glass, 2 ft by 3 mm i.d. and 6 ft by 3 mm i.d., and were operated isothermally in accordance with parameters specified in this earlier investigation. The data processing equipment, complete with teletype terminal and paper tape punch, and accessed by means of a telephone acoustical coupler, permitted the reference spectra to be stored as a file

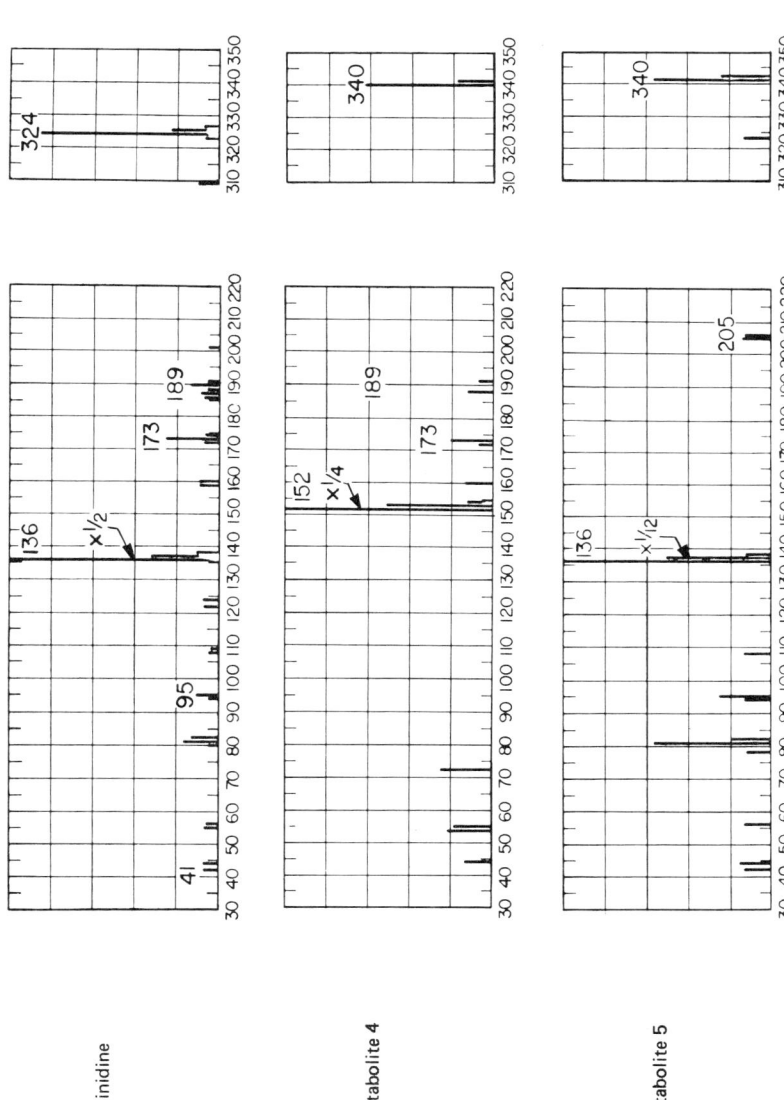

Figure 1.11. Mass spectra of quinidine, metabolite 4, and metabolite 5. Adapted from Palmer et al. [56].

and manipulated by using three computer programs written in time-share basic language. The programs enabled the analyst to list the data as an alphabetical index or as a base peak index (both indices for quinidine shown below), search the file for identification purposes, and add new data to the file or modify the existing data.

Alphabetical Index

QUINIDINE
MØL. WT. 324   BASE PEAK 136

42	55	67	81	95	117	122	136	158	173	174	189
214	226	240	253	269	283	295	309	324	0	0	0
0	0	0	0	0	0						

Base Peak Index

QUINIDINE
MØL. WT. 324   BASE PEAK 136

In their system, the mass spectrum of the peak was obtained via the oscillographic recorder. It was numerically coded by first noting the atomic mass unit value of the base peak, and then recording in sequence the m/e of the most intense peak in each group of 14 amu beginning at mass 34 and continuing through mass 453. If the parent peak was present and recognized, then the molecular weight of the material could be considered. In their system, two tables provided the necessary means for rapid manual search but, alternatively, the coded spectrum could be typed into the computer and the search-identification routine effected automatically.

As noted by the authors, an identification was accepted only if all of the analytical information was in consonance, that is, chemical extraction characteristics, GC relative retention time, and base peak, molecular weight, and digital code of the mass spectrum.

In 1974, Finkle et al. [58] published supplementary data to the earlier 1972 report, which gives revised GC-MS reference data for toxicological and biomedical purposes including chemical ionization data for 450 drugs and metabolites and the facility of an interactive minicomputer by which the library can be manipulated. A master alphabetical list of library compounds is cross-indexed with an electron-impact base peak table (for EI spectral data) and a molecular-weight table (for CI spectral data) which are rapid and simple to use. The data can be used manually by time-share computer or through a dedicated interactive data system. The EI spectra are presented in a digital code unique to each compound with matching GC relative retention times, and the CI spectra as the protonated molecular ion and most abundant ions. As noted by Finkle et al.:

The protonated molecular ion (MH^+) is clearly evident in most methane CI mass spectra of drugs and drug metabolites. Often it is the most intense peak in the spectrum and it is nearly always accompanied by a characteristic pattern of the alkyl adduct ions. If the drug molecule contains an aliphatic amine, there will always be a prominent $(M-H)^+$ ion. Any prominent fragment ions should correspond to loss of reasonable neutral molecules such as H_2O, ROH, AcOH, HNR_2, etc., from the protonated molecular ion.

After determining the molecular weight of the compounds, final identification can usually be achieved by comparing the m/e and relative intensities of the fragment ions observed in the CI mass spectrum with those listed for compounds of the same molecular weight. Occasionally additional information will be needed for a conclusive identification. The needed additional information may be furnished by the GC relative retention time, or EI mass spectrum.

In comparing CI mass spectral data, it should be kept in mind that the ion source temperature can have a dramatic effect on relative ion intensities [60,61].

Other factors such as the reactant gas and sample pressures in the ion source and the ion repeller voltage can also affect relative ion intensities. Consequently, the major consideration in attempting to identify drugs from CI mass spectra is usually the presence or absence of certain ion peaks rather than a quantitative comparison of ion intensities.

In addition to EI mass spectral data given for quinidine, this report, together with that of Foltz et al. [62], contained CI mass spectral information for several antiarrhythmic agents as given below.

Methane CI-MS Data

Compound	M.W.	MH^+ (RI)	Prominent fragment ions > m/e 50
Lidocaine metabolite	206	207 (100)	169 (44), 205 (20)
Lidocaine	234	235 (100)	233 (15), 132 (2), 148 (2)
Diphenylhydantoin	252	253 (100)	175 (25), 210 (7), 225 (4)
Atropine	289	290 (2)	124 (100), 288 (1)

Moffat [59] suggested the use of SE-30 as a stationary phase for the identification of drugs based on retention indices alone. In compiled retention index data for 480 drugs, several antiarrhythmic drugs were included whose retention indices were reported as follows: atropine, 2175; isoproterenol, 1720; lidocaine, 1860; procainamide, 2230; propranolol, 2145.

In 1973, Smith, Barkan, Ross, Maienthal, and Levine [63] investigated methods for the detection and measurement of possible contaminants in quinidine and quinine and their pharmaceutical preparations to establish the actual composition of quinidine and quinine on the market at that time. Since no single TLC or GC procedure separated all of the compounds under consideration, multiple systems encompassing them were used to characterize the samples. Chromatographic and fluorometric techniques were applied to the analysis of a wide variety of samples of quinidine, quinine, and pharmaceutical preparations. In all of the 75 samples examined, the dihydro analogs were found, and the desmethoxy analogs (cinchonine and cinchonidine) were present in approximately half of the samples. The level of the dihydro alkaloids was higher in quinidine than in quinine (usually 5 to 9% in quinidine and 3 to 6% in quinine); the level of the desmethoxy analog, however, was higher in quinine than in quinidine (about 0.0 to 0.5% in quinidine as compared to 1 to 2% in quinine). In this investigation, no epi-alkaloid, quininone, or quinotoxine was detected in any sample.

As noted by the authors, the system described separates the vinyl alkaloids from their dihydro analogs. It does not resolve the quinidine-quinine, dihydroquinidine-dihydroquinine, cinchonidine-cinchonine, and dihydrocinchonidine-dihydrocinchonine pairs, but it did resolve these pairs from each other.

The GC separations were performed with a Varian Aerograph model 1200 gas chromatograph equipped with a flame ionization detector, an electronic integrator, and a 6.1-m by 3-mm-i.d. glass column packed with 3% OV-225 coated on Gas Chrom Q. The silyl derivatives of the various alkaloids were prepared with either 0.1 ml of N-methyl-N-trimethylsilyl-trifluoroacetamide or bis-(trimethylsilyl)-trifluoroacetamide added to approximately 0.1 mg of the alkaloid; the mixture was then heated at 60°C for about 45 min. From this reaction solution, a 3 μl aliquot was withdrawn and injected into the chromatograph operated in the following manner: injector temperature, 235°C; column temperature, 225°C; nitrogen carrier-gas flow rate, 30 ml/min. Using these GC conditions, Figure 1.12 is a typical chromatogram of the alkaloids in a quinidine sulfate sample, whereas in Table 1.12 are the retention times observed for the silyl derivatives.

Midha and Charette [64] described a method for the quantitative estimation of quinidine in plasma and whole blood. In their GC method, after the addition of approximately 2 μg of cinchonidine (internal standard) to 1 ml of either plasma or whole blood, the specimen is extracted at pH 12.0 with 10 ml of benzene. After the benzene extract is evaporated to dryness at

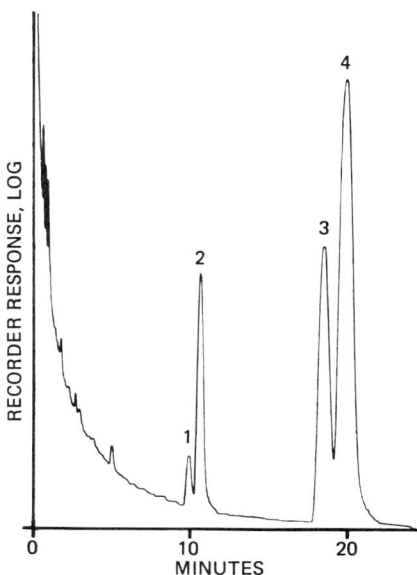

Figure 1.12. GLC chromatogram of the trimethylsilyl derivatives of the alkaloids in a quinidine sulfate sample. Key: 1, dihydrocinchonidine; 2, cinchonine; 3, dihydroquinidine; and 4, quinidine. From Smith et al. [63], courtest of the Journal of Pharmaceutical Sciences.

75°C under a stream of nitrogen, the residue is dissolved with 25 μl of a methanolic solution of trimethylanilinium hydroxide (0.2 M). From this basic solution, a 1- to 2-μl aliquot is withdrawn and injected into a Perkin-Elmer F-11 gas chromatograph equipped with a flame ionization detector and a 1.2-m by 0.3-cm-o.d. stainless steel column packed with OV-7 (percent loading not specified) on 80-100 mesh Chromosorb W. Using operating conditions of injector temperature, 350°C; column temperature, 270°C; detector temperature, 350°C; nitrogen carrier-gas flow rate, 20 ml/min, the retention times of flash-methylated quinidine and cinchonidine were 6.9 and 4.4 min, respectively, whereas the methyl derivatives of 2-hydroxyquinidine (XVI) and monohydroxyquinidine (XVII) (both metabolites of quinidine) gave retention times of 12.1 and 10.6 min, respectively.

As noted by the authors, "the response of the flame ionization detector was linear with concentrations in the 0.2- to 12.0-μg/ml range. The overall recoveries of quinidine and cinchonidine from plasma at pH 12.0 by extraction with benzene were 98.27 ± 3.61 and 81.63 ± 2.84%, respectively. The ratio of the peak heights of quinidine to the internal standard plotted

TABLE 1.12

Retention Times of TMSi Derivatives of Cinchona Alkaloids[a]

Alkaloid	Ret. time (min)
Cinchonidine	11.6
Cinchonine	11.6
Dihydrocinchonidine	10.5
Dihydrocinchonine	10.5
Epiquinidine	17.8
Epiquinine	19.9
Dihydroquinidine	19.5
Dihydroquinine	19.5
Quinidine	21.0
Quinine	21.0
Quininone	17.4
Quinotoxine (quinicine)	32.0
Thioglycerol adduct of quinidine	~282.0

[a]Adapted from Smith et al. [63].

against concentration in the 0.2- to 12.0-µg/ml range gave a straight line passing through the origin (r = 1). A mean slope value of 0.295 ± 0.008 was obtained. The overall coefficient of variation was 4.61%."

Applied to the determination of quinidine plasma levels in a healthy male volunteer and a dog, the plasma profiles obtained are illustrated in Figure 1.13.

The structures of the methylated derivatives of quinidine and cinchonidine were confirmed using an integrated Parker-Elmer model 900 gas chromotograph interfaced with a Hitachi-Perkin-Elmer model RMSU mass spectrometer. From their data, Midha and Charette postulated the mass spectral fragmentation of flash-methylated quinidine and cinchonidine as shown in Figure 1.14, noting that:

The mass spectrum of methylated quinidine showed a molecular ion at m/e 338. Characteristic ions at m/e 323, 308, 203, 202, 188, 186, 173, 172, 159, 158, 136, 129, 108, and 81 were tentatively assigned the structures illustrated [see Fig. 1.14]. These

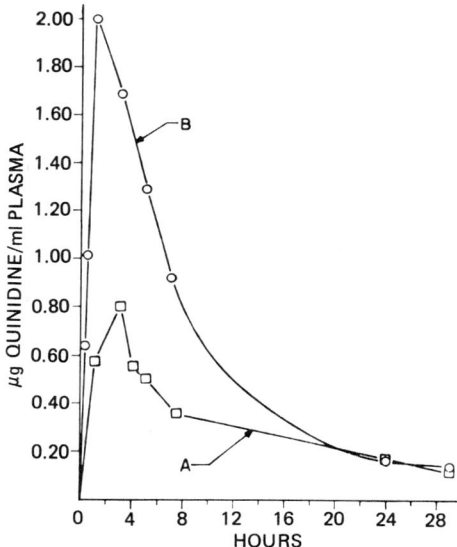

Figure 1.13. Plasma profile of quinidine. Key: (A), healthy male volunteer (73 kg) receiving a 200-mg tablet of quinidine sulfate; and (B), dog receiving 10 mg quinidine sulfate/kg. From Midha and Charette [64], courtesy of the Journal of Pharmaceutical Sciences.

fragmentations suggest that flash-methylated quinidine has Structure Ia. The mass spectrum of flash-methylated cinchonidine showed a molecular ion at m/e 308 and other major ions at m/e 293, 278, 173, 172, 156, 143, 142, 136, 129, 128, 108, and 81. Structures for these ions were postulated, indicating that flash-methylated cinchonidine has Structure Ib.

In 1976, Valentine, Driscoll, Hamburg, and Thompson [65] assayed by GC quinidines (quinidine and hydroquinidine) in human plasma using a procedure that had been evaluated over a 0.5- to 10.0-μg/ml range which gave an overall precision and accuracy of ±4.5% (RSD and RE). The recommended extraction procedure consisted of the following:

To 1 ml of plasma was added 0.5 ml of 5% NaOH and 5 ml of methylene chloride. This solution was mixed thoroughly for 10 to 15 sec and then allowed to stand for 1 min. The lower organic phase was removed, and the plasma layer was reextracted with 5 ml of methylene chloride. In general, this second extraction was centrifuged at 2500 rpm for 5 min to give separation of layers.

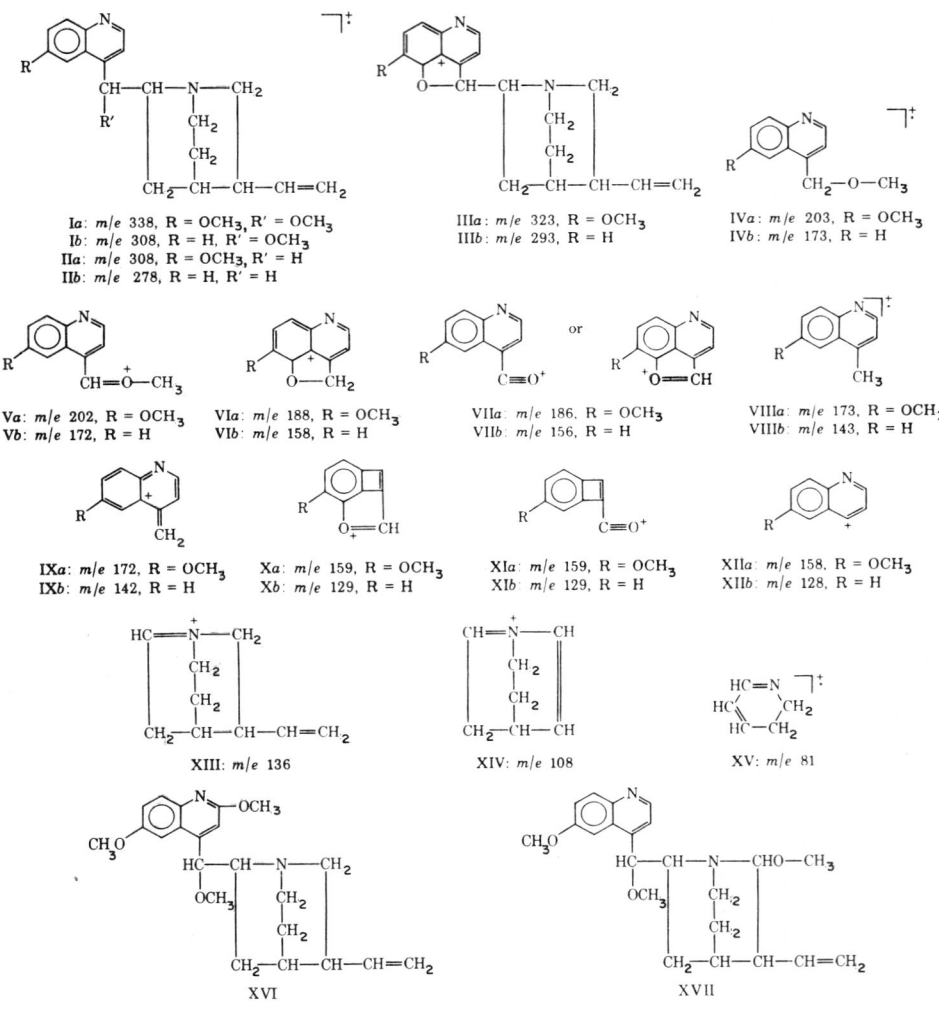

Figure 1.14. Postulated mass spectral fragmentation of flash-methylated quinidine and cinchonidine. From Midha and Charette [64], courtesy of the Journal of Pharmaceutical Sciences.

The lower layer was removed again and combined with the first extract, to which was added 0.5 ml of the cinchonine internal standard solution (4 μg/ml). This solution was evaporated to dryness under a stream of nitrogen at 50°C. To the resultant residue was added 30 µl of 0.2 M trimethylanilinium hydroxide in methanol, followed by mixing. Then 1 µl of this solution was analyzed by GC.

For this investigation, Valentine et al. used a Packard model 419 gas chromotograph equipped with a hydrogen flame ionization detector and a 1.83-m by 2-mm-i.d. glass-coiled column packed with 3% OV-17 coated on 80-100 mesh Chromosorb W-HP. The separation of the methylated derivatives was performed at specified GC operating conditions: injector temperature, 220°C; detector temperature, 200°C; column temperature, programmed from 255 to 280°C with an initial isothermal period of 4 min, a temperature rise of 5°C/min, a final isothermal period of 5 min; nitrogen carrier-gas flow rate, 14.5 ml/min. Using these conditions, the retention times of quinidine, hydroquinidine, and cinchonine were 9.1, 9.1, and 5.9 min, respectively. Although their method does not distinguish between quinidine and hydroquinidine, the overall recovery of quinidine added to plasma over a concentration range of 0.5 to 10.0 µg/ml was 99.9%.

In 1976, Huffman and Hignite [66] determined serum quinidine concentrations in patients on chronic therapeutic doses; a study in which a comparison of fluorescence (method 1: protein precipitate procedure described by Brodie and Udenfriend [67]; method 2: extraction method of Hartel and Korhonen [68] as modified by Kessler et al. [52]), gas chromatographic, and gas chromatographic-mass spectrometric methods was made.

With regard to the GC procedure, Huffman and Hignite noted that:

We used a modification of the flash methylation procedure of Midha and Charette [64]. To duplicate 1-ml serum samples, 1 ml of water containing the internal standard, cinchonidine (2 µg/ml), 0.5 ml of NaOH (1 mole/liter), and 5 ml of benzene were added. The mixture was shaken for 10 min, centrifuged, and the benzene layer transferred to a conical tube and evaportated at 70°C under air. The residue was reconstituted in 25 µl of trimethylanilinium hydroxide (0.2 mole/liter in methanol). Two microliters of the TMAnH solution were injected into a Varian Aerograph model 2400 gas chromatograph equipped with a hydrogen flame detector. Nitrogen was the carrier gas, with a flow rate of 30 ml/min. The column was a 180-cm glass column packed with 3% OV-17 on Gas Chrom Q, 80-100 mesh. The temperatures of the injection port, column, and detector were 320, 245, and 285°C, respectively. Under these conditions, the retention times for methylated cinchonidine and quinidine were 4.25 and 7.20 min, respectively.

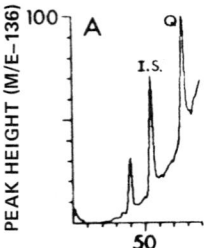

Figure 1.15. Mass chromatograms for m/e 136, the base peak in the mass spectra of the methylated products of both quinidine (Q) and cinchonidine (IS) for a 5-μg/ml quinidine standard. Adapted from Huffman and Hignite [66].

With the above GC procedure, the sensitivity limit for serum quinidine concentration was 50 ng/ml. The quinidine levels were determined by the peak-height ratio for quinidine and the internal standard over a 1.0- to 7.0-μg/ml concentration range.

For further verification of the GC method, portions of selected samples were also examined by an integrated GC-MS-COMP system, a Finnigan 3300 GC-MS, operated on line with a Finnigan 6000 data system. Using column conditions identical to the GC analyses except that helium was the carrier gas (30 ml/min) and the column temperature was programmed from 220 to 320°C at 10°C/min, the electron impact (EI) mass spectra were continuously monitored throughout the complete PTGC analysis, five to ten mass spectra being recorded for each effluent component. For the determination of quinidine in each specimen, the mass chromatogram for m/e 136, the base peak in the mass spectra of the methylated products of both quinidine and cinchonidine, was used. Quantitative data were obtained via the computer system based on the areas of the peaks in the mass chromatogram for both quinidine and internal standard. Figure 1.15 is a typical mass chromatogram for m/e 136, the base peak in the mass spectra of the methylated products of both quinidine (Q) and cinchonidine (IS).

Based on their comparative data, they summarized their findings as follows:

> Although results were higher by a protein precipitate-fluorescence method as compared to a specific extraction fluorescence method, there was substantial correlation between results by the two methods ($r = 0.945$, $p < 0.001$). We established the specificity of the extraction method by a methylation gas chromatographic method and by a

gas chromatographic-mass spectrometric method in which the base peak in the mass spectra of the methylated products of both quinidine and cinchonidine, the internal standard, was monitored. We conclude that the protein precipitate method should be discarded.

B. Procainamide

Procainamide [p-amino-N-(2-diethylaminoethyl)-benzamide] differs structurally from procaine merely in replacement of the ester linkage by the amide moiety. Although a large percentage of the drug is excreted unchanged by man, a small amount, 2 to 10%, is excreted either as p-aminobenzoic acid via the hydrolysis metabolic pathway or as N-acetylprocainamide (NAPA) via the acetylation route; these metabolic pathways are shown in Figure 1.16.

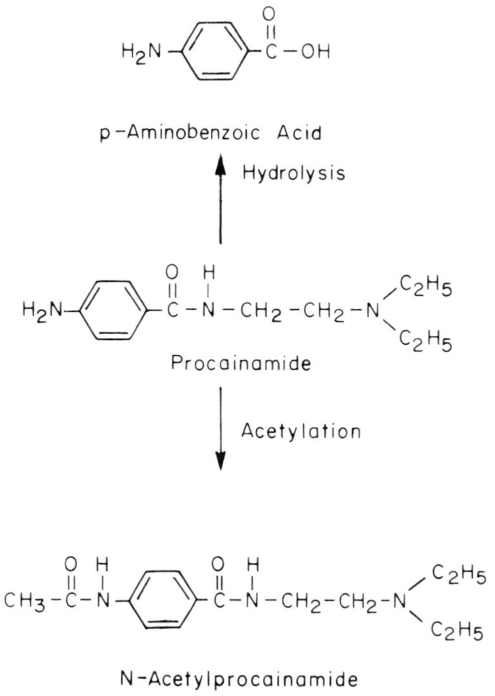

Figure 1.16. Biotransformation of procainamide via two metabolic pathways.

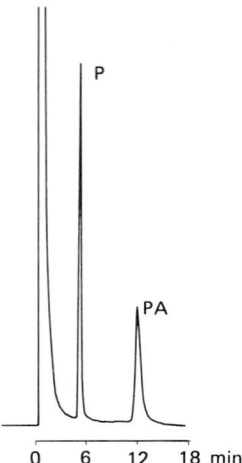

Figure 1.17. Separation of procaine (P) and procainamide (PA) on an OV-17 glass column. Adapted from Kern et al. [69]

Procainamide and its metabolites have been analyzed by either GC or GC-MS in recent years [28,59,69-89]. As noted by Kern et al. [69], both procaine (see Chapter 2, Volume 5, for details of its analysis) and procainamide have been used in clinical arrhythmia since 1951. Used primarily as an alternative to quinidine, both compounds can be easily separated without derivatization as illustrated in Figure 1.17. This separation was performed with a Varian Aerograph model 2100 equipped with flame ionization detection and 4-ft by 1/4-in.-o.d. glass columns packed with 3% OV-17 coated on 100-120 mesh Chromosorb W-HP. To obtain the retention times for both compounds indicated in Figure 1.17, the column was maintained isothermally at 230°C with a nitrogen carrier-gas flow rate of 45 ml/min.

In 1972, Atkinson et al. [70] developed a rapid GC method for measuring procainamide in plasma. Sample preparation for GC analysis consisted of adding to 1 ml of plasma contained in a 15-ml glass-stoppered conical centrifuge tube 1 ml of internal standard solution [the dipropyl analog of procainamide, p-amino-N-(2-dipropylaminoethyl)-benzamide prepared in a concentration of 5 mg/liter of water], 0.2 ml of 5 M NaOH, and 3 ml of methylene chloride. Following centriguation at 1600 X g for 3 min, the methylene chloride phase was transferred to a 5-ml pear-shaped flask where it was subsequently evaporated at 350 mm Hg in a water bath at 25°C. The residue was dissoved in 50 μl of ethyl acetate, and from the extract solution a 5-µl aliquot was withdrawn and injected into the gas chromatograph. For quantitative investigations, a standard curve was constructed by plotting the peak-height ratio of procainamide to internal standard versus the procainamide concentration in each standard sample.

For this study, the GC analyses were performed with a Varian series 1400 gas chromatograph equipped with a flame ionization detector and a 2-m by 2-mm-i.d. glass-coiled column packed with 0.2% OV-17 on 100-120 mesh Corning GLC-110 textured glass beads. To obtain retention times for procainamide and the internal standard of approximately 3.92 and 5.95 min, respectively, the following operating conditions were used: injector temperature, 230°C; column temperature, 225°C; detector temperature, 240°C; nitrogen carrier-gas flow rate, 30 ml/min. At the conditions specified, N-acetylprocainamide had a retention time about 3.9 times that of the parent drug or about 15.3 min. As noted by the authors, "the efficiency of the extraction of procainamide from plasma was 80%. The precision of the method, determined by analyzing standard plasma solutions of procainamide at least five times in duplicate, averages less than 8% for procainamide concentrations ranging from 1 to 20 mg/liter. This standard deviation is comparable to the precision for the most widely used gas-chromatographic method for measuring lidocaine [90], but is greater than the standard deviation (1.8% to 3.2%) reported for the spectrophotometric and spectrofluorometric methods for procainamide."

GC-MS investigations were carried out with a Finnigan model 3000 instrument equipped and operated as follows: 2-m by 2-mm-i.d. stainless steel column packed with 3% OV-17 coated on 80-100 mesh Chromosorb W-HP; GC injector temperature, 250°C; GC column temperature, 230°C; helium carrier-gas flow rate, 20 ml/min; GC-MS transfer-line temperature, 225°C; MS ionizing energy, 70 eV. Used to monitor and confirm the identity of the peaks emerging from the GC column, they noted that the most prominent ion, or base peak, for procainamide and the internal standard occurred at m/e 86 and 114, respectively.

Meola [71] described in 1973 a GC procedure utilizing a stabilized OV-17 liquid phase on glass beads for the determination of lidocaine and procainamide at therapeutic and toxic levels in serum. The procedure used to isolate both drugs from serum was as follows:

1. Transfer 1 ml of serum to a 15-ml glass-stoppered centrifuge tube. Add 1 ml of internal standard solution (either chlordiazepoxide for procainamide or mepivacaine for lidocaine analysis) followed by 2 ml of carbonate-buffer (pH 11.0 prepared by dissolving 21 g of sodium carbonate and 420 mg of sodium bicarbonate in 1 liter of water). Add 10 mg of Norit A (neutral charcoal).

2. Mix briefly on a Vortex mixer and then centrifuge at 2000 rpm for 4 min.

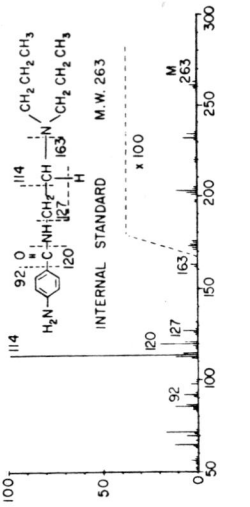

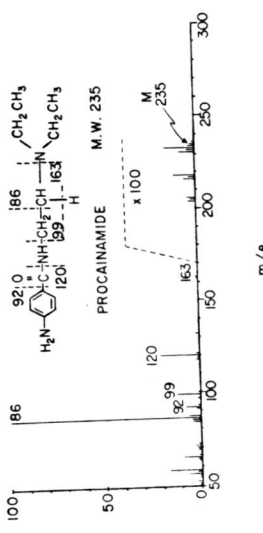

3. After the removal of the supernatant by aspiration, disperse the charcoal over the wall of the tube using the Vortex mixer. Extract the charcoal with 2 ml of chloroform (shake the tube's contents vigorously).
4. Decant the chloroform into a small glass tube and evaporate it to dryness at room temperature using a stream of nitrogen.
5. After dissolving the residue in 20 μl of chloroform, a 1-μl aliquot is injected into the chromatograph.

The gas chromatograph used consisted of a Perkin-Elmer model 900 instrument equipped with dual flame ionization detectors and a 6-ft by 0.08-in. i.d. glass column packed with 0.2% OV-17 on 100-120 mesh Corning GLC-110 textured glass beads (the OV-17 liquid phase was stabilized by the addition of 0.2% Silanox). The helium carrier-gas flow rate, injector temperature, and detector temperature were maintained at 20 ml/min, 270°C, and 300°C, respectively. The column temperature was slightly varied, depending on the analysis to be performed: 255°C for procainamide and 220°C for lidocaine. Under these operating conditions, the retention times of procainamide to chlordiazepoxide and lidocaine relative to mepivacaine were 0.465 and 0.482, respectively.

Meola summarized his findings as follows:

Detection limits as low as 1 μg/ml of lidocaine and 5 μg/ml for procainamide are attained with good accuracy of quantitation. The coefficient of variation for replicate lidocaine and mepivacaine determinations carried out on the same day is close to 5% at the 5- and 10-μg/ml levels. For procainamide it is 12% at the 5-μg/ml level and 5.7% at the 10-μg/ml level. Recoveries range from 60% for procainamide to 75% for lidocaine and mepivacaine, at levels from 5 μg/ml to 20 μg/ml. The procedure for procainamide shows excellent correlation with a spectrophotometric method ($r = 0.92$).

Sterling et al. [73] developed a procedure for the analysis of procainamide in plasma based on the reaction of procainamide with fluorescamine and subsequent determination of the derivative by spectrophotofluorometry. The accuracy and precision of results were compared to those obtained using colorimetric and GC methods.

In their comparative study, the extraction of procainamide from plasma was carried out in the following manner:

Two milliliters of plasma was mixed with pH 9.5 borate buffer (1 ml), extracted with 16.0 ml of methylene dichloride, and centrifuged at

2000 rpm for 3 min. The extract was passed through phase-separating filter paper. An aliquot (6.0 ml) was removed, evaporated to dryness, and reconstituted with pH 5.5 phosphate buffer. Fluorescence of the solution was determined against a reagent blank.

An aliquot (6.0 ml) of the remaining methylene dichloride extract was combined with 3.0 ml of internal standard solution (dibucaine, 8.5 µg/ml of chloroform as solvent), evaporated to dryness, reconstituted with 50 µl of carbon disulfide, and injected into the chromatograph.

GC analyses were performed with a Varian model 575 gas chromatograph equipped with a flame ionization detector and a 1.82-m spiral-shaped borosilicate column packed with 0.5% Versamid 900 and 6% (3,3,3-trifluoropropyl)-methylsilicone coated on 100-120 calcined diatomite. For the quantitative determination of procainamide (peak areas determined using an automatic electronic integrator), the GC conditions used were injector temperature, 270°C; column temperature, 235°C; detector temperature, 280°C; nitrogen carrier-gas flow rate, 40 ml/min; hydrogen flow rate, 40 ml/min; air flow rate, 225 ml/min. Maintaining these conditions, the retention times of procainamide and dibucaine were 4.02 and 5.85 min, respectively.

As noted by the authors, calibration curves for the GC assay were prepared on ten consecutive days, and the standard deviation of the curve slope was 1.6%. The average correlation coefficient was 1.022, and the average y intercept was +0.007. Results of the investigation of the extraction efficiency as determined by spectrophotofluorometry and GC are shown in Table 1.13, whereas the data from the study designed to examine day-to-day accuracy and precision of each of the three analytical procedures are listed in Table 1.14. Finally, the specificity of the fluorometric and colorimetric methods was studied by assaying the apparent procainamide concentration in plasma of patients and comparing these results with those obtained by GC; the comparative data are given in Table 1.15.

In 1975, Simons and Levy [76] presented a GC method for the determination of procainamide (PA) in which a dipropyl analog of procainamide was used as an internal standard such that both compounds could be chromatographed directly, yielding linear calibration curves and a sensitivity that allows quantitative determination of concentrations as low as 0.1 µg/ml.

Using an extraction procedure that was carefully modified to avoid hydrolysis of N-acetylprocainamide (APA), a 1 to 3 µl aliquot of the final chloroform solution containing the extract and internal standard (p-amino-N-[2-(dipropylamino)ethyl]-benzamide) was injected directly into a Varian Aerograph model 200 equipped with a flame ionization detector and a 0.91-m by 2-mm-i.d. glass-coiled column packed with 10% OV-7 on 60-80 mesh Gas Chrom Q and operated isothermally at 245°C with the p-Amino-N-[2-(dipropylamino)ethyl]-benzamide

injector and detector temperatures maintained at 280 and 300°C, respectively. Using a helium carrier-gas flow rate of 40 ml/min, the retention times of PA, the internal standard, and APA were approximately 2.91, 4.36, and 8.40 min, respectively.

Daily calibration curves prepared by plotting peak height ratios against PA concentration (μg/ml) yielded a linear regression equation y = 0.229x - 0.002 (r = 1.000). With regard to the precision of the method, for amounts

TABLE 1.13

Efficiency of Extraction of Procainamide from Plasma as Determined by GLC and Spectrophotofluorometry[a]

Method	Procainamide		Recovery (%)	SD (%)[b]
	Added (μg)	Recovered (μg)		
GLC	2.00	1.97	98.50	5.43
Spectrophotofluorometry	2.00	2.02	101.00	2.73
GLC	4.00	4.13	103.75	4.51
Spectrophotofluorometry	4.00	3.96	98.75	2.30
GLC	8.00	7.85	98.12	1.84
Spectrophotofluorometry	8.00	7.93	99.12	1.94
GLC	12.00	12.31	102.58	2.47
Spectrophotofluorometry	12.00	12.11	101.16	2.11
GLC	16.00	15.53	97.06	4.14
Spectrophotofluorometry	16.00	15.74	98.30	1.76
GLC	20.00	21.06	105.33	5.91
Spectrophotofluorometry	20.00	20.40	102.00	2.14

[a]From Sterling et al. [73], courtesy of the Journal of Pharmaceutical Sciences.
[b]n = 10.

TABLE 1.14

Accuracy and Precision of Three Methods of
Procainamide Determination[a]

Method	Procainamide Quantity (μg)	Procainamide Found (μg)	Recovery (%)	SD (%)[b]
GLC	2.00	1.94	97.00	7.57
Spectrophotofluorometry	2.00	2.02	101.00	3.41
Colorimetry	2.00	2.09	104.50	9.84
GLC	4.00	4.23	105.75	6.90
Spectrophotofluorometry	4.00	4.13	103.25	4.11
Colorimetry	4.00	3.81	95.25	8.72
GLC	8.00	8.31	103.87	5.74
Spectrophotofluorometry	8.00	8.07	100.87	3.02
Colorimetry	8.00	8.39	104.87	6.59
GLC	12.00	12.60	105.00	6.94
Spectrophotofluorometry	12.00	11.71	97.59	3.17
Colorimetry	12.00	11.55	96.25	6.87
GLC	16.00	16.03	100.19	8.42
Spectrophotofluorometry	16.00	15.87	99.19	2.54
Colorimetry	16.00	15.34	95.88	7.22

[a]From Sterling et al. [73], courtesy of the Journal of Pharmaceutical Sciences.
[b]$n = 30$.

ranging from 1 to 10 μg, coefficients of variation ranged from 3.6 to 9.5%, whereas the standard deviation of the slope of nine routine calibration curves over 8 months was 4.0%.

Simons and Levy noted that "the recovery of PA from spiked plasma samples was determined to be 37.3%, and the recovery from urine samples was 82.8%. The low recovery in the double-extraction procedure is due to several factors: (a) the unfavorable solvent ratio of 8 ml of ether to 0.2 ml of phthalate buffer (pH 3), (b) the transfer of this small volume from test tubes to the vials, and (c) the necessity of two extractions at pH 10.8 (procainamide pK_a 9.23) to prevent hydrolysis of N-acetylprocainamide."

TABLE 1.15

Procainamide Concentration in Plasma as Determined by Three Methods[a]

Sample	Other drugs	Apparent Procainamide Concentration[b]		
		GLC	Spectrophoto-fluorometry	Colorimetry
1	Nitrofurantoin, methaqualone	5.40	5.12	5.59
2	Digoxin, glutethimide	7.21	6.84	7.36
3	Chlordiazepoxide, codeine	2.74	2.92	4.16
4	Tolbutamide, diazepam	6.14	6.23	5.71
5	Aspirin, phenacetin, caffeine, propoxyphene	2.10	2.34	2.61
6	Dicumarol, erythromycin	6.41	6.29	6.53
7	Aspirin, codeine, chlordiazepoxide	5.37	5.54	8.97
8	Methaqualone, chlorothiazide	10.74	9.96	10.92

[a]From Sterling et al. [73], courtesy of the Journal of Pharmaceutical Sciences.
[b]Expressed in micrograms per milliliter.

On the other hand, "a study of the hydrolysis of N-acetylprocainamide in 1 N HCl revealed 77.5% hydrolysis in 8 hr at 50°C and 26.3% hydrolysis in 18 hr at 25°C. In 1 N NaOH, 83.0% of N-acetylprocainamide was found in 8 hr at 50°C. Control studies on procainamide showed no hydrolysis in either 1 N HCl or 1 N NaOH in 8 hr at 50°C. There was, however, no hydrolysis of N-acetylprocainamide between pH 3 and 10 for up to 40 hr at 50°C. Therefore, buffers at pH3 (phthalate buffer) and pH 10.8 (2 N Na_2CO_3) were substituted for the 2 N HCl and 2 N NaOH solutions, respectively, used in the procedure of Mather and Tucker [91]. Analysis of solutions of N-acetylprocainamide by this method showed no more procainamide present than control solutions of N-acetylprocainamide injected directly into the gas chromatograph without extraction."

Frislid et al. [77], realizing the need for and value of controlling the plasma concentrations of the active drug, compared the fluorometric and GC methods for the determination of PA. For this purpose, the plasma PA concentration of 20 patients on PA therapy was monitored by the fluorometric method by Koch-Weser and Klein [44], using a Perkin-Elmer fluorescence spectrophotometer (model MPF 2A) whereas, for comparison, a modified Atkinson et al. GC procedure [70] was used for specific and concomitant analysis of PA and APA in the same samples. In the GC method, the analyses were performed with Varian model 2100 gas chromatograph equipped with a flame ionization detector and a 1-m by 2-mm-i.d. silanized glass column packed with 5% OV-17 on 100-120 mesh Gas Chrom Q. Using standard solutions containing 2, 5, and 10 μg each of PA and APA per milliliter (prepared in drug-free human sera), sample preparation for GC studies was as follows:

Volumes of 0.1 ml of p-amino-N-(2-dipropylaminoethyl)-benzamide (internal standard, 50 μg/ml of distilled water), 0.5 ml of 2 M NaOH, and 8 ml of dichloromethane were carefully mixed with 1 ml of sample for 10 min in a 12-ml stoppered tube. After centrifugation, 5 ml of the dichloromethane layer was evaporated at 20°C under a stream of nitrogen, the residue redissolved in 50 μl of ethyl acetate, and a 3-μl sample injected into the chromatograph. Under the conditions described, the peak-height ratios between the drugs and the internal standard plotted versus the drug concentration gave a linear relationship.

The extraction recoveries of PA and APA were 90 and 97%, respectively, whereas their respective coefficients of variation for the modified GC procedure were 3.3 and 8.2% (n = 15). The standard deviation for PA using the fluorometric method was reported to be 3.2% [44].

As shown in Table 1.16, the PA values by both methods were rather equal, despite some tendency for higher results in most fluorometric determinations. Frislid et al. theorized that this could be due to the presence of APA, which has a fluorescence spectrum very close to that of PA (excitation maximum, 300 and 295 nm; emission maximum, 336 and 355 nm, respectively) and, at the emission maximum of PA, a fluorescence intensity of about 6% of that of PA.

As noted by the authors:

Recovery of APA when extracted with benzene under the conditions of the fluorometric method was, however, only about 50%. Thus, at equal plasma concentrations of the two substances, APA might add about 3% to the apparent PA concentration as determined fluorometrically. As seen from Table [1.16], the concentration ratio of

TABLE 1.16

PA and APA Concentrations in Plasma from 20 Patients on Maintenance Therapy, as Analyzed by the Gas Chromatographic (Both) and the Fluorometric (PA) Methods[a]

Fluorometric method PA	Gas chromatographic method		
	PA (mg/liter)	APA	APA/PA
8.7	8.8	10.5	1.19
8.6	8.6	6.2	0.72
6.4	6.0	7.6	1.27
5.4	5.3	3.0	0.57
4.9[b]	5.1	3.0	0.59
4.8	4.6	5.6	1.30
4.6	4.4	9.4	2.14
4.0	3.6	5.7	1.58
3.9	4.1	3.2	0.78
3.5	3.5	6.5	1.90
3.3	3.1	6.1	1.96
3.2[b]	3.3	7.7	2.33
3.0	2.8	8.5	3.05
2.7	2.5	3.8	1.52
2.7	2.5	7.6	3.04
1.7	1.3	2.0	1.67
1.7	1.6	1.6	1.00
1.5	1.3	3.2	2.46
1.4	1.0	1.5	1.56
0.9	0.8	4.3	4.80

[a]From Frislid et al. [77], courtesy of Clinical Chemistry.
[b]Patients with manifest SLE syndrome.

APA and PA in plasma varied from 0.57 to 4.80. In the patient with the highest ratio (the last listed) it would be expected that APA could add 12 to 14% to the PA concentration as determined fluorometrically.

Based on their findings, Frislid et al. concluded that the fluorometric method was adequate for routine control of procainamide therapy but, since APA also possesses significant antiarrhythmic activity in man, the wide interindividual variation in the APA/PA plasma ratio may require concomitant GC determination of both substances to ensure optimal therapy.

Drayer et al. [89] discussed the role of GC-MS in a clinical pharmacology program in 1976, using as an example the metabolic fate in vivo of procainamide, and others in the past several years have studied the pharmacokinetics of both procainamide [79,81,86-88,92] and N-acetylprocainamide [80,82-85,93].

Using GC-MS for the qualitative identification of drug metabolities from biological fluids, Drayer et al. [89] reviewed its role in a clinical pharmacology environment, describing an experimental procedure to ascertain PA in vivo metabolism as reported by Drayer et al. [75] in 1974. In their approach to APA identification, its presence was confirmed based on a comparison of GC retention time (about 5.47 min using a Varian Aerograph model 1840 gas chromatograph equipped with a 6-ft by 1/4-in. glass column packed with 0.2% OV-17 on Corning textured glass beads maintained isothermally at 230°C with a nitrogen carrier-gas flow rate of 30 ml/min) and mass spectrum with that of an authentic sample. As did Drayer et al. [75] and Elson et al. [93], they noted that APA plasma levels were higher than simultaneously measured PA concentrations. The reference mass spectrum (similar to that shown in an earlier section of this chapter by Atkinson et al. [70]) was obtained on a Finnigan 3000 quadrupole GC-MS unit equipped with a 2-m by 2-mm-i.d. glass column containing 3% SE-30: OV-17 (6:1 ratio, respectively) and operated in the following manner: injection port temperature, 250°C; column temperature, 245°C; transfer-line temperature, 180°C; ionizing potential, 70 eV. Using a novel MS technique that combines temperature-controlled evaporation of a sample (removed from a TLC plate) from a solid-probe inlet system with selective ion monitoring of mass spectral ions, in this particular study compound identification was based on the time at which compound vaporization is maximal (about 2.60 to 2.74 min) during a programmed increase in direct-probe temperature and on the relative intensity of two selected mass spectral ions (m/e ions 162:86 having a ratio between 0.0239 to 0.0243).

Using spectrofluorometric [44] and spectrophotometric [94] methods for the determination of unchanged PA in plasma [44] and urine [94] and the GC procedure of Karlsson [72] for estimating APA levels in urine which employed a glass column containing 3% OV-17 on 100-120 mesh Gas Chrom Q with hexatriacontane as internal standard, Graffner et al. [79]

studied the pharmacokinetics of PA in healthy volunteers after single doses intravenously and orally as conventional and slow-release tablets and after repeated oral doses at steady state. From their investigation, they noted that:

> The initial distribution after intravenous administration was rapid and the overall elimination in the β-phase corresponded to $t_{1/2}$ of 2.7 hr. The mean volume of the central compartment (based on a two-compartment open model) was small and only 4% of $V_{d(\beta)}$, which was 2.3 liters/kg of body weight. About 65% was excreted unchanged after intravenous administration and about 55% after a single oral dose of 500 mg [a typical plot of PA level versus time is shown in Fig. 1.18A]. The recovery of the APA metabolite was 12% after both routes of administration. Procainamide was completely adsorbed from the gastrointestinal tract and the first-pass elimination was very limited. The rates of absorption from the tablet compositions were well correlated to the in vitro dissolution properties. Administration of slow-release tablets every 8 hr gave about the same mean plasma level as steady state as ordinary tablets given every 4 hr [see Fig. 1.18B], and the availability was the same from both preparations. The occasional high plasma concentration peaks after ordinary tablets were not observed after the slow-release tablets. Renal clearance was about 500 ml/min, indicating an active secretion in the tubules.

The rate of formation of total metabolites after intravenous administration was determined by combining Eqs. (1.2) and (1.3),

$$k_{el} = k_f + k_e \tag{1.2}$$

$$\frac{M_u^\infty}{X_u^\infty} = \frac{k_f}{k_e} \tag{1.3}$$

where M_u^∞ is the amount of total metabolites and X_u^∞ the amount of unchanged drug excreted in urine within infinite time, respectively; k_f is the rate constant for formation of total metabolites; and k_e is the urinary elimination rate constant of unchanged drug from the central compartment. Based on four male volunteers receiving 500 mg of procainamide administered intravenously, the mean elimination rate constants as well as urinary excretion obtained were X_u^∞ (mg), 332; M_u^∞ (mg), 167; k_{el} (hr^{-1}), 4.0; k_e (hr^{-1}), 2.6; k_f (hr^{-1}), 1.4. From these data, the rate of formation of metabolites corresponded to a $t_{1/2}$ of approximately 30 min whereas the average urinary elimination rate of unchanged PA yielded a $t_{1/2}$ of about 20 min.

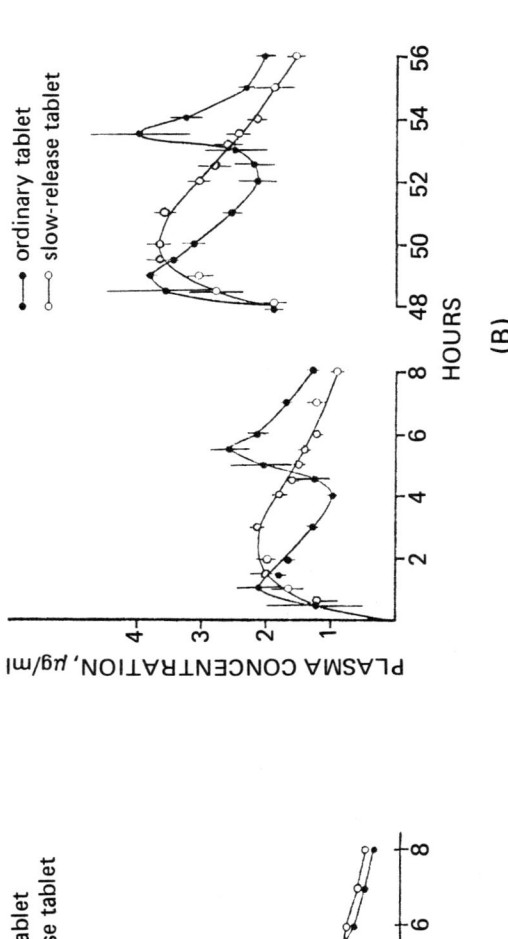

Figure 1.18. Typical individual plasma PA concentrations after a single 500-mg oral dose (A) and after repeated doses of slow-release and conventional tablets administered every 8 and 4 hr, respectively (B). Adapted from Graffner et al. [79].

In 1975, Simons et al. [81] reinvestigated the pharmacokinetics of PA in normal subjects using GC because previous studies using colorimetric and fluorometric methods for the determination of drug concentrations in plasma and urine were suspect in view of recent evidence that APA, the major metabolite in humans, is hydrolyzed during these assay procedures. As a result, a specific GC method [Ref. 76, previously discussed in this chapter] was used for the determination of PA in biological fluids.

The experimental data points were fitted to a biexponential equation,

$$C_p = Ae^{-\alpha t} + Be^{-\beta t} \tag{1.4}$$

where C_p represents the plasma concentration at any time t, A and B are the zero time intercepts, and α and β are the hybrid time constants. This suggested that the pharmacokinetics of PA minimally should be described by a two-compartment open model as indicated below:

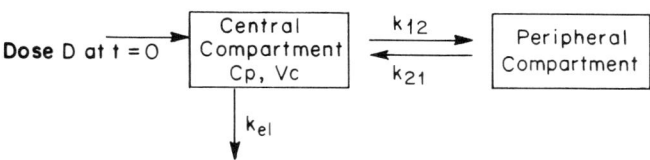

Following the administration of a 3.5-mg/kg dose of PA by slow intravenous injection over a 5-min period to seven healthy, drug-free volunteers, urine and plasma specimens were taken for analysis at specified time intervals. Using the GC data, kinetic parameters for plasma specimens were calculated as shown in Table 1.17. Simons et al. noted that the values of half-life, volume of distribution, and total body clearance found in this study differed from those previously reported; these differences ascribed to differences in assay specificity. The discrepancies attributed to methodology are also shown in Table 1.17, where kinetic parameters calculated for one normal subject from GC and colorimetric (values shown in parentheses) data are compared.

Analysis of urine specimens yielded a calculated mean biological half-life ($t_{1/2}$) of 2.22 ± 0.36 hr, which was in good agreement with the value determined from plasma measurements.

Galeazzi et al. [86,87] reported their findings in 1976 for two studies: (1) the renal elimination of PA and (2) the relationship between the pharmacokinetics and pharmacodynamics of PA.

In the investigation of renal elimination of PA [86], analyses for PA and APA concentrations were performed with a Varian 1400 gas chromatograph equipped with a hydrogen flame ionization detector and a 6-ft

TABLE 1.17

Average PA Kinetic Parameters (Plasma)[a,b]

No. of subjects	α (hr^{-1})	$t_{1/2}$ (β, hr)[c]	k_{el} (hr^{-1})	V_c (liters/kg)[d]
7	10.0 ± 4.8	2.1 ± 0.5	1.7 ± 0.9	0.9 ± 0.5
1		1.9 (2.7)		0.5 (0.4)

[a]Adapted from Simons et al. [81].
[b]Creatinine clearance, 122.9 ± 34.4 ml/min; serum creatinine, 0.91 ± 0.2 mg%.
[c]$t_{1/2} = 0.693/\beta$.
[d]Volume of central compartment.
[e]Volume of distribution.

by 1/8-in. o.d. glass coiled column packed with 3% OV-7 coated on 100-120 mesh Gas Chrom Q. Maintaining specified GC operating conditions (column temperature, 260°C; injector temperature, 240°C; detector temperature, 285°C; nitrogen carrier-gas flow rate, 30 ml/min), the retention times of PA, internal standard [p-amino-N-(2-dipropylaminoethyl)-benzamide], and APA were 7.5, 11.0, and 23.5 min, respectively. To obtain quantitative data, standard curves of PA and APA were prepared from standard solutions containing PA, APA, and internal standard and their respective digital readings obtained with an electronic integrator.

Galeazzi et al. summarized this study as follows:

> The question of pH or flow dependence for the renal elimination of procainamide was studied under four conditions in each of four subjects. Each subject received 500 mg of procainamide intravenously at weekly intervals while in a state of (1) acid load (NH$_4$Cl) and water deprivation, (2) acid load and water excess, (3) alkali load (NaHCO$_3$) and water deprivation, and (4) alkali load and water excess. Plasma and urine were collected at frequent intervals for procainamide and N-acetylprocainamide analysis. Urine flow rates varied markedly between the water deprivation and water excess states (approximately 1.5 vs. 5.0 ml/min, respectively), and pH varied markedly between the acid and alkali load states (pH = ca. 5 vs. 8, respectively). Despite this marked variation, there were no significant changes in procainamide renal clearance or

Vd_B (liters/kg)[e]	Total body clearance, (ml/min)	Drug in urine (%)	Renal clearance (ml/min)
4.3 ± 0.6	1344 ± 238	42.3 ± 8.2	580.7 ± 187.5
4.6 (2.5)	1472 (698)		811 (393)

24-hr procainamide or N-acetylprocainamide excretion. If passive diffusion of procainamide were taking place, such flow and pH changes would have caused marked changes in procainamide clearance were the pH partition hypothesis true. We therefore conclude that passive diffusion is not an important mechanism in the renal elimination of procainamide in man and that there must be tubular secretion. The implication for the clinical use of the drug is that dose adjustments need not be made in response to variations in urine flow and pH.

In the subsequent study performed by Galeazzi et al. [87], which used the GC procedure described above to determine the relationship between the pharmacokinetics and pharmacodynamics of procainamide, the investigation and findings were described as follows:

The kinetics of a measure of pharmacologic effect (prolongation of the QT interval of the EKG) of procainamide, as well as the kinetics of the plasma concentration, urine excretion, and saliva concentration of the drug were investigated in 14 trials in four subjects. A single 500-mg dose was given by rapid intravenous infusion, and frequent subsequent determinations of the above variables were made. A two-compartment pharmacokinetic model with a third compartment for the saliva was used to fit the plasma, urine, and saliva data simultaneously. Analysis of the data reveals that the kinetics of the drug concentrations in saliva and of the pharmacologic effect are indistinguishable. They both must be considered to be different from those of the drug concentration in plasma. Thus, in normal individuals under the conditions of this study, saliva concentrations more precisely indicate the time-course of drug at a cardiac site of action, although they do not parallel plasma drug concentrations until 6 hr or more after a rapid intravenous infusion. The following average pharmacokinetic parameters for plasma were found: terminal half-life, 2.9 hr; total clearance, 828 ml/min; renal clearance, 334 ml/min; and steady-state volume of distribution, 180 liters. Average distribution pseudoequilibrium half-life ($t_{1/2}\ \alpha$) was 5.2 min from an initial volume of distribution of 36.6 liters.

The procedure used to prepare samples for GC analysis involved first the alkalinization of the sample followed by the addition of the internal standard (dipropyl analog of PA). The sample was then diluted with water and extracted with dichloromethane; the extract was then back-titrated into an acid aqueous layer, alkalinized, and reextracted with dichloromethane. This last solvent extract was evaporated to dryness, redissolved in dichloromethane, and finally analyzed by gas chromatography.

In 1976, Atkinson et al. [88] reported their clinical and pharmacokinetic observations for a woman (67 years old) who ingested approximately 7 g of procainamide and developed severe hypotension, renal insufficiency, and life-threatening toxicity. Using a GC procedure developed by Elson et al. [83] to study the antiarrhythmic potency of N-acetylprocainamide, Atkinson et al. concluded from their data that:

Hemodialysis doubled the rate of procainamide elimination and increased fourfold the clearance of N-acetylprocainamide, the acetylated metabolite of procainamide. Observations of procainamide and N-acetylprocainamide plasma levels during the patient's recovery suggest that lethargy and profound hypotension can be expected when these levels total 60 μg/ml and that severe cardiac toxicity should be anticipated with levels totaling 42 μg/ml or more. Hemodialysis also permitted investigation of the effects of hypotension on the pharmacokinetics of these compounds. The apparent volume of procainamide distribution was reduced from a normal value of 2 liters/kg to 0.76 liter/kg and that of N-acetylprocainamide from 1.4 liters/kg to 0.63 liters/kg. The elimination of $t_{1/2}$ of procainamide was prolonged from the normal of 3 hr to 10.5 hr, and that of N-acetylprocainamide from 6 to 35.9 hr. Procainamide absorption was also slowed in this clinical setting, causing procainamide plasma levels to continue rising for some time after toxicity was first recognized.

ANTIARRHYTHMIC AGENTS

In this study, dialysance of procainamide and N-acetylprocainamide was calculated using Eq. (1.5), whereas dialytic clearance for each dialysis period was determined by Eq. (1.6). As noted by the investigators, these dialysance and clearance values, given in Table 1.18, were not corrected for procainamide protein binding, which usually averaged 15% [45], or for N-acetylprocainamide protein binding of 11% [95].

$$\text{dialysance} = (\text{flow}) \times \left(\frac{\text{arterial concentration - venous concentration}}{\text{arterial concentration - bath concentration}} \right) \quad (1.5)$$

$$\text{clearance} = \frac{(\text{bath concentration}) \times (\text{bath volume/time})}{(\text{mean arterial concentration})} \quad (1.6)$$

Although not listed in Table 1.18, the dialytic clearances of urea and creatinine averaged 69.2 ml/min and 67.0 ml/min, respectively.

Finally, in 1977, Baer and Barkus [92] studied the disposition of PA and APA in beagle dogs; their objectives being (1) to study the pharmacokinetic behavior of PA in beagles, (2) to determine the effect of urinary pH on renal excretion of PA, and (3) to compare the pharmacokinetics of PA with APA.

To obtain analytical data, plasma PA levels were measured spectrophotometrically by the method of Mark et al. [94] as modified by Sitar, Graham, Rango, Dufresne, and Ogilvie [96]. Urine samples were assayed for PA as above and also by a modification of the Atkinson et al. [70] GC procedure. Duplicate samples of the methylene chloride extract were analyzed for hydrolyzable metabolite (1 N HCl, 100°C, 1 hr). Plasma APA levels were approximated spectrophotometrically after acid hydrolysis. Urinary APA concentrations were analyzed after hydrolysis by both the GC and spectrophotometric methods; furthermore, the deacetylated metabolite was also measured. Whereas the sensitivity of the spectrophotometric and GC methods were reported to be 0.10 μg/ml and 1-2 μg/ml, respectively, the respective recoveries of both species using their procedure were 98% and 97%.

Based on the results found, their data showed that urinary alkalinization (pH between 8.0 and 8.8):

1. Increased $t_{1/2}$ values from 136 to 336 min

2. Decreased renal clearance from 6.50 to 1.80 ml/min/kg

3. Decreased total body clearance from 10.30 to 4.19 ml/min/kg

4. Had very little effect on the apparent body volume at distribution equilibrium (2.09 versus 2.11 liters/kg)

5. Decreased the percentage of PA excreted unchanged in the urine from 60.4% to 42.2%

TABLE 1.18

Dialysis of Procainamide and N Acetylprocainamide[a,b]

Bath number	Time (min)	Concentration (μg/ml)			Bath total (mg)	Dialyzer blood flow (ml/min)	Dialysance (ml/min)	Dialytic clearance (ml/min)
		Arterial plasma	Venous plasma	Bath				
Procainamide								
1	0	25.7	12.7	0	0	100	50.6	
	120	19.7	12.4	2.4	240	100	42.2	87.8
2	0	19.7	12.4	0	0	100	37.1	
	120	15.5	10.0	1.0	100	100	38.0	47.1
							Mean: 42.0	67.5
NAPA								
1	0	47.0	29.2	0	0	100	37.9	
	120	39.8	29.1	2.8	280	100	28.9	53.5
2	0	39.8	29.1	0	0	100	26.9	
	120	35.5	27.8	1.9	190	100	19.9	41.9
							Mean: 28.4	47.7

[a]Adapted from Atkinson et al. [88].
[b]Dialysis data for urea and creatinine concentrations were also determined; expressed in mg/dl.

On the other hand, acid hydrolysis of the urine collected caused a 17% increase in the amount of PA measured. As noted by Baer and Barkus, this hydrolyzable substance was found not to be N-acetylprocainamide and, when i.v. N-acetylprocainamide was administered in crossover fashion to some of the beagles, it exhibited a longer $t_{1/2}$ than PA. In Table 1.19 are compared the PA and APA pharmacokinetic parameters observed in the same dogs as well as human kinetic data reported in the literature for PA [45,79,82,87,97]. As noted, the mean beagle/human set of figures suggests that the beagle may be an adequate model of pharmacokinetics in man because of the similarity of renal and nonrenal clearance dependencies.

In 1975, Gibson et al. [82] assessed the extent of the acetylation of procainamide in man and its relationship to isonicotinic acid hydrazide acetylation phenotype. For the analysis of PA and APA in urine, a Hewlett-Packard model 5750 gas chromatograph equipped with flame ionization detectors and 4-ft by 2-mm-i.d. glass columns packed with 3% OV-17 on 80-100 mesh Gas Chrom Q was used. To obtain retention times of 1.99 and 4.61 min for PA and APA, respectively, the following chromatographic conditions were maintained: injector temperature, 240°C; column temperature, programmed, initial temperature of 230°c held for 3 min after sample injection and then increased at a rate of 50°C/min to the upper limit of 280°C where it was kept isothermally for 2 min; type of carrier and its flow rate not specified. On the other hand, the isonicotinic acid hydrazide (INH) phenotype of each subject was assessed by determining the serum $t_{1/2}$ of INH using the method of Scott and Wright [98] following a single oral dose of 4 mg/kg. Using the $t_{1/2}$ INH data, subjects were classified into two categories: those with $t_{1/2}$ of less than 2 hr were called fast acetylators while those with $t_{1/2}$ values greater than 2 hr were considered slow acetylators [98].

For GC analysis of PA and APA using calibration curves prepared by plotting average integrated peak area versus concentrations, sample preparation involved the addition of 1 ml of the urine specimen to a test tube containing 250 mg of sodium chloride and 250 µl of 2.5 N sodium hydroxide. This mixture was then extracted into 10 ml of redistilled benzene by shaking for 1 min. After centrifugation for 10 min at 800 X g, 9 ml of the benzene phase was transferred to an Addis tube and evaporated to dryness in a 50°C water bath under a stream of nitrogen. After washing down the dried extract with 500 µl of methanol and then drying it again in a vacuum oven at 56°C (10 mm Hg), the final extract residue was redissolved in a measured volume of methanol. From this alcohol solution, an aliquot was withdrawn and injected into the gas chromatograph. Using this procedure, the recoveries of PA and APA added to urine were 97 ± 4% and 87 ± 96%, respectively.

After single doses of 500 mg of PA were administered to 14 subjects with normal renal function, all urine voided for 96 hr was saved and levels of PA and APA measured by gas chromatography. The mean results of this study are shown in Table 1.20 [82].

TABLE 1.19

Comparative Pharmacokinetics of PA and APA in Beagles (Study A) and PA in Beagles and Man (Study B)[a,b]

Drug species	$t_{1/2}$ (min)	C_B (ml/min/kg)	C_R (ml/min/kg)	Vd_{area} (liters/kg)	Excreted unchanged (%)	Urinary metabolites	Ratio (%)
Study A							
PA	142 ± 18	13.77 ± 1.12	7.39 ± 1.65	2.82 ± 0.44	52.7 ± 8.8	16.8% acid hydrolyzable	53.6
APA	235 ± 21	6.29 ± 0.24	3.72 ± 0.31	2.12 ± 0.12	60.1 ± 4.1	3.5% deacetylated	59.2
Study B							
PA (mean values)							
Man	192			2.30			53.6
Dog	144			2.82			53.6

[a] Adapted from Baer and Barkus [92].
[b] $t_{1/2}$, plasma disappearance half-life; C_B, total body clearance; C_R, renal clearance; Vd_{area}, apparent body volume at distribution equilibrium.

TABLE 1.20

Mean PA and APA Test Results[a]

INH acetylation phenotype	Number of subjects	C_{CR}[b] (ml/min)	PA, dose (mg/kg)	PA, $t_{1/2}$ (hr)	INH[c] k_e	Percent dose excreted		
						PA	APA	Ratio[d]
Slow	10	118.7 ± 4.8	6.2 ± 0.2	3.3 ± 0.2	0.202 ± 0.033	53.1 ± 3.6	12.4 ± 1.4	19.0 ± 2.0
Fast	4	124.0 ± 9.8	6.5 ± 0.2	3.4 ± 0.3	0.449 ± 0.029	49.8 ± 4.0	23.4 ± 3.4	31.7 ± 2.8
Fast and slow	14			3.3 ± 0.2		52.2 ± 2.7	15.6 ± 1.9	

[a]Adapted from Gibson et al. [82].
[b]C_{CR} is creatinine clearance.
[c]k_e is INH elimination rate constant, where $k_e = 0.693/t_{1/2}$.
[d]Ratio = % APA/(% APA + % PA).

Gibson et al. summarized their findings by noting that "the 14 subjects eliminated 52 ± 4% of the dose as procainamide and 16 ± 2% of the dose as N-acetylprocainamide. Four fast INH acetylators eliminated 23 ± 3% of the dose as APA as compared to 12 ± 1% by the slow acetylators (p < 0.05). The amount of unaltered procainamide excreted by the fast and slow INH acetylators was not significantly different, 50 ± 4% and 53 ± 4%, respectively. Of the total amount of drug recovered from the urine of the fast and slow acetylators, APA accounted for 32% and 19%, respectively (p < 0.01). There appears to be a positive correlation between the ability to acetylate INH and the ability to acetylate procainamide."

In 1974, discussing the antiarrhythmic potency of APA, Elson et al. [93] noted that Drayer and co-workers had shown that APA had antiarrhythmic activity in mice and dogs. Elson et al. also found that patients treated with PA often showed APA plasma levels several times greater than their PA concentrations. In their investigation, as a first step in assessing the significance of these plasma levels in patients, the potency of PA and APA were compared in mice. In this animal model, their data confirmed that PA and APA injected intraperitoneally into 42- to 49-day-old male mice were able to prevent coarse ventricular fibrillation caused by inhaled chloroform and hypoxia 10 min after drug administration. The ED_{50} for PA was 122 mg/kg and 130 mg/kg for APA; these results suggest that PA and APA were equally potent antiarrhythmic agents. Their data showed that blood levels following the ED_{50} dose of PA averaged 65.1 µg/ml of PA and 3.6 µg/ml of APA, whereas levels following the ED_{50} dose of APA averaged 92.4 µg/ml of APA. Based on these results, APA appears to be only 73% as potent as PA on a weight basis and 86% as potent on a molar basis.

Shortly thereafter, in 1975, Elson et al. [83] reported that, compared to procainamide in an animal arrhythmia model, the antiarrhythmic potency of APA was 92% with respect to dose and 70% with respect to plasma level. Using a modification of a GC method for measuring plasma procainamide concentration [70], plasma levels of both PA and APA were determined with a Varian series 1440 gas chromatograph equipped with a flame ionization detector and a 1.6-m by 1-mm-i.d. coiled glass column packed with 3% OV-17 on Chromosorb W-HP. Using the specified GC conditions (injector temperature, 255°C; column temperature, programmed from 210 to 250°C at a rate of 2°C/min; nitrogen carrier-gas flow rate, 40 ml/min), the areas of the peaks corresponding to PA, APA, and the two internal standard compounds [p-amino-N-(2-dipropylaminoethyl)-benzamide and N-acetyl-p-amino-N-(2-dipropylaminoethyl)-benzamide] were measured and plasma concentrations of PA and APA estimated from standard curves. The analytical precision for PA over the concentration range of 1 to 20 µg/ml and for APA over a 1- to 30-µg/ml range was 4% and 5%, respectively.

Based on their data, they concluded that "the antiarrhythmic effects of combinations of the drugs were additive. Measurements of procainamide and N-acetylprocainamide plasma levels needed to suppress ventricular extrasystoles suggested that both compounds are nearly equipotent in patients as well. The average plasma level required for arrhythmia control in these patients was equivalent to 5.1 µg/ml of procainamide. Since patients on long-term procainamide therapy have plasma concentrations of N-acetylprocainamide that are usually comparable to, and occasionally greater than, their procainamide levels, dose regimens based on procainamide levels alone need revision to include consideration of the levels of this metabolite."

Graffner [80] studied the elimination rate of APA after a single intravenous dose of procainamide hydrochloride in man. To determine the APA concentration in urine samples, a GC method was employed [72, 79] and to obtain an estimate of the elimination rate of APA, two pharmacokinetic compartment models were used to derive a mathematical description of the excretion process since metabolites could be formed by parallel processes (system I) or via a consecutive reaction (system II), as shown below,

System I:

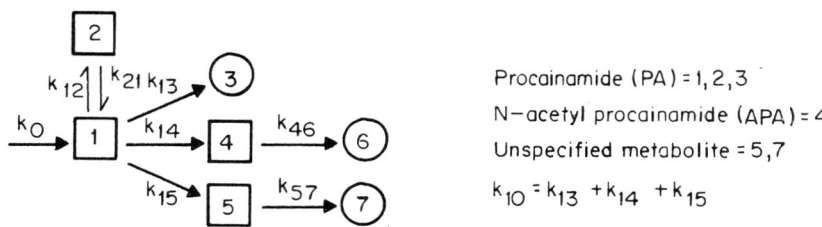

Procainamide (PA) = 1, 2, 3
N-acetyl procainamide (APA) = 4, 6
Unspecified metabolite = 5, 7
$k_{10} = k_{13} + k_{14} + k_{15}$

System II:

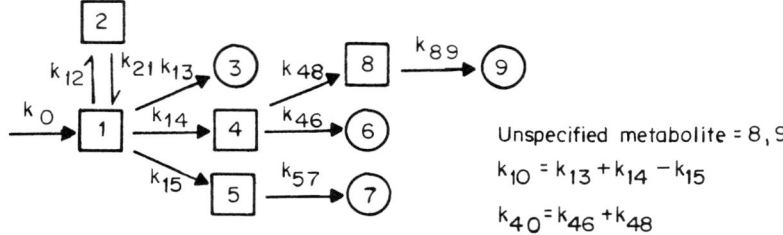

Unspecified metabolite = 8, 9
$k_{10} = k_{13} + k_{14} - k_{15}$
$k_{40} = k_{46} + k_{48}$

where the transfer processes are presumed to obey first-order kinetics and the pharmacokinetics of APA are capable of being properly described by the one-compartment model.

As noted by Graffner, in both systems I and II, the squares and circles represent body compartments and urinary excretion compartments, respectively. The equations derived by Graffner to describe the rate of change of APA in the body via either system are given below.

1. System I:

$$\frac{dQ_4}{dt} = (k_{14}Q_1 - k_{46}Q_4) \tag{1.7}$$

where the Q's are the amount of each form in their respective compartments, k_{14} equals the rate of APA formation (Q_4) from PA (Q_1), and k_{46} is the APA urinary excretion rate constant.

By integration, it follows that

$$Q_4 = A_1 e^{-k_{46}t} + A_2 e^{-\alpha t} + A_3 e^{-\beta t} \tag{1.8}$$

where

$$A_1 = \left[\frac{k_0 k_{14}(1 - e^{-k_{46}\tau})(k_{21} - k_{46})}{-k_{46}(\alpha - k_{46})(\beta - k_{46})}\right] \tag{1.9}$$

and the other coefficients have the symmetrical form as originally described by Benet [99]. The infusion time is designated by τ, and t is the clock time from the start of the experiment.

In either system, the APA urinary excretion rate can be expressed as

$$\frac{dQ_6}{dt} = k_{46} Q_4 \tag{1.10}$$

Because preliminary data showed the so-called α rate constant to be rather large (6.2 hr^{-1} to 9.6 hr^{-1}), Graffner noted that the term vanished after 1 hr so that now one can use a biexponential equation to describe the excretion rate process for system I:

$$\frac{dQ_6}{dt} = k_{46}(A_1 e^{-k_{46}t} + A_3 e^{-\beta t}) \tag{1.11}$$

Integration of Eq. (1.11) gives

$$Q_6^\infty - Q_6^t = A_1 e^{-k_{46}t} + \frac{k_{46}A_3}{\beta} e^{-\beta t} \qquad (1.12)$$

where Q_6^∞ is the fraction of the dose excreted in urine specimens as APA and $Q_6^\infty - Q_6^t$ is the amount remaining to be excreted at time t.

Thus, from system I:

$$Q_6^\infty = \frac{k_0 K_{14} k_{46} k_{21} \tau}{\alpha \beta k_{46}} \qquad (1.13)$$

$$= \frac{D k_{14}}{k_{10}} \qquad (1.14)$$

Finally, the overall APA elimination rate constant for system I, k_{el}, can be expressed as

$$k_{el} = k_{46} \qquad (1.15)$$

Whereas the expression describing the elimination of APA from urine is the same for systems I and II, Graffner reemphasizes the fact that the overall rate constant reflects only the APA excretion rate in system I but, in system II, both this excretion rate constant for APA and the formation rate constant for the unknown metabolite are included.

In like manner, the equations associated with system II are given below:

$$\frac{dQ_4}{dt} = (k_{14} Q_1 - k_{40} Q_4) \qquad (1.16)$$

where k_{40} is the overall elimination constant for APA and is the sum of k_{46} (APA urinary excretion rate constant) and k_{48} (the metabolic rate constant).

$$Q_4 = B_1 e^{-k_{40}t} + B_2 e^{-\alpha t} + B_3 e^{-\beta t} \qquad (1.17)$$

where

$$B_1 = \left[\frac{k_0 k_{14}(1 - e^{-k_{40}\tau})(k_{21} - k_{40})}{-k_{40}(\alpha - k_{40})(\beta - k_{40})}\right] \quad (1.18)$$

$$\frac{dQ_6}{dt} = k_{46}(B_1 e^{-k_{40}t} + B_3 e^{-\beta t}) \quad (1.19)$$

$$Q_6^\infty - Q_6^t = \left[\frac{k_{46}}{k_{40}}\right]B_1 e^{-k_{40}t} + \left[\frac{k_{46}}{\beta}\right]B_3 e^{-\beta t} \quad (1.20)$$

$$Q_6^\infty = \frac{k_0 k_{14} k_{46} k_{21} \tau}{\alpha \beta k_{40}} \quad (1.21)$$

$$= \frac{D k_{14} k_{46}}{k_{10} k_{40}} \quad (1.22)$$

A summary of pharmacokinetic parameters (average values based on intravenous administration of 500 mg of ^{3}H-procainamide to four healthy subjects) determined by Graffner from the analytical data is given in Table 1.21.

Strong et al. [84] also studied the pharmacokinetics of N-acetylprocainamide in three normal subjects who received 500 mg of this compound by timed intravenous injection. Plasma APA concentrations and urine excretion were measured by quadrupole mass fragmentography, and a three-compartment pharmacokinetic model was used for data analysis. N-Acetylprocainamide elimination half-life and total distribution volume averaged 6.0 hr and 1.39 liters/kg, respectively. Renal excretion of unchanged APA accounted for 81% of its elimination, and the mean renal APA clearance was 179 ml/min. Approximately 2% of the injected APA was deacetylated to procainamide. The fate was not determined of 17% that was estimated to have been eliminated during the 16-hr study period.

For GC-MS analysis, sample preparation consisted of placing 2 ml of plasma in a 15-ml glass-stoppered glass tube and then adding 1 ml of internal standard solution [N-acetyl-p-amino-N-(2-dipropylaminoethyl)-benzamide, 5 µg/ml of distilled water], 0.1 ml of 5 N NaOH, and 5 ml of ethyl acetate. After mixing for 15 sec and centifuging at 800 X g for 5 min, the ethyl acetate phase was removed and evaporated to dryness in a 10-ml pear-shaped flask. The extract residue was redissolved in 30 µl of benzene and from the solution a 2-µl aliquot was removed and injected into a

TABLE 1.21

Procainamide Pharmacokinetic Parameters
(Average Values)[a]

Parameter	Average value[b]
Dose (mg/kg)	7.1
A (μg/ml)	80
B (μg/ml)	3.0
α (hr^{-1})	8.7
β (hr^{-1})	0.26
k_{10} (hr^{-1})	4.0
Percent of dose in 0- to 48-hr urine as	
Total radioactivity	101
Unchanged procainamide	67
N-Acetylprocainamide	12
k_{el} (APA) (hr^{-1})	0.5
k_2 (hr^{-1})	0.20
k_1 (hr^{-1})	0.7

[a]Adapted from Graffner [80].
[b]Average data from four healthy subjects.

Finnigan model 3000 GC-MS instrument equipped with a model 240-01 automatic peak selector and a 1.5-m by 1-mm-i.d. glass column packed with 3% OV-17 on Chromosorb W-HP. For the elution of APA and the internal standard, the following GC-MS conditions were maintained: injector, column, and separator temperatures, 255°C; transfer-line temperature, 230°C; helium carrier-gas flow rate, 5 ml/min; ionizing potential, 70 eV.

By monitoring the base peak of APA (m/e 86) and the internal standard (m/e 114) and fragment ion m/e 120 (common to both compounds), the ratio of the areas of APA to the internal standard was used to determine the plasma APA levels from a standard curve prepared by analyzing blank plasma samples to which known amounts of APA had been added. The areas of both m/e ions were simultaneously calculated by a Hewlett Packard model 3352B laboratory data system interfaced to the peak selector.

For urine analysis, APA was assayed by the above method, whereas PA was determined by a GC procedure described previously in this chapter [83]. In addition to these two compounds, p-aminobenzoic acid and its acetylated analog, N-acetyl-p-aminobenzoic acid or p-acetamidobenzoic acid, were determined quantitatively. To determine the latter compound, this was accomplished by acidifying 2 ml of urine with 0.25 ml of 3 N HCl and extracting this acidic solution with two 5-ml portions of dichloromethane. After separating the organic phase and evaporating it to approximately 0.5 ml, an excess of diazomethane in ether was added [reacted with p-acetamidobenzoic acid (PABA)] and then this solution was evaporated to dryness. This residue was then dissolved in 25 µl of benzene and a 1-µl aliquot was analyzed by GC for the methyl ester of PABA.

On the other hand, p-aminobenzoic acid in urine was determined by acidifying 2 ml of urine with 2 ml of 0.3 M NaH_2PO_4 buffer (pH 4.5) and extracting with 5 ml of diethyl ether. After separating and evaporating the organic phase to dryness, the residue was dissolved in 0.25 ml of methyl alcohol; this solution was then reacted with diazomethane as above. The residue resulting from the reaction mixture was dissolved in 50 µl of ethyl acetate and a 1-ul aliquot was analyzed for the methyl ester of p-aminobenzoic acid (PABA).

For the three subjects studied, the average pharmacokinetic data calculated based on a three-compartment model are listed in Table 1.22, which also includes values derived by Koch-Weser and Klein [44] for comparison.

Strong et al. [85] determined by a novel stable isotope method the absolute bioavailability in man of N-acetylprocainamide. In this investigation, the internal standard for APA analysis was p-(acetamido-d_3)-N-(2-diethylaminoethyl-1,1-d_2)-benzamide (APA-d_5). To prepare the specimen for GC-MS analysis, 1 ml of diluted aliquots of urine or undiluted plasma was placed in a 10-ml glass-stoppered centrifuge tube together with 5 ml of 4:1 benzene:chloroform containing 7 µg of APA-d_5 and 0.2 ml of 5 N NaOH. After shaking and then centifuging the mixture for 3 min at 800 X g, the organic phase was transferred to a 10-ml pear-shaped flask and evaporated to dryness in a 25°C water bath at 25 mm Hg. Having dissolved the residue in 50 µl of tetrahydrofuran, a 5-µl aliquot was injected into an integrated GC-MS instrument, the Finnigan model 3200E instrument equipped with a 0.6-m by 1-mm-i.d. glass column packed with 3% OV-17 coated on Chromosorb W-HP (100-120 mesh). GC-MS conditions were as follows: methane carrier-gas flow rate, 9 ml/min; column temperature, 245°C; injector temperature, 270°C; GC-MS transfer-line temperature, 290°C; ion source temperature, 50°C; ion source pressure, 0.5 torr of methane; analyzer region pressure, 2×10^{-5} torr; ionizing energy, 150 eV. Using these conditions, the stable isotope-labeled internal standard made it possible to reduce the retention time for APA to 2.5 min from the 12 min required with a conventional internal standard [84].

TABLE 1.22

Results of Pharmacokinetic Analyses[a]

Parameter	This study	Koch-Weser and Klein[b]
Weight (kg)	71	68
Vd_{ss}[c] (liters)	99.7	119.5
Vd_{ss} (liters/kg)	1.38	1.76
$t_{1/2}$ (elimination) (hr)	6.0	2.9
Plasma clearance (ml/min)	222	517
Plasma clearance (ml/min/kg)	3.09	7.60
Renal clearance (ml/min)	179	179-309[d]
Renal clearance (ml/min/kg)	2.51	
Percent renal elimination	81	40-54[d]
Q_{fast}[e] (liters/min)	1.74	17.2
Q_{slow} (liters/min)	0.909	4.73

[a]Adapted from Strong et al. [84].
[b]Results calculated from Koch-Weser and Klein [44].
[c]Total apparent volumes of APA and PA distribution are the sums of the individual compartment volumes.
[d]Range of values reported by Koch-Weser and Klein.
[e]Permeability coefficients [100] or intercompartmental clearances.

As noted by Strong et al.:

Plasma and urine concentrations of APA and APA-^{13}C were measured by the technique of quadrupole mass fragmentography. The intensity of the quasimolecular ions of APA, APA-^{13}C, and the APA-d_5 internal standard, at m/e 278, 279, and 283, respectively, were monitored with a modified Finnigan Automatic Peak Selector interfaced to a Hewlett-Packard Laboratory Data System which calculated the chromatographic retention time and area for each selected ion peak. Quantitation was based on the internal standard method after the measured peak areas were corrected to reflect the actual concentrations of administered APA and APA-^{13}C in the samples. An initial correction was made by subtracting the contribution to m/e 278 and 279 from the synthesized APA-d_5. Then the intensity of the m/e 279 peak was corrected for the natural abundance of ^{13}C in APA, and m/e 278 was corrected for the contribution to m/e 278 from mass spectral fragmentation of synthesized APA-^{13}C. Since the standard curves were prepared from the same APA-^{13}C that was administered intravenously, this provided an internal correction for the APA contained in the synthesized APA-^{13}C.

As in a previous report [84], a three-compartment mamillary system was used to model the distribution kinetics of APA after intravenous injection. The plasma APA levels were analyzed with the SAAM 23 digital computer program for multicompartmental analysis developed by Berman and Weiss [101]. In their study, by deconvoluting the plasma level versus time curves resulting from intravenous and oral drug administration, and also by comparing the relative percentage of APA and APA-^{13}C excreted unchanged in the 24-hr urine after simultaneous administration, bioavailability was assessed. Using this approach for determining pharmacokinetic data, Table 1.23 lists for subject 3 the pharmacokinetics of APA distribution, elimination, and oral absorption.

TABLE 1.23

Pharmacokinetics of APA Distribution, Elimination, and Oral Absorption[a]

A. APA Distribution and Elimination

Weight (kg)	77
$V_{central}$ (liters)	7.8
V_{fast} (liters)	18.4
V_{slow} (liters)	103.4
Vd_{ss} (liters/kg)	1.68
Elimination $t_{1/2}$ (hr)	5.9
Plasma clearance (ml/min/kg)	3.99
Renal clearance (ml/min/kg)	3.28
Nonrenal clearance (ml/min/kg)	0.72
Percent renal elimination	82
Q_{fast} (liters/min)	1.81
Q_{slow} (liters/min)	1.04

ANTIARRHYTHMIC AGENTS

TABLE 1.23 (continued)

B. APA Oral Absorption

Oral dose (mg)	443
Initial lag (min)	40
k_s (min^{-1})	0.0399
k_p (min^{-1})	0.0228
k_t (min^{-1})	0.0150
k_d (min^{-1})	0.00197
k_o (min^{-1})	0.000002
Percent dose absorbed	
12 hr	89.3
Maximum	100.0
Proximal	60.2
Distal	39.8
Oral/I.V. APA excretion	
Observed (%)	78.1
Predicted (%)	91.5

[a]Adapted from Strong et al. [85].

C. Lidocaine

A prominent antiarrhythmic agent in common use in the treatment of ventricular arrhythmias and capable of developing antiarrhythmic action very rapidly after intravenous administration, lidocaine has been successfully analyzed as well as its metabolic products by GC and GC-MS methods, many of which have been discussed in detail in Volume 5, Chapter 2 [102-136] or referred to or mentioned in earlier sections of this chapter [28, 57-59, 62, 69, 71, 90].

D. Diphenylhydantoin

Diphenylhydantoin, which exerts antiepileptic activity without causing general depression of the central nervous system, also possesses antiarrhythmic activity, decreasing automaticity, but its action on conduction velocity and refractory period are the opposite of those of quinidine [1].

In addition to the various GC and MS procedures for its analysis reported in detail in Volume 2, Chapter 3 [28,57,58,62,102,137-189], other studies have appeared in the literature [190-216]; some of these are discussed in this section.

In 1975, Horning et al. [198] noted that gas-phase methods are ideally suited for the study of drug metabolism in the neonate because multicomponent analysis can be carried out on very small biological samples of blood, urine, and breast milk. GC procedures are very satisfactory for qualitative studies such as the comparison of drug profiles of the mother and her neonate, whereas GC-MS-COMP systems, with selective ion detection, are preferred for identification and quantitation.

Horning et al. noted that*

> During our studies of the human neonate, it was sometimes necessary to administer drugs (barbiturates and anticonvulsants) to newborn infants for medical reasons. Urine samples were collected from several infants who had received secobarbital, diphenylhydantoin, and phenobarbital during the first few days (1-5) after birth. None of the drugs administered to the infants had been given to the mothers. The expected hydroxylated metabolites, which included hydroxysecobarbital, dihydroxysecobarbital, ketohydroxysecobarbital, hydroxyphenobarbital, hydroxydiphenylhydantoin [5-(4-hydroxyphenyl)-5-phenylhydantoin] and the dihydrodiol of diphenylhydantoin [5-(3,4-dihydroxy-1,5-cyclohexadien-1-yl)-5-phenylhydantoin] were identified (GC-MS) in neonatal urines [217]. The glucuronides of hydroxyphenobarbital and hydroxydiphenylhydantoin were also detected in neonatal urines.
>
> Figure [1.19] shows the urinary drug profile of a 5-day-old infant who received a total of 70 mg of secobarbital both intramuscularly and intravenously on days 1-3 after birth, and a total of 100 mg of diphenylhydantoin intramuscularly on days 1-6. Phenobarbital had been given to the mother before delivery. A 24-hr urine sample was collected from the infant on the fifth day. Hydroxysecobarbital (HO-SECO), dihydroxysecobarbital [$(HO)_2$-SECO], and p-hydroxydiphenylhydantoin (HO-DIL) and the glucuronide of p-hydroxydiphenylhydantoin were identified in the urine. From these results it is apparent that almost from the day of birth the neonate has active enzyme systems for carrying out aromatic and aliphatic hydroxylation, epoxidation, hydration, and also conjugation with glucuronic acid [217].

---

*Portions of text and selected figures reproduced with permission of National Institute of General Medical Sciences (HEW).

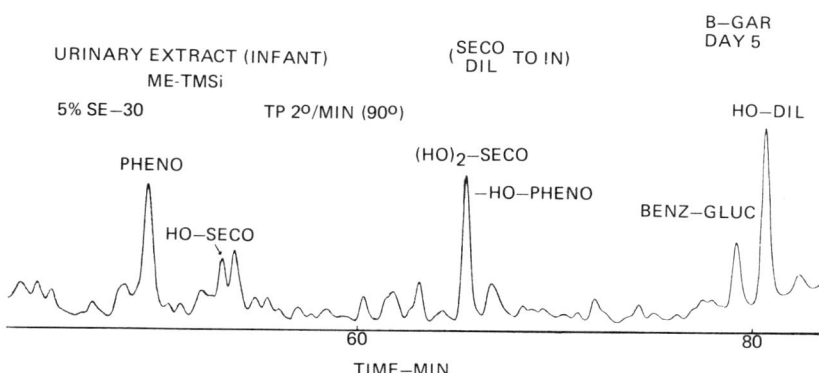

Figure 1.19. Gas chromatographic separation of the ME-TMSi derivatives of drugs and metabolites present in a solvent extract of urine. The compounds identified were phenobarbital (PHENO), hydroxyphenobarbital (HO-PHENO), hydroxysecobarbital (HO-SECO), dihydroxysecobarbital [(HO)$_2$-SECO], hydroxydiphenylhydantoin (HO-DIL), and benzoyl glucosiduronic acid (BENZ-GLUC). Secobarbital and diphenylhydantoin had been given directly to the infant, while phenobarbital had been given to the mother. A 24-hr urine collection was made on day 5. The separation conditions were the same as those for Figure 1.21. From Horning et al. [198], courtesy of National Institute of General Medical Sciences (HEW).

Only a few studies of the half-life of drugs in the newborn have been reported [217-223]. Since the half-lives of many drugs are prolonged in the infant, it is important to recognize that active drugs may persist in neonatal tissues for weeks, and perhaps months. As a result, drugs deposited in fetal tissues may influence neonatal behavior for relatively long periods after birth. The length of time that transplacentally acquired drugs persist in the neonate after birth can be followed by analyzing serial urine samples collected every second or third day after birth. Metabolites of aspirin, phenobarbital, and diphenylhydantoin have been identified in urines 7-8 days after delivery by the use of standard gas chromatographic procedures [217,224]. When analyses were carried out by selective ion detection [225-227] with GC-MS-COMP systems in order to increase the sensitivity of detection, it was possible to quantify phenobarbital in urine collected 22 days after birth. The concentration of phenobarbital declined from 13.2 μg/ml on day 1, to 0.13 μg/ml on day 22. Hydroxyphenobarbital was also identified on day 22 but was not quantified because a satisfactory internal standard was not available.

The exposure of the infant to pharmacologically active agents

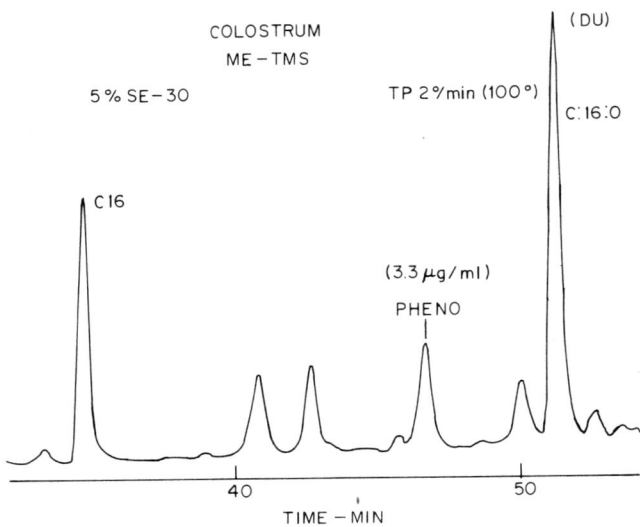

Figure 1.20. Gas chromatographic analysis of the isopropanol extraction of human colostrum collected 58 hr after delivery from a mother (Fig. 1.21) maintained on phenobarbital (195 mg/day). The compounds were separated as the methylated derivatives, under conditions described in Figure 1.21, with temperature programming (TP) from 100°C. The peaks identified by GC-MS were phenobarbital (PHENO) and palmitic acid (C:16:0). From Horning et al. [198], courtesy of National Institute of General Medical Sciences (HEW).

initiated in utero may continue for several months after birth if the neonate is breast fed while the mother is receiving drugs. A gas chromatographic analysis of an extract of breast milk is shown in Figure [1.20]. This mother [Fig. 1.21] was on chronic phenobarbital therapy. The concentration of phenobarbital was 3.3 μg/ml. Although the concentration may seem low, the quantities of drug ingested by the neonate may approach amounts that exert therapeutic action if the infant consumes 750-1000 ml of milk per day [228,229].

It is possible to quantify some drugs in plasma and breast milk by the use of standard gas chromatographic procedures [Fig. 1.20]; however, usually greater sensitivity and selectivity are required. For example, it was not possible to quantify diphenylhydantoin by GC in the analysis shown in Figure [1.22] because the peak was not homogeneous. The concentration of diphenylhydantoin, however, in this sample was quantified with a GC-MS-COMP system by the use of

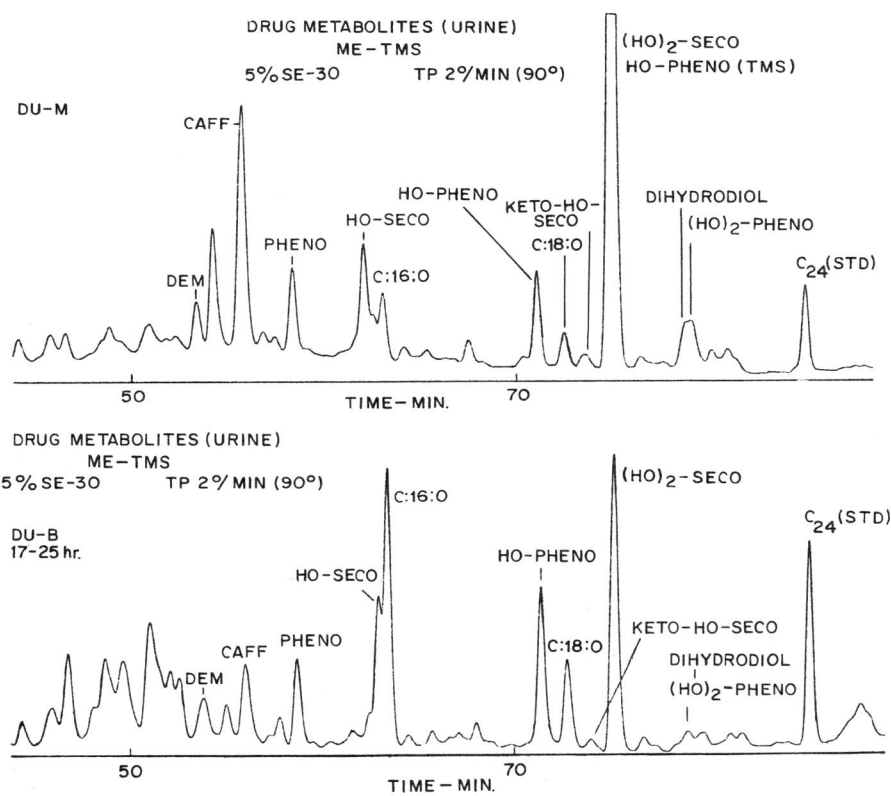

Figure 1.21. Gas chromatogratographic separation of the methylated and silylated (ME-TMS) derivatives of a urinary fraction containing neutral and basic metabolites. The urine sample was collected from the neonate (DU-B) 17-25 hr after birth; a random sample of urine was collected from the mother (DU-M) at delivery. The metabolites identified were Demerol (DEM), caffeine (CAFF), phenobarbital (PHENO), hydroxysecobarbital (HO-SECO), p-hydroxyphenobarbital as the p-methoxy derivative (HO-PHENO), ketohydroxysecobarbital (KETO-HO-SECO), dihydroxysecobarbital [(HO)$_2$-SECO], p-hydroxyphenobarbital as the p-trimethylsilyloxy derivative [HO-PHENO(TMS)], the dihydrodiol of phenobarbital (DIHYDRODIOL), and dihydroxyphenobarbital [(HO)$_2$-PHENO]. Palmitic (C:16:0) and steric (C:18:0) acids were also present. Tetracosane (C$_{24}$STD) was added as an internal standard for quantification. The compounds were separated on a 5% SE-30 column by temperature programming at 2°C/min from 90°C. Demerol, caffeine, phenobarbital, and secobarbital had been ingested by the mother. From Horning et al. [198], courtesy of National Institute of General Medical Sciences (HEW).

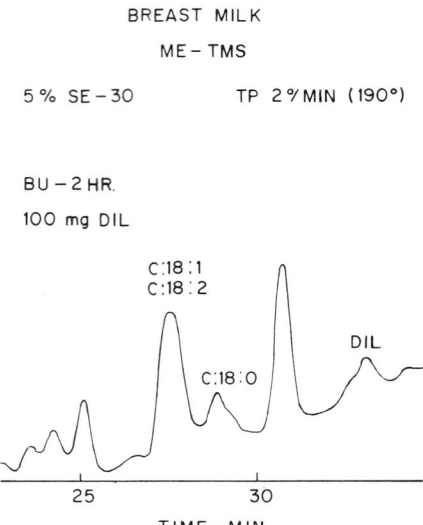

Figure 1.22. Gas chromatographic analysis of the isopropanol extract of human breast milk collected 19 days after delivery. The mother was maintained on 300 mg of diphenylhydantoin (DIL) per day. The compounds were separated as the methylated derivatives, under the conditions described in Figure 1.21, with temperature programming (TP) from 190°C. The peaks identified by GC-MS were C:18:1, oleic acid; C:18:2, linoleic acid; C:18:0, stearic acid; and DIL, diphenylhydantoin. From Horning et al. [198], courtesy of National Institute of General Medical Sciences (HEW).

selective ion detection. With such systems, the mass spectrometer is used as a detector.

Two GC-MS-COMP systems are in use in our laboratory, an LKB 9000-PDP 8/I operated in a chemical ionization mode [176]. A third system, an atmospheric pressure ionization (API) mass spectrometer-computer [230], has also been used in these studies.

For high-sensitivity detection, internal reference compounds are added to biological samples before the isolation of drugs and drug metabolites is initiated. Stable isotope-labeled analogs are the most satisfactory internal reference compounds, although structurally related compounds (homologs) can be used. If suitable standards are not available, a calibration curve can be made each day using a reference solution of the drug to be measured [231].

Figure [1.23] shows the electron impact spectra of the N-methylated derivatives of diphenylhydantoin and $(2,4,5\text{-}^{13}C_3)$-diphenylhydantoin obtained with a LKB 9000-PDP 12 system. The molecular ions at 266 and 269 were monitored for purposes of quantification. The base peak (m/e 180) in the spectrum of diphenylhydantoin was not used for selective ion detection because

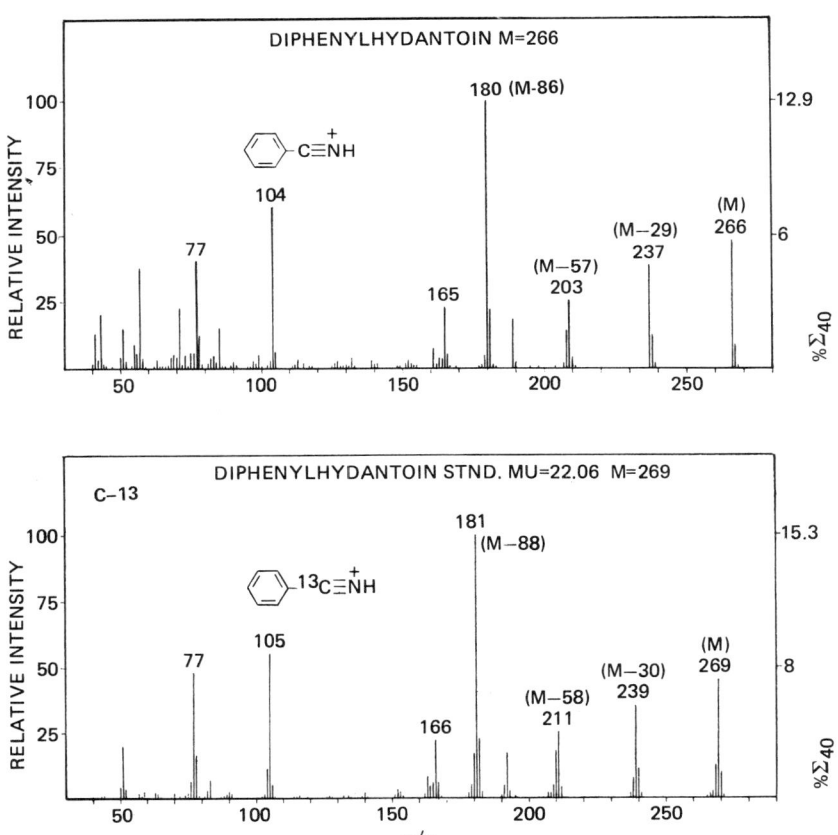

Figure 1.23. Electron impact spectra (LKB 9000) of the N-methyl derivative of diphenylhydantoin and $(2,4,5\text{-}^{13}C_3)$ diphenylhydantoin. From Horning et al. [198], courtesy of National Institute of General Medical Sciences (HEW).

the corresponding peak in the spectrum of the labeled drug occurred at m/e 181, and this ion would have a contribution due to the natural abundance of ^{13}C in the unlabeled drug.

The chemical ionization spectra of diphenylhydantoin and $(2,4,5-^{13}C_3)$-diphenylhydantoin obtained with a Finnigan 1015-PDP 8/I are shown in Figure [1.24]. The protonated molecular (MH$^+$, N-methyl derivative) of the drug (m/e 267) and the internal standard (m/e 270) were monitored. The ion at 269 in the spectrum of the ^{13}C-labeled compound was due to a protonated molecular species containing two instead of three labeled carbon atoms in the heterocyclic ring. The ratio of the ion at m/e 270 to that at m/e 269 was 4:1. Suitable corrections were made, therefore, when calculating plasma concentrations since 1 μg of the internal standard contained 0.8 μg of the triply labeled diphenylhydantoin (MH$^+$ = 270).

The sensitivity of detection of the two systems in their present configuration for barbiturates and anticonvulsant drugs is approximately the same. The sensitivity of the Finnigan system is illustrated in Figure [1.25]. It is possible to measure as little as 80 pg of phenobarbital with a precision of ±5% when a reference solution of the drug is employed. When a plasma extract is used, slightly larger samples are needed (150-200 pg). Increasing the voltage on the multiplier increases the sensitivity of detection. This can be seen by comparing the peak areas or peak heights obtained for 400 pg with multiplier settings of 2400 and 2500 V [Fig. 1.25].

The time required for a single analysis with either system is about 10-15 min. This includes the time necessary to purge the column before injecting the next sample. Thus, between 20 and 40 analyses can be carried out daily. Preliminary results with the API system indicate that quantification may be possible with femtogram to picogram samples [232]. The time for analyses is 1-5 min.

These methods have been used to quantify drugs in plasma and breast milk. Figure [1.26] shows a comparison of diphenylhydantoin in human plasma and breast milk following ingestion of 10 mg of the drug by a patient who was no longer nursing her infant and had not previously taken the drug. Diphenylhydantoin was transferred from the maternal circulation to breast milk. The drug was cleared more rapidly from plasma than from breast milk, although the concentration was lower in breast milk than plasma.

Figure [1.27] shows a comparison of phenobarbital concentrations in maternal plasma, breast milk, neonatal plasma, and neonatal urine for a mother-infant pair. This mother, who was on chronic therapy, received 60 mg of phenobarbital every 3-4 hr. Phenobarbital was transferred from the maternal circulation to breast milk, and as a result of breast feeding, phenobarbital was present in the plasma and urine of her infant.

The concentration of phenobarbital in neonatal plasma varied from 90 to 240 ng/ml. The concentration in urine averaged 40 ng/ml for the sample collected 2-6 hr and 20 ng/ml for the sample collected 6-10 hr after the first morning dose. The concentration of the drug in maternal plasma and colostrum were much higher [Fig. 1.27]. In this particular study the drug was extracted from 75-200 μl of plasma and 1-2 ml of urine. The amount of drug injected into the GC-MS-COMP (Finnigan 1015-PDP 8/I) system varied from 2-50 ng.

When greater sensitivity of detection of drugs in biological samples is required, the API mass spectrometer is used. The limiting sensitivity of detection of this system with reference compounds is 50-100 fg, and the quantity of drug normally measured is 5 to 500 pg [232].

An analysis of plasma obtained from a patient maintained on diphenylhydantoin is shown in Figure [1.28]. The scan was carried out over a limited mass range (245-260 amu) with unit resolution. The peaks at m/e 251 and 254 corresponded to the M-1 peaks of diphenylhydantoin and diphenylhydantoin-2,4,5-^{13}C, respectively. One microliter taken from 5 ml of a methylene chloride extract of plasma was injected directly into the ion source without concentration or derivatization. This was equivalent to 0.04 μl of plasma. The total time required for extraction and instrumental analysis was 30 min.

In 1975, Walle [199] described the alkylation of barbituric acids and diphenylhydantoin with pentafluorobenzyl bromide; the reaction being quantitative in the presence of an excess of triethylamine.

On a micro scale, the di-PFB derivatives of phenobarbital and barbital, and the mono-PFB derivatives of mephobarbital, hexobarbital, and diphenylhydantoin were prepared as follows:

To 5 μg each (about 3×10^{-8} mole) of barbituric acids and diphenylhydantoin dissolved in 100 μl of methanol (containing 5 μg of 9-bromophenanthrene as internal standard) were added triethylamine (1 to 50×10^{-5} mole) and PFB bromide (5 to 50×10^{-6} mole), and the reaction mixture was heated for 5 to 120 min at 50°C before gas chromatography with FID. The percentage yield was obtained from a standard curve prepared from known amounts of synthetic derivative and internal standard.

In this study, Walle used two GC instruments. For electron capture detection, a Pye series 104, model 84, gas chromatograph equipped with a 10-mCi ^{63}Ni electron capture detector and a 160-cm by 4-mm-i.d. borosilicate glass column packed with 3% of liquid stationary phase (OV-1, OV-17 and NPGS) supported on 80-100 mesh Chromosorb W was used in

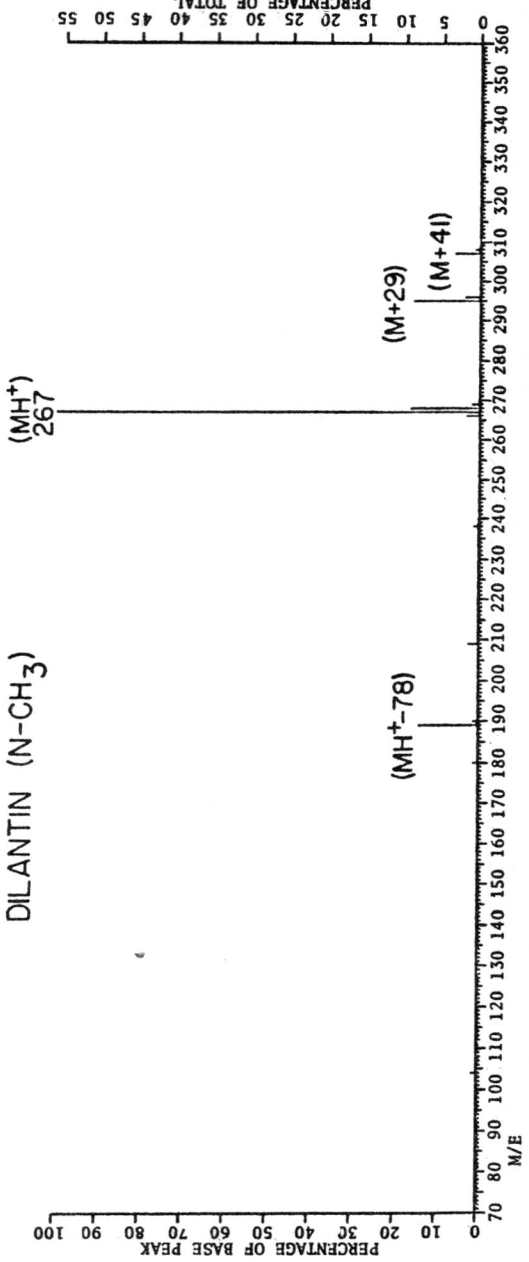

Figure 1.24. Chemical ionization spectra (Finnigan 1015-PDP 8/I) of the N-methyl derivative of (a) diphenylhydantoin and (b) (2,4,5-$^{13}C_3$) diphenylhydantoin. The ion at m/e 269 is the MH$^+$ ion of doubly labeled diphenylhydantoin. From Horning et al. [198], courtesy of National Institute of General Medical Sciences (HEW).

ANTIARRHYTHMIC AGENTS

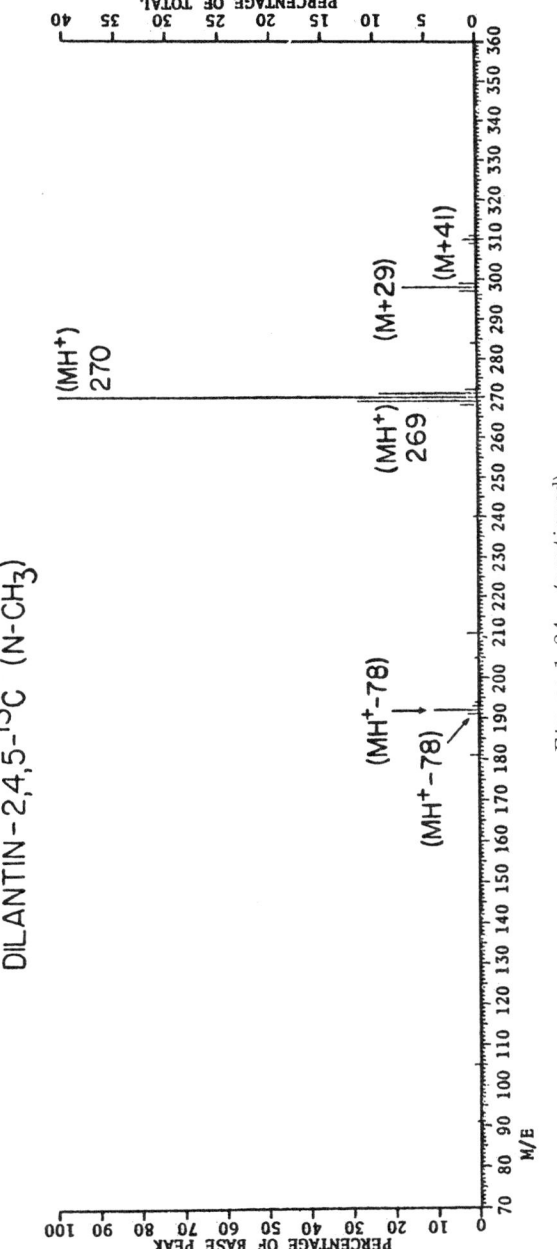

Figure 1.24. (continued)

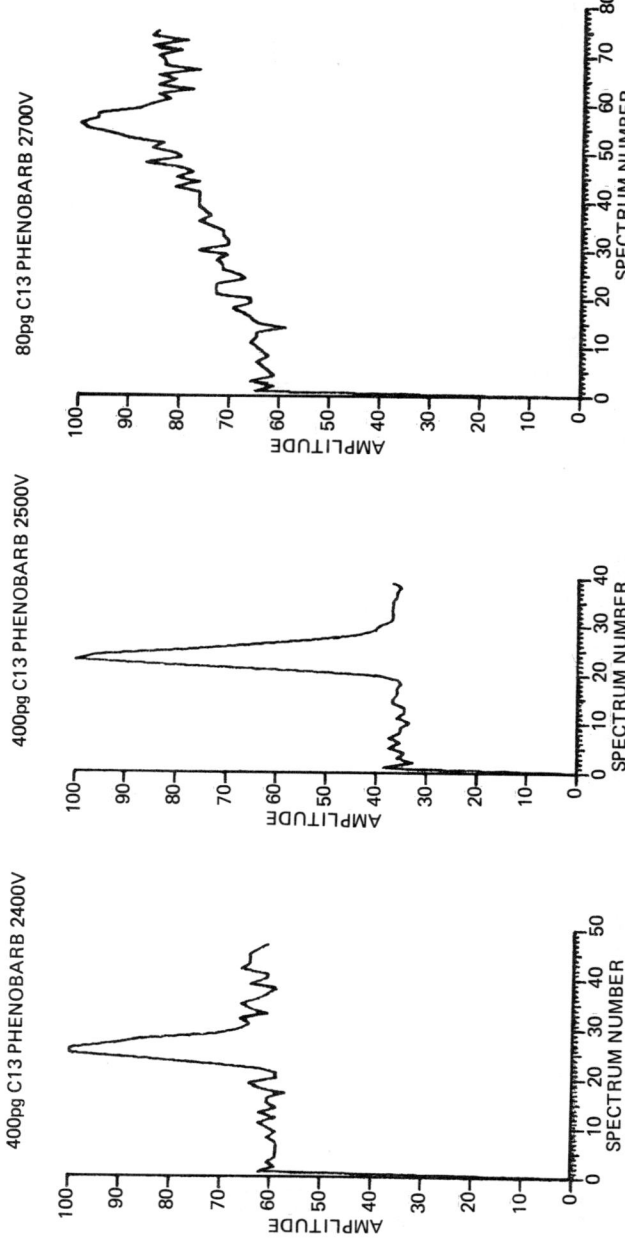

Figure 1.25. Response of the Finnigan 1015-PDP 8/I (chemical ionization mode) to 400 pg (2400 V and 2500 V) and 80 pg (2700 V) of (2,4,5-$^{13}C_3$) phenobarbital monitoring the ions at m/e 263-266. From Horning et al. [198], courtesy of National Institute of General Medical Sciences (HEW).

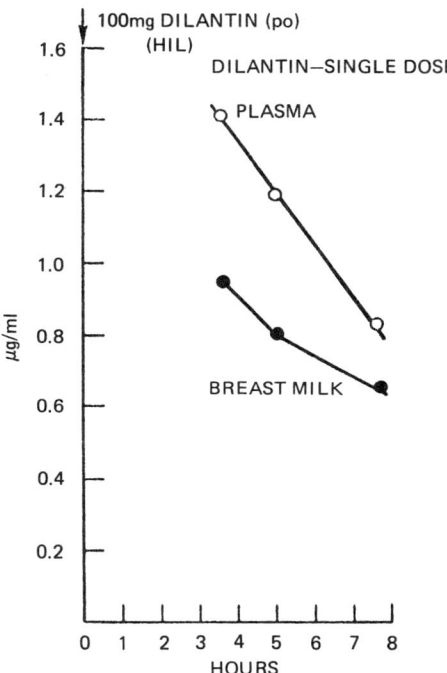

Figure 1.26. Analysis of ammonium carbonate-ethyl acetate extracts of 200 µl of plasma and 500 µl of breast milk by SID (Finnigan system). The ions at 267 (MH^+, diphenylhydantoin-2,4,5-^{13}C) were monitored. From Horning et al. [198], courtesy of National Institute of General Medical Sciences (HEW).

conjunction with the following GC operating conditions: detector temperature, 250°C; pulse amplitude, 50 V; pulse period, 500 µsec; pulse width, 0.75 µsec; nitrogen carrier-gas flow rate, 80 ml/min. Based on a signal three times the background noise level and adjusting column temperature conditions so as to elute each derivative in approximately 3 min on a column with 3600 theoretical plates, the minimum detectable amount of derivative were reported as follows: di-PFB barbital, 0.05 pg (2.2×10^{-17} mole/sec); di-PFB phenobarbital, 0.07 pg (2.6×10^{-17} mole/sec); mono-PFB mephobarbital, 0.11 pg (3.6×10^{-17} mole/sec); mono-PFB hexobarbital, 0.10 pg (3.4×10^{-17} mole/sec); mono-PFB diphenylhydantoin, 0.25 pg (8.2×10^{-17} mole/sec).

For monitoring the derivatization procedure, a Varian Aerograph model 600D gas chromatograph equipped with a model 240 F&M

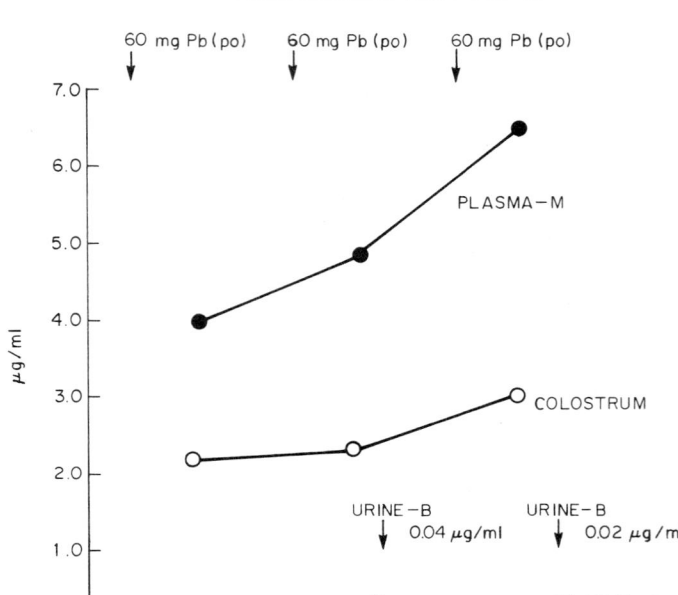

Figure 1.27. Analysis of ammonium carbonate extracts of maternal plasma (200 μl), colostrum (500 μl), neonatal plasma (50-150 μl), and neonatal urine (1-2 ml) by SID (Finnigan system). The ions at m/e 261 (MH$^+$, phenobarbital) and 264 (MH$^+$, phenobarbital-2,4,5-^{13}C) were monitored. From Horning et al. [198], courtesy of National Institute of General Medical Sciences (HEW).

temperature programmer and 150-cm by 2-mm-i.d. glass columns packed with 3% of stationary phase (OV-1, OV-17 or NPGS) on 80-100 mesh Chromosorb W was used with a nitrogen flow rate of 40 ml/min.

The structure of the derivatives were confirmed with a LKB 9000 CG-MS instrument equipped with a 180-cm by 4-mm-i.d. glass column packed with 1% OV-17; the operating conditions used were ion source temperature, 270°C; trap current, 60 μA; ionizing voltage, 70 eV; scan time, 10 sec. As listed by Walle, the molecular ions and major fragment ions characteristic of several barbituric acid derivatives and diphenylhydantoin were as follows:

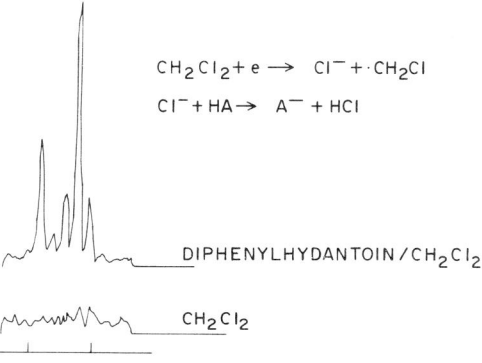

Figure 1.28. Narrow-range scan of negative ions (245-260 amu) of the plasma extract. From Horning et al. [198], courtesy of National Institute of General Medical Sciences (HEW).

1. Mono-PFB diphenylhydantoin: base peak, m/e 180; other main fragments m/e 181 (41%), m/e 432 (M^+, 33%), m/e 403 (M-29, 18%), m/e 355 (M-77, 11%), and m/e 251 (M-181, 8%)

2. Mono-PFB mephobarbital: m/e 398 (M-28, 100%, with m* 371.8), m/e 181 ($C_6F_5CH_2$, 58%), and m/e 426 (M^+, 20%)

3. Di-PFB barbital: m/e 181 ($C_6F_5CH_2$, 100%), m/e 516 (M-28, 56% with m* 489.4), m/e 292 (24%), m/e 278 (20%), m/e 544 (M^+, 17%), m/e 501 (M-43, 17%, with m* 486.4)

4. Di-PFB phenobarbital: m/e 181 ($C_6F_5CH_2$, 100%), m/e 564 (M-28, 76%, with m* 537.3), m/e 592 (M^+, 25%)

Least et al. [200] described a sensitive and precise GC method in which benzylmalonate methylester monoamide was used as the internal standard for the simultaneous determination of primidone, phenylethylmalonamide, carbamazepine, and diphenylhydantoin. The trimethylsilyl derivatives were well separated from each other and from normal serum constituents. As reported, the lower limit of detection for each compound studied was 0.5 mg/liter when 1 ml of serum was analyzed. Within-run precision (coefficient of variation), established by analyzing ten replicates, was as follows: diphenylhydantoin (6.6 mg/liter), 3.8%; carbamazepine (10.4 mg/liter), 3.2%; primidone (5.4 mg/liter), 2.6%; and phenylethylmalonamide

(5.5 mg/liter), 1.6%. In their investigation, 50 specimens were analyzed for primidone and 35 for diphenylhydantoin by a standard GC method involving on-column methylation [168] and by the present procedure. Least et al. summarized their findings, noting that "serum concentrations of primidone ranged from 1.0 to 34.0 mg/liter. The mean value observed with the on-column alkylation procedure was 9.3 mg/liter and with our procedure was 9.6 mg/liter. When values for our assay were regressed against values for the standard method the slope of the weighted linear least-squares regression line was 0.936, the intercept was 1.00 μg/ml, and the coefficient of correlation was 0.939. Our procedure for the determination of primidone gave a coefficient of variation of 2.6% at a concentration of 5.4 mg/liter, compared to 7.6% obtained by the method employing on-column methylation. Serum concentrations of diphenylhydantoin ranged from 1.0 to 51.4 mg/liter. The mean value observed for diphenylhantoin by on-column methylation was 12.6 mg/liter and with our procedure was 12.6 mg/liter. When values for our assay were regressed against values for the standard method, the slope of the weighted linear least-squares regression line was 0.944, the intercept was 0.3 μg/ml, and the coefficient of correlation was 0.988."

Following a prescribed procedure for extraction and silylation of the anticonvulsants, GC analyses were performed with a Hewlett-Packard model 5710A instrument equipped with dual flame ionization detectors and 122-cm by 2-mm-i.d. glass columns packed with 3% OV-17 coated on 100-120 mesh Gas Chrom Q. Using the specified instrumental conditions (injector temperature, 250°C; detector temperature, 300°C; column temperature, programmed from 150 to 260°C at 16°C/min; nitrogen carrier-gas flow rate, 40 ml/min), the approximate retention times of the silylated derivatives of primidone, benzylmalonate methylester monoamide, phenylethylmalonamide, diphenylhydantoin, and carbamazepine were 2.17, 2.58, 2.92, 5.42, and 5.84 min, respectively. Whereas some drugs did not interfere when assayed by the proposed method (dimethadione, trimethadione, ethosuximide, mesantoin, metharbital, and mebaral), methsuximide and phensuximide had retention times that were identical to those for the silyl derivatives of primidone and the internal standard, respectively.

By comparing the ratio of corrected peak heights of extracted serum samples (spiked with the drug being studied) to those of nonextracted standards, the recoveries of drugs determined were carbamezepine, about 100%; primidone, 42%; diphenylhydantoin, 95%; and phenylethylmalonamide, 47%.

Hoppel et al. [202] described a method for the mass fragmentographic determination of diphenylhydantoin and its major metabolite, 5-(4-hydroxyphenyl)-5-phenylhydantoin, in human plasma as their dimethyl and trimethyl derivatives, respectively. The derivatives are formed via an extractive alkylation technique (the optimal conditions for the metabolite being 1 N NaOH in the presence of 0.2 M tetrabutylammonium hydrogen sulfate using an extraction time of 30 min with the organic phase containing 100 µl of methyl iodide in 5 ml of methylene chloride). With recoveries for diphenylhydantoin and the metabolite reported to be in excess of 99%, the above extractive alkylation method could be used successfully to analyze, in addition to the two compounds mentioned, 4-methyldiphenylhydantoin, 3-hydroxydiphenylhydantoin, 2,4-dihydroxydiphenylhydantoin, 3-methoxy-4-hydroxydiphenylhydantoin, 4-hydroxy-4'-methyldiphenylhydantoin, and 4,4'-dihydroxydiphenylhydantoin.

Using pentadeuterated 4-hydroxydiphenylhydantoin [5-(4-hydroxyphenyl)-5-(2,3,4,5,6-pentadeuterophenyl)hydantoin] as the internal standard and following acidic hydrolysis of the plasma sample [0.05 ml of plasma sample, 0.05 ml of internal standard (10 µg/ml), and 0.1 ml of 10 N HCl heated in a 95°C water bath for 60 min], conjugated 4-hydroxydiphenylhydantoin and, indirectly, the dihydrodiol metabolite, 5-(3,4-dihydroxy-1,5-cyclohexadien-1-yl)-5-phenylhydantoin, could be measured with a LKB 9000 integrated GC-MS instrument equipped with a 1.2-m by 2-mm-i.d. glass column packed with 3% OV-17 on 80-100 mesh Gas Chrom Q. With the specified settings (ionizing voltage, 20 eV; injector temperature, 270°C; column temperature, either 250 or 270°C; carrier-gas and its flow rate not specified), for mass fragmentography (multiple ion detection), the m/e ions used for the various methyl derivatives studied were diphenylhydantoin, 280; 3-hydroxydiphenylhydantoin, 310; 4-hydroxydiphenylhydantoin, 310; 5-(4-hydroxy-3,5-dideuterophenyl)-5-phenylhydantoin, 312; 5-(4-hydroxyphenyl)-5-(2,3,4,5,6-pentadeuterophenyl)hydantoin, 315; 3,4-dihydroxydiphenylhydantoin, 340; 2,4-dihydroxydiphenylhydantoin, 340; 3-methoxy-4-hydroxydiphenylhydantoin, 340, dihydrodiol-diphenylhydantoin, 342. With a column temperature of 270°C, Hoppel et al. noted that 3-hydroxydiphenylhydantoin and 4-hydroxydiphenylhydantoin could be separated and measured with injection of samples every 1.5 min. To detect diphenylhydantoin also, only a decrease in column temperature to 250°C was required. Using 100-µl plasma samples, the lower limit of detection was about 10 ng/ml (0.03 nmole/ml).

In addition to diphenylhydantoin, other commonly used hydantoins investigated by GC and reported in Volume 2, Chapter 3, are 5-(4-hydroxyphenyl)-5-phenylhydantoin [57,58,138,152,173,187], 5-(4-methylphenyl)-5-phenylhydantoin [145,146,152,170,178,184-186,188], 5-ethyl-5-phenylhydantoin [139,144,184,233], 5-ethyl-3-methyl-5-phenylhydantoin [28,57,58,139,144,154,162,165,167,178,188,233,234], methetoin [57,58, 62], 3-ethyl-5-phenylhydantoin [28,57,58,62,165,167,188,234], and 3-allyl-5-isobutyl-2-thiohydantoin [154]. Mass spectra of selected hydantoins via chemical ionization [62,235] or electron impact [58,62,236] are also included.

Midha et al. [203] developed an improved GC procedure for the simultaneous determination of phenytoin (diphenylhydantoin) and its predominat metabolite, 5-(4-hydroxyphenyl)-5-phenylhydantoin, in plasma and urine following enzyme hydrolysis.

Prior to GC analysis, sample preparation consisted of the following steps:

To 2-ml plasma or urine samples in screw-capped centrifuge tubes (15 ml) were added 0.2 ml of 1 M acetate buffer (pH 5.0) and 50 µl of β-glucuronidase. Then the samples were incubated for 4 hr at 37°C. To the hydrolyzed samples were added 1 ml of the internal standard, 5-(4-methylphenyl)-5-phenylhydantoin (2.5 µg/ml), and 2 ml of 1 N HCl. The samples were then extracted with 5 ml of ether by shaking for 10 min at 50 rpm followed by centrigugation at 2500 rpm for 10 min.

Four-milliliter portions of the ether layer were transferred into a centrifuge tube (20 ml) containing 5 ml of 0.2 M phosphate buffer (pH 11.2). The tubes were mixed for 10 min followed by centrifugation for 10 min, and the organic extracts were then discarded. The remaining aqueous solution was acidified with 2 ml of 2 N HCl and extracted twice with 5-ml portions of ether (mixed for 10 min and centrifuged for 10 min).

Four milliliters of the first extract and 5 ml of the second extract were transferred into an evaporating tube, and the combined ether extracts were evaporated to dryness at 50°C under a stream of dry nitrogen. The dried extracts were dissolved by mixing with 25 µl of methanolic trimethylanilinium hydroxide (0.2 M), and aliquots (1 to 2 µl) were injected into the gas chromotograph.

For this study, Midha et al. used a Perkin-Elmer model F-10 gas chromatograph equipped with a metal sleeve injector port, a flame ionization detector, and 1.83-m by 3-mm-i.d. coiled glass columns packed with 5% OV-17 on AW-DMCS-treated, 80-100 mesh Chromosorb W. Using prescribed GC conditions (injector temperature, 310°C; column temperature, 215°C; detector temperature, 280°C; nitrogen carrier-gas flow rate, 60 ml/min), the retention times of the methylated products of diphenylhydantoin, the internal standard, and the metabolite were 4.9, 6.9, and 11.9 min, respectively. Using gas chromatography-mass spectrometry, the structures of the methylated derivatives were established. The degree of methylation and the predominant m/e ions observed in the mass spectrum of the derivatives were as follows: 1,3-dimethyl-5,5-diphenylhydantoin with the molecular ion at 280 and diagnostic ions at m/e 251, 223, 203, 194, 165, 152, 146, and 118; 1,3-dimethyl-5-(4-methylphenyl)-5-phenylhydantoin with the molecular ion at 294 and other characteristic ions at m/e 279, 265, 251, 237, 217, 208, 203, 194, 165, 132, 118, and 91; 1,3-dimethyl-5-(4-methoxyphenyl)-5-phenylhydantion, which had a molecular ion at 310 and other major m/e ions at 280, 233, 224, 203, 148, and 118.

Using peak height ratios (drug or metabolite/internal standard) versus drug concentration calibration curves, the recovery of diphenylhydantoin, the metabolite, and the internal standard from plasma was 76, 64, and 65%, respectively, whereas the method's sensitivity for the drug and its metabolite were reported as being 150 ng/ml and 125 ng/ml, respectively. A comparison of diphenylhydantoin concentrations by the proposed GC procedure and a UV procedure [237], as modified previously [238,239], following a single oral dose of two 100-mg tablets of diphenylhydantoin to a human volunteer (84 kg) is shown in Figure 1.29A. In Figure 1.29B the diphenylhydantoin and 5-(4-hydroxyphenyl)-5-phenylhydantoin levels in the plasma of the same volunteer are compared.

In 1976 also, Abraham and Joslin [206] reported their findings using a newly developed simple, sensitive GC procedure capable of determining simultaneously phenobarbital, diphenylhydantoin, carbamazepine, and primidone in serum.

Following a detailed extraction procedure which yielded a residue upon evaporation, the residue was reconstituted with 100 μl of a trimethylphenylammonium hydroxide solution from which 1 to 2 μl were withdrawn and injected into a Fisher model 2400 gas chromatograph equipped with dual flame ionization detectors and 200-cm by 2-mm-i.d. borosilicate glass columns packed with 3% SP 2250 on 100-120 mesh Supelcoport. With the specified GC conditions maintained (injector temperature, 310°C; detector temperature, 250°C; column temperature, programmed from 190 to 300°C at a rate of 15°C/min, the program being started after the sample extract was injected; nitrogen carrier-gas flow rate, 160 ml/min), the retention times of the methylated species of phenobarbital, carbamazepine, primidone, diphenylhydantoin, and the internal standard, 5-(4-methylphenyl)-5-phenylhydantoin, were about 4.85, 6.33, 6.93, 8.67, and 9.39 min, respectively, whereas the between-day analytical recoveries (n = 31) of drug added to plasma were phenobarbital, 99%; diphenylhydantoin, 99%; primidone, 101%; and carbamazepine, 104%. Requiring only 0.20 ml of serum and less than 30 min of analysis time, the lower limit of detection for each of the drugs was 0.5 mg/liter.

Shortly thereafter, in 1977, Abraham and Gresham [213] described a modified GC method for simultaneously determining phenobarbital, diphenylhydantoin, primidone, carbamazepine, ethosuccinimide, methsuccinimide, and phensuccinimide in 1 ml of plasma or serum in less than 1 hr. Using two internal standards, 5-(4-methylphenyl)-5-phenylhydantoin and fluorene, and instrumental conditions as described by Abraham and Joslin [206] with two exceptions [two column temperature programs were used: (1) isothermal heating at 150°C for 1 min, increased to 300°C at a rate of 20°C/min; (2) temperature programmed from 180 to

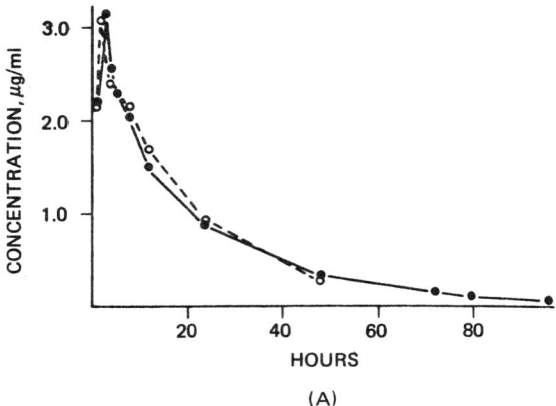

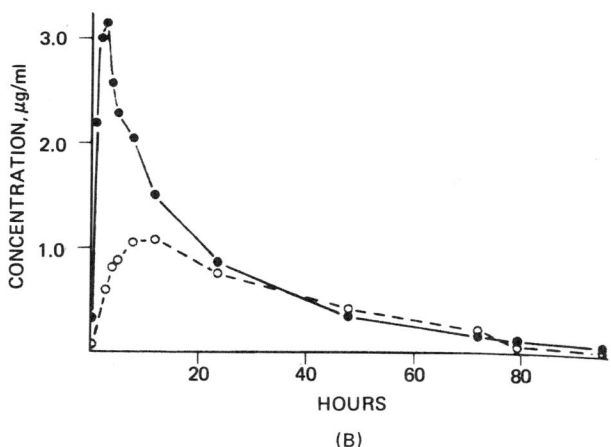

Figure 1.29. A. Comparison of phenytoin plasma concentrations by the GLC method (●) and a UV method (O) following a single oral dose of two 100-mg tablets of phenytoin to a human volunteer (84 kg). B. Phenytoin (●) and the metabolite (O) concentrations in the plasma of a human volunteer (84 kg) following a single oral dose of 200 mg of phenytoin. Adapted from Midha et al. [203], courtesy of the Journal of Pharmaceutical Sciences.

300°C at a rate of 10°C/min], the on-column methylated derivatives formed by reaction of each drug with trimethylphenylammonium hydroxide yielded with chromatographic condition (2) retention times of 4.90, 5.50, 5.78, 7.55, and 8.05 min, respectively, for phenobarbital, carbamazepine, primidone, diphenylhydantoin, and 5-(4-methylphenyl)-5-phenylhydantoin. Using chromatographic conditions (1), the retention times of ethosuccinimide, fluorene, methsuccinimide, and phensuccinime were approximately 2.39, 4.63, 5.56, and 6.00 min, respectively.

Schwartz et al. [209] determined "the solubility of diphenylhydantoin in pH 7.4 and 5.4 phosphate buffers at five temperatures; in hydroalcoholic solutions, 0 to 4% methanol; and in pH 4.8-8.4 buffer solutions. From the temperature data, the enthalpy and entropy of solution of this nonideal system were calculated and were similar at both pH values. The data obtained from the buffer solutions were used to calculate the apparent dissociation constant, pKa', of diphenylhydantoin as 8.06. A GC method with on-column methylation was used to quantitate diphenylhydantoin with 5-(4-methylphenyl)-5-phenylhydantoin as an internal standard. The assay uses chloroform for extraction of the drug from aqueous solutions. The ratio of peak heights was adjusted for weights of aqueous and organic layers, and results were calculated in micrograms per gram of sample and mole fraction of diphenylhydantoin."

The methylated derivatives of diphenylhydantoin and the internal standard using trimethylanilinium hydroxide as reagent were separated and analyzed with a Varian model 2100 gas chromatograph equipped with dual flame ionization detectors and 183-cm by 2-mm-i.d. U-shaped borosilicate glass columns packed with 3% OV-17 coated on 100-120 mesh Chromosorb W-HP. For routine analysis of diphenylhydantoin, the GC operating conditions were injector temperature, 250°C; column temperature, 230°C; detector temperature, 250°C; nitrogen carrier-gas flow rate, 30 ml/min. Retention times of the methylated diphenylhydantoin and internal standard were about 8 and 12 min, respectively.

In this study, Schwartz et al. expressed the total solubility, S, as a function of the hydrogen ion concentration, solubility of the unionized form, S^0, and the dissociation constant, K_a:

$$S = S^0 + P^- = S^0 + \frac{K_a S^0}{(H^+)} \tag{1.23}$$

which, in turn, was transformed into the more customary pH and pKa notation,

$$\log\left[\frac{S}{S^0} - 1\right] = pH - pK_a \tag{1.24}$$

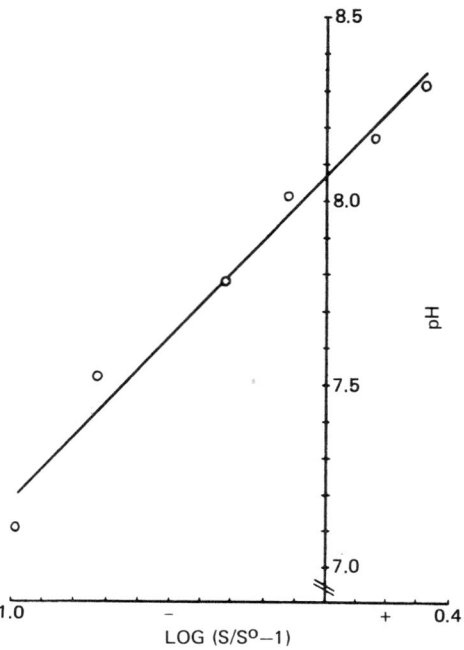

Figure 1.30. Plot of log (S/S^0-1) for phenytoin as a function of pH, r = 0.977. The intercept on the pH axis is the apparent pK_a. From Schwartz et al. [209], courtesy of the Journal of Pharmaceutical Sciences.

such that a plot of pH versus the logarithmic term yielded a straight line intersecting the pH axis at the pKa as illustrated in Figure 1.30. On the other hand, values for the enthalpy and entropy of solution were determined from the slope and the intercept of the plot of log mole fraction solubility versus the reciprocal absolute temperature as shown in Figure 1.31 for pH 5.4.

To suppress the partial hydrolytic cleavage of phenobarbital during on-column methylation procedures with the formation of N-methyl-α-phenylbutyramide (earlier designated as the early phenobarb peak by some investigators), Serofontein and De Villiers [210] showed that the hydrolytic reaction could be drastically reduced by decreasing the pH of the solution injected into the chromatograph when buffer solution (pH 8-10) was used for the extraction of barbiturates and hydantoins from the initial toluene extract.

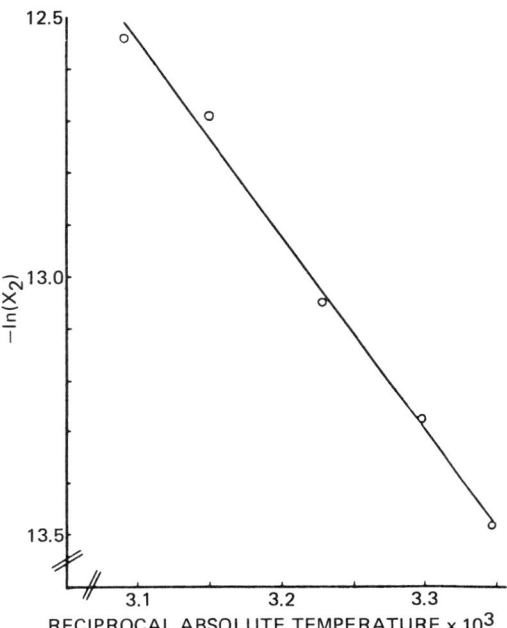

Figure 1.31. Van't Hoff plot for solubility of phenytoin at pH 5.4, r = 0.995. From Schwartz et al. [209], courtesy of the Journal of Pharmaceutical Sciences.

As noted by Serfontein and De Villiers:

The general procedure for the determination of barbiturates and diphenylhydantoin was similar to that previously described by Mac Gee [240] and Kananen et al. [168], in which the primary toluene extract was vortexed with 100 μl of 0.2 M trimethylanilinium hydroxide solution and 20 μl of water. After centrifugation, the lower, aqueous phase (approximately 50 μl) was transferred into a second nipple tube (10-ml ground-glass stoppered tube with the bottom portion drawn out) and 20 μl of "acid buffer" (freshly prepared) were added. After thorough mixing with a syringe, 1.5 μl of the mixture were injected slowly (6 sec) into the gas chromatograph.

GC analyses were performed with a Varian Aerograph 1400 gas chromatograph fitted with a flame ionization detector and a 1-m by 3-mm-i.d.

glass column packed with 3% OV-17 on 100-120 mesh Gas Chrom Q. To obtain retention times of approximately 0.26, 0.57, and 0.93 for N-methyl-α-phenylbutyramide, phenobarbital, and diphenylhydantoin, respectively, relative to the internal standard, the following GC conditions were maintained: injector temperature, 270°C; column temperature, programmed from 150 to 280°C at 15°C/min; nitrogen carrier-gas flow rate, 30 ml/min.

In a similar manner, they noted that the "early phenobarb peak" was less pronounced when methyl iodide and dimethyl sulfoxide were added to the unbuffered trimethylanilinium hydroxide extracts immediately before injecting the extracts into the gas chromatograph. The presence of these two compounds presumably creates a strongly methylating environment in the gas phase, which also tends to enhance the formation of the fully methylated product.

Hill and Latham [211] described a quantitative GC method for the determination of blood levels of ethosuximide, diphenylhydantoin, phenobarbital, and primidone; all four compounds being determined using 1 ml of serum. In their procedure, reported in 1977, a simple, direct extraction technique was employed which consisted of the following steps:

> Serum or plasma (1 ml) is added to a 50-ml glass tube fitted with a PTFE-lined screw cap, acidified with 0.5 ml of 0.5 N HCl and extracted with 10 ml of chloroform containing the internal standards [α,α-dimethyl-β-methylsuccinimide was the I.S. for ethosuximide, hexobarbital for phenobarbital, while 5-(4-methylphenyl)-5-phenylhydantoin served for primidone and diphenylhydantoin]. The extraction for 10 min (Buchler Omnishaker) is followed by centrifugation at 500g for 5 min. The aqueous phase is removed by aspiration and the chloroform decanted into a disposable glass tube (15 ml). The solution is taken to dryness by warming under a stream of dry nitrogen, and the residue dissolved in a few drops of methanol. If ethosuximide is part of the analysis, 2 μl of this solution are injected onto the OV-225 column and chromatographed isothermally at 150°C. The remaining material is derivatized by adding 100 μl of 0.2 M trimethylanilinium hydroxide in methanol and flash heating at 100°C for 10 min. The residue is redissolved in a small volume of methanol (about 50 μl) and 1 μl is injected onto the OV-17 column of the gas chromatograph.

Hill and Latham performed their separations and quantitative analyses with a Hewlett-Packard model 5780 gas chromatograph equipped with dual flame ionization detectors and two 6-ft by 1/8-in.-o.d. coiled glass columns, one packed with 3% OV-17 on 100-120 mesh Gas Chrom Q and the other with 4% OV-225 on 100-120 mesh Gas Chrom Q. Using detector and injector temperatures of 300°C and a nitrogen carrier-gas flow rate of 22 ml/min on each column, ethosuximide was analyzed isothermally at 150°C on the OV-225 column whereas the methyl derivatives of diphenylhydantoin, phenobarbital, and primidone were analyzed with the OV-17 column operated at 205°C for 8 min and then linearly programmed to 220°C at 4°C/min where the final temperature was held constant for 10 min until all compounds had been eluted. With the OV-225 column, the retention time of underivatized α,α-dimethyl-β-methylsuccinimide and ethosuximide were 7.17 and 9.00 min, respectively, whereas the methylated derivatives of hexobarbital, phenobarbital, primidone, diphenylhydantoin, and 5-(4-methylphenyl)-5-phenylhydantoin on the OV-17 column, which was temperature-programmed, were eluted in 2.54, 2.94, 6.67, 12.28, and 15.60 min, respectively.

As emphasized by Hill and Latham, there are several features of this method worthy of attention: (1) The one-step extraction procedure requires little time; (2) the inclusion of the internal standards in the extraction chloroform minimizes the number of operations in the procedure; (3) the method of derivative preparation is also important for the accurate analysis of barbiturates; and (4) the routine sample size is 1 ml.

In 1977, Gordos et al. [215] described a GC method for the determination of diphenylhydantoin in micro samples of blood plasma. After a double extraction with chloroform containing an analog of diphenylhydantoin, 5-(4-methylphenyl)-5-phenylhydantoin, as internal standard, the drug and standard are N,N-dimethylated in alkaline aqueous solution with methyl iodide followed by extraction into acetone. These compounds were chromatographed and identified as 1,3-dimethyl-5,5-diphenylhydantoin and 1,3-dimethyl-5-(4-methylphenyl)-5-phenylhydantoin, respectively. Using this double extraction and derivatization procedure, the total recoveries for the drug and internal standard were 64% (coefficient of variation = 3.5%) and 68% (coefficient of variation = 4.5%), respectively.

The methylated derivatives were separated and determined quantitatively with a Pye Unicam GCV gas chromatograph equipped with flame ionization detection and a 5-ft by 2-mm-i.d. glass column packed with 3% OV-225 on 100-120 mesh Chromosorb W-HP, conditioned for 24 hr at 245°C with nitrogen at a flow rate of 20 ml/min. The retention times of N,N-dimethylated diphenylhydantoin and the internal standard were approximately 2.98 and 3.78 min, respectively, using the following GC conditions: nitrogen carrier-gas flow rate, 35 ml/min; injector temperature, 200°C; column temperature, 234°C; detector temperature, 300°C. Using a standard calibration curve for diphenylhydantoin (prepared by plotting peak area ratios of the dimethylated drug to internal standard versus drug concentration, which yielded a linear response in the range of 0.26 to 2.6 µg of diphenylhydantoin), the lowest concentration of drug that could be quantitatively determined in plasma using a 100-µl sample was 0.5 to 1.00 µg/ml. If drug plasma levels in known samples were evaluated by means of a simultaneously produced working standard curve, rather favorable results were obtained, as shown in Table 1.24.

TABLE 1.24

Determination of Drug Plasma Levels in Known Samples[a]

Sample	Known conc. (µg/ml)	Found conc.[b] (µg/ml)	Percent recovery	
			As is	Corrected[c]
1	15.0	14.7	98.2	96.8
2	4.0	4.0	100.0	95.0
3	8.0	7.5	93.8	91.3
4	33.1	33.4	101.0	100.3
5	0.0[d]	0.2		
6	1.0	1.4	140.0	120.0
7	26.5	24.9	94.0	93.4
8	12.0	11.8	98.3	96.8
9	20.1	19.8	98.6	98.0

[a]Adapted from Gordos et al. [215].
[b]Average (mean) of three determinations.
[c]Corrected for plasma blank of 0.2 µg/ml.
[d]Plasma blank value.

Using the mass fragmentographic method previously described by Hoppel et al. [202] to analyze unconjugated and conjugated 5-(4-hydroxyphenyl)-5-phenylhydantoin (4-OH-DPH), 5-(3-hydroxyphenyl)-5-phenylhydantoin and, indirectly, the 5-(3,4-dihydroxyl-1,5-cyclohexadien-1-yl)-5-phenylhydantoin metabolites of diphenylhydantoin, Hoppel et al. [216] in 1977 determined unconjugated and conjugated 4-OH-DPH in plasma of patients being treated with diphenylhydantoin. They noted that "the plasma concentration of unconjugated 4-OH-DPH is stable at steady state for diphenylhydantoin and the level does not change during the dose interval. Most patients (82.5%) have plasma concentrations of unconjugated 4-OH-DPH between 0.04 and 0.20 µg/ml at concentrations of diphenylhydantoin between 5 and 30 µg/ml. Interindividual differences in the ratio between plasma concentration of unconjugated 4-OH-DPH and diphenylhydantoin were noted in a wide range of doses. Dosage adjustments of diphenylhydantoin in patients were not associated with major changes in the plasma level of unconjugated 4-OH-DPH. The plasma concentration of conjugated 4-OH-DPH also showed interindividual differences and varied between 1.2 and 4.5 µg/ml in patients with diphenylhydantoin concentrations between 5 and 30 µg/ml. The data are consistent with the concept of Michaelis-Menten kinetics for diphenylhydantoin metabolism." Also reported was the fact that the plasma concentration of dihydrodiol-diphenylhydantoin ranged from 0.02 to 0.45 µg/ml in patients with diphenylhydantoin levels of 5 and 30 µg/ml and showed marked interindividual variation.

In the period between 1975 and 1977, several investigations were performed using nitrogen-selective detectors for the analysis of anticonvulsants [208,214], whereas enzymatic immunoassay procedures for the determination of diphenylhydantoin [201,204,205] and phenobarbital [201, 205] were compared with gas chromatographic methods. In addition to the above, a rapid micromethod for measuring anticonvulsant drugs in serum by high-performance liquid chromatograph [207] was described; its results comparing favorably with GC data.

Vandemark and Adams [208] described a procedure for determining phenobarbital, primidone, and diphenylhydantoin simultaneously in 50 µl of serum by gas chromatography and a detector with heightened sensitivity and selectivity for nitrogenous compounds. The drugs, together with an internal standard, 5-allyl-5-phenylbarbituric acid, were extracted by the procedure of MacGee [145], converted to their methyl derivatives with tetramethylammonium hydroxide by a modification of the method proposed by Greeley [241], and then analyzed with a Perkin-Elmer model 910 gas chromatograph equipped with dual flame ionization detectors, one of them modified with the nitrogen-phosphorus detector, a 91.4-cm by 2-mm-i.d. glass column packed with 3% OV-1 on 100-120 mesh Chromosorb W-HP (the column effluent split, half going to each detector for simultaneous comparison), and the PEP-2 data processor for automatic data reduction based on peak areas of the drugs. To achieve method reproducibility of about 7% and sensitivities of 0.5 mg/liter for 50-μl serum samples, the following conditions were maintained: injector temperature, 260°C; column temperature, programmed from 170°C with an initial hold of 1 min to 220°C at 16°C/min and held for 2 min, then 270°C for 2 min; detector temperature, 290°C; helium carrier-gas flow rate, 30 ml/min. From known standards, they noted that the degree of enhancement of the nitrogen detector over the flame ionization detector for free anticonvulsants as a ratio of peak areas were 13X for phenobarbital, 54X for primidone, and 18X for diphenylhydantoin, while for the methylated compounds the enhancement was 125X for phenobarbital, 122X for primidone, and 87X for diphenylhydantion. Absolute recoveries of drugs were calculated by comparing peak area ratios of extracted serum to nonextracted standard; recoveries for the drugs studied were phenobarbital, 49 to 54%; primidone, 28 to 34%; and diphenylhydantoin, 53 to 57%. As described, the GC procedure with the nitrogen-selective detector gives an analyst a significant advantage in terms of sensitivity and selectivity if the sample is suitably pretreated.

Sengupta and Peat [214] reported a simple and rapid technique for the simultaneous extraction of eight commonly prescribed anticonvulsant drugs [ethotoin (3-ethyl-5-phenylhydantoin), ethosuximide, carbamazepine, pheneturide, phenobarbital, diphenylhydantoin, primidone, and sodium valproate]; seven of these drugs were chromatographed simultaneously using an alkali flame ionization detector whereas the remaining drug, sodium valproate, was analyzed using a flame ionization detector.

Sample preparation was rather simple and straightforward: A 1-ml sample of plasma containing 20 μg each of heptabarbital (internal standard for ethotoin, ethosuximide, carbamazepine, pheneturide, and phenobarbital) and 5-(4-methylphenyl)-5-phenylhydantoin (internal standard for primidone and diphenylhydantoin) and 100 μg of cyclohexane carboxylic acid (internal standard for sodium valproate) was acidified with two drops of 1 M HCl and extracted with 5 ml of diethyl ether. The organic phase was evaporated to dryness and the residue redissolved in 100 μl of methanol. Using a 1-μl aliquot of this final residue in methanol, which was injected after flash methylation with 1 μl of freshly prepared tetramethylammonium hydroxide (20% TMAH in methanol diluted 1:10 with methanol before use), the methylated derivatives of phenobarbital, diphenylhydantoin, primidone, pheneturide, carbamazepine, ethosuximide, and ethotoin were determined with a Varian 1400 gas chromatograph equipped with an alkali flame ionization detector and a 4-ft by 1/4-in.-o.d. glass column packed with 1% OV-17 on 80-120 mesh Gas Chrom Q and temperature programmed from 110 to 240°C at 8°C/min. With the injector and detector temperatures maintained at 240 and 280°C, respectively, and the nitrogen carrier-gas flow rate set at 50 ml/min, the retention times of ethosuximide, pheneturide, ethotoin, phenobarbital, heptabarbital, carbamazepine, primidone, and diphenylhydantoin relative to that of 5-(4-methylphenyl)-5-phenylhydantoin (RRT = 1.000) were calculated to be 0.203, 0.455, 0.650, 0.682, 0.723, 0.770, 0.813, and 0.927, respectively. On the other hand, sodium valproate (salt of 2-propylpentanoic acid) was analyzed using a Varian model 2400 gas chromatograph fitted with a flame ionization detector and a 1-ft by 1/4-in.-o.d. glass column packed with 2% SP-1000 on 85-100 mesh Universal support. For this analysis, a 2-μl aliquot of the underivatized final methanol extract solution was injected into the GC unit operated at the following conditions: injector temperature, 200°C; column temperature, 120°C; detector temperature, 240°C; nitrogen carrier-gas flow rate, 40 ml/min. With the GC instrument operated as described, the retention time of sodium valproate relative to that of cyclohexane carboxylic acid (RRT = 1.000) was 0.744. For the analysis of diphenylhydantoin in plasma, the mean recovery of drug over a 5.5 to 25.0 μg/ml concentration range was 99.7 ± 3.3% (n = 9).

For comparative purposes, Booker and Darcey [201] measured phenobarbital and diphenylhydantoin in serum by an enzyme immunoassy procedure ("EMIT") in which the enzyme, glucose-6-phosphate dehydrogenase, had been coupled to the drug to be analyzed; the drug/enzyme complex retaining its enzymatic activity. In turn, the antibody binds with both the "free" drug and drug/enzyme complex. In the reaction of enzyme with substrate (glucose-6-phosphate), NAD^+ is converted to NADH with the change in concentration of NAD^+ measured spectrophotometrically at 340 nm.

Using a modified version of the procedure of Evenson et al. [147], the GC method of analysis was performed with a Hewlett-Packard model 402 gas chromatograph equipped with hydrogen flame ionization detectors and 150-cm by 2-mm-i.d. U-shaped glass columns packed with 3% OV-17 on 80-100 mesh Chromosorb W. To obtain retention times of 1.1, 6.0, 7.1, and 9.3 min for phenobarbital, primidone, diphenylhydantoin, and 5-(4-methylphenyl)-5-phenylhydantoin (internal standard), respectively, the GC conditions used were nitrogen carrier-gas flow rate, 50 ml/min; injector temperature, 290°C; column temperature, 260°C; and detector temperature, 290°C.

Sample preparation for GC analysis consisted of adding 1 ml of an aqueous solution of 5-(4-methylphenyl)-5-phenylhydantoin to 1 ml of each standard and unknown, acidfying the serum with 0.5 ml of 0.5 M HCl, extracting the drugs with chloroform, evaporating the chloroform, and finally dissolving the residue with carbon disulfide. From this CS_2 solution, an aliquot was removed and injected onto the gas chromatographic column.

With regard to the EMIT procedure, the method requires less than

5 min and no more than 50 µl of serum per determination. It is simple; only four steps (pipetting and diluting with an automatic pipettor-dilutor) are required before spectrophotometry. Twenty replicate analyses of a serum containing phenobarbital and diphenylhydantoin gave results with a coefficient of variation of 6.8% and 9.1%, respectively.

With regard to precision studies for both analytical techniques, Booker and Darcey reported that:

> Within-day reproducibility of the gas chromatographic method was determined by the repeated analysis (20 times) of a serum containing phenobarbital (25 mg/ml) and diphenylhydantoin (12.5 mg/ml). The average phenobarbital concentration was 24.99 mg/liter, with a standard deviation of 0.98 and a coefficient of variation of 3.9%. The average diphenylhydantoin concentration was 12.52 mg/liter, with a SD of 0.28 and a CV of 2.2%.
>
> Within-day reproducibility of the EMIT system was determined by 20 replicate analyses of a serum containing phenobarbital (20 mg/liter) and diphenylhydantoin (10 mg/liter). For phenobarbital the average concentration was 19.8 mg/liter, with a SD of 1.34 and a CV of 6.8%. For diphenylhydantoin the average concentration was 9.95 mg/liter, with a SD of 0.91 and a CV of 9.1%. Day-to-day variation was determined by analyzing on 25 days a calibration serum containing phenobarbital (30 mg/liter) and diphenylhydantoin (15 mg/liter). The average phenobarbital concentration was 31.1 mg/liter, with a SD of 2.27 and a CV of 7.3%. The average diphenylhydantoin concentration was 15.3 mg/liter, with a SD of 0.87 and a CV of 5.7%.

To compare GC/immunoassay data, 197 specimens containing diphenylhydantoin and 202 specimens containing phenobarbital were examined by both methods; for phenobarbital (Fig. 1.32), $r = 0.97$, $R^2 = 3.8$ mg/liter, intercept = 2.15 mg/liter, and slope = 0.79. For diphenylhydantoin (Fig. 1.33), $r = 0.98$, $R^2 = 1.80$ mg/liter, intercept = -0.90 mg/liter, and slope = 1.09. As stressed by the investigators, no false negatives or false positives were encountered using the EMIT procedure.

In 1973, a radioimmunoassay for diphenylhydantoin was developed by Tigelaar, Rapport, Inman, and Kupferberg [242] which, however, was nonspecific, detecting the main metabolite, 5-(4-hydroxyphenyl)-5-phenylhydantoin, as sensitively as the parent drug. Shortly thereafter, Cook, Kepler, and Christensen [243] developed an immunoassay that was specific for diphenylhydantoin and showed little cross-reactivity with either 5-(4-hydroxyphenyl)-5-phenylhydantoin or with drugs structurally similar to diphenylhydantoin, such as primidone or phenobarbital. Using the Cook et al. procedure with a few modifications, Orme et al. [204]

ANTIARRHYTHMIC AGENTS

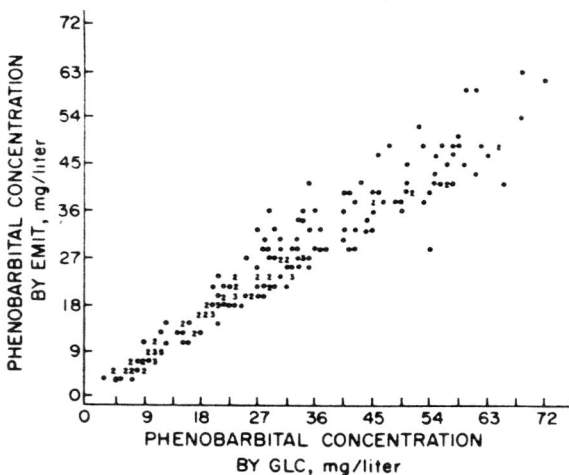

Figure 1.32. Serum phenobarbital concentrations as measured by two methods. Single data points are indicated by the dots. Numbers in the body of the figure replace some dots and are the number of data points at that particular position. From Booker and Darcey [201], courtesy of Clinical Chemistry.

measured concentrations of diphenylhydantoin by both radioimmunoassay and an improved version of the method of Berlin et al. [193], a microadaptation of the principles outlined in the method by MacGee [145], including on-column methylation of diphenylhydantoin with trimethylanilinium hydroxide and use of 5-(4-methylphenyl)-5-phenylhydantoin as internal standard.

In their evaluation of the data obtained, Orme et al. found that:

> There was an excellent correlation between values obtained by the two methods ($r = 0.983$), and in only 11 plasma samples did the results differ by more than 20%. Of the investigated samples, 105 were obtained from uremic patients. For these, an equally good agreement was obtained between the two methods ($r = 0.993$, $n = 105$, with the equation of the line being $y = 0.94x + 0.04$). Within-assay variance was 3.1% for the immunoassay and 3.3% for the gas chromatographic procedure. Without automatic pipetting equipment, the radioimmunoassay procedure took twice as long as the chromatographic assay, and the cost of chemicals was considerably higher. Nevertheless, the better sensitivity of the radioimmunoassay makes

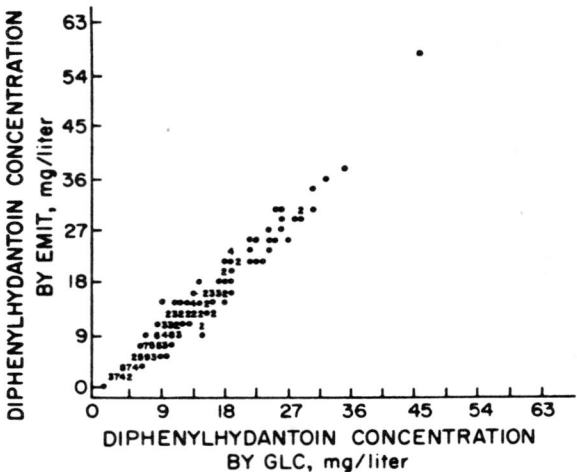

Figure 1.33. Serum diphenylhydantoin concentrations as measured by two methods. Single data points are indicated by the dots. Numbers in the body of the figure replace some dots and are the number of data points at that particular position. From Booker and Darcey [201], courtesy of Clinical Chemistry.

it of great value, especially in children, because plasma samples of 10 and 20 µl can be used.

As reported, the average time for immunoassay of 20 unknown plasma samples was 8.2 hr (not including counting time), while the average time for the determination of the same samples by GC was 4.6 hr. The cost of chemicals (excluding the costs for antiserum and ^{3}H-diphenylhydantoin) via the immunoassay was $1.50 per plasma sample (based on 20 plasma sample assays), whereas the cost of the GC analysis was less than $0.25 per plasma sample. Furthermore, capital costs of the immunoassay are also likely to be greater, because a liquid scintillation counter is usually much more costly than a gas chromatograph.

Spiehler et al. [205] compared radioimmunoassay, enzyme immunoassay, spectrophotometry, and gas chromatography for the determination of phenobarbital and diphenylhydantoin. Whereas the manufacturer's protocol was used for radioimmunoassay (RIA) and enzymatic immunoassay (EMIT) of both drugs, spectrophotometric analyses of phenobarbital and diphenylhydantoin were performed according to the method of Goldbaum [244] as modified by Bogan and Smith [245] and the procedure of Wallace

[246] as modified by Dill et al. [237], respectively. On the other hand, the method of Perchalski et al. [194] was used to assay both drugs by gas chromatography.

In the GC method, methylene chloride was substituted for ethyl ether as the solvent extractant, trimethylanilinium hydroxide was used to methylate the drugs via an on-column injection, and 5-(4-methylphenyl)-5-phenylhydantoin was used as internal standard. The GC separations and quantitative results were performed with a Hewlett-Packard model 5710A gas chromatograph equipped with a 1.82-m by 2-mm-i.d. glass column packed with 3% OV-17 on Gas Chrom Q.

In their study, Spiehler et al. compared quantitative results obtained by RIA and EMIT to each other and to the results on aliquots of the same sample by GC and ultravoilet spectrophotometry (SPECT). For diphenylhydantoin, the correlation coefficients were RIA versus EMIT, 0.953; RIA versus GC, 0.951; EMIT versus GC, 0.957; RIA versus SPECT, 0.862; EMIT versus SPECT, 0.898. As noted, the immunoassays could be substituted for GC or SPECT without changing the resulting clinical interpretations.

A statistical comparison of RIA, EMIT, GC, and SPECT for the determination of diphenylhydantoin is shown in Table 1.25. If calculated from the least-squares regression parameters, immunoassays for diphenylhydantoin would yield average values of 27.8 mg/liter (RIA) and 24.2 mg/liter (EMIT) for a GC value of 20 mg/liter and/or average values of 25.2 mg/liter (RIA) and 25.4 mg/liter for a SPECT value of 20 mg/liter.

In 1976, Soldin and Hill [207] described an assay system for measuring phenobarbital, diphenylhydantoin, primidone, ethosuximide, and carbamazepine in 25 µl of serum. This high-performance liquid chromatographic procedure involved precipitation of proteins with an acetonitrile solution containing cyheptamide as an internal standard and reverse-phase chromatography on a 30-cm by 4-mm column containing "micro-Bondapak C 18." The anticonvulsants were eluted with an equivolume mixture of potassium phosphate buffer (10 mmoles/liter, pH 8.0) and acetonitrile at a flow rate of 0.8 ml/min, detected by their absorbance at 200 nm, and quantitated by measuring peak areas. When measurement of primidone is not required, a 254-nm detector may be used. When compared with gas chromatography [240,247,248], the correlation coefficients varied between 0.77 and 0.98 as shown in Figure 1.34. For diphenylhydantoin, the correlation coefficient was 0.98.

E. Propranolol and Isoproterenol

The GC and/or GC-MS methods for propranolol analysis have been previously reported in Chapter 2 of Volume 4 [249-261]. In addition to its

TABLE 1.25

Statistical Comparison of RIA, EMIT, GC, and SPECT for Determining Diphenylhydantoin[a]

Methods compared	m[b]	b[c]	S_{xy}[d]	r[e]	n	t	PE[f]
1. RIA vs. EMIT	1.110	-0.120	2.78	0.953	59	23.76	11.0
2. RIA vs. GC	0.661	1.610	2.19	0.951	47	21.16	33.9
3. EMIT vs. GC	0.786	0.976	2.04	0.957	60	26.47	21.4
4. RIA vs. SPECT	0.718	1.78	1.93	0.862	33	14.52	28.2
5. EMIT vs. SPECT	0.711	1.98	1.63	0.898	36	11.89	28.9

[a]Adapted from Spiehler et al. [205].
[b]m (mg/liter) = slope of the least-squares regression line.
[c]b (mg/liter) = intercept of the least-squares regression line = constant error.
[d]S_{xy} (mg/liter) = standard of the estimate = random error.
[e]r = correlation coefficient.
[f]PE = proportional error = $(1.000 - m) \times 100$.

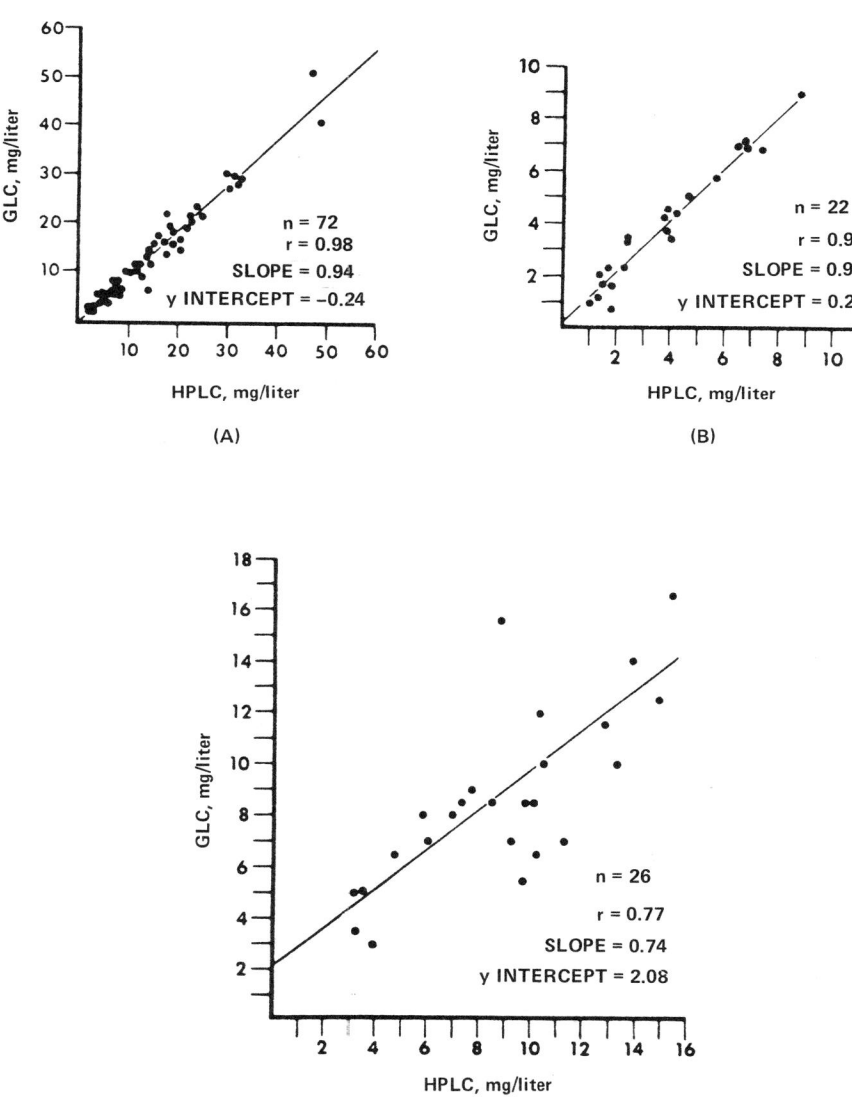

Figure 1.34. Comparison of the HPLC method with the GC method for diphenylhydantoin (A), carbamazepine (B), primidone (C), ethosuximide (D), and phenobarbital (E). Adapted from Soldin and Hill [207].

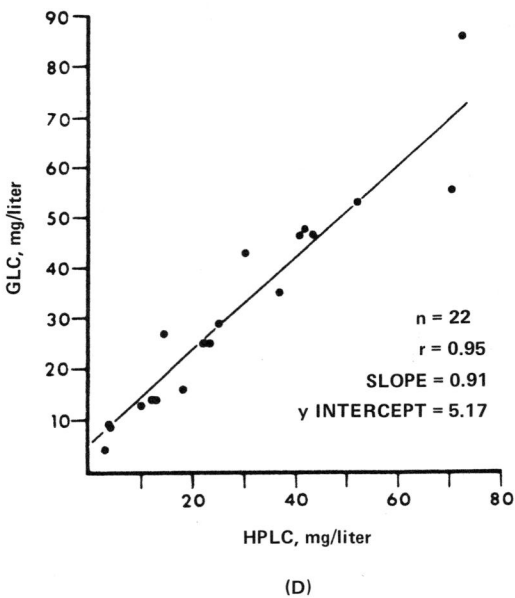

(D)

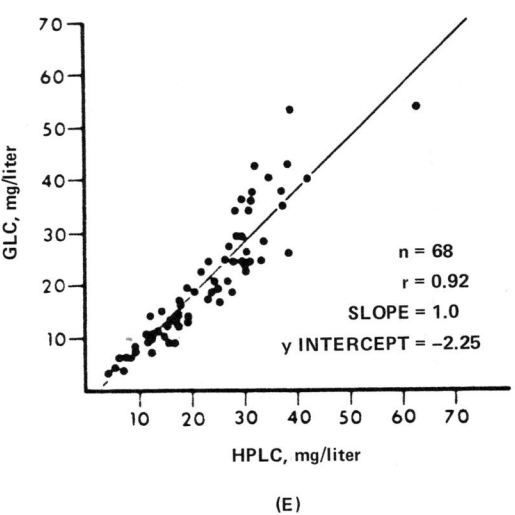

(E)

Figure 1.34. (continued)

β-adrenergic blocking action, propranolol has direct quinidine-like actions on the heart. Useful in atrial tachyarrhythmias in which its effect on A-V transmission may control the ventricular rate, Abramson [262] discussed its analysis using a "second-generation" mass fragmentography technique which he appropriately named "functional group mass spectrometry." In this pragmatical approach to mass spectrometry, the analyst monitors one mass which is indicative of a structural feature common to multiple compounds. The single mass chromatogram which results is the representation of all the compounds in the sample containing this structural moiety. Using only one mass, functional group mass spectrometry does not, therefore, require any additional hardware and is straightforward to set up instrumentally. As noted by Abramson:*

> The difficulty is in finding appropriate compounds and derivatives to direct fragmentation away from the R-group. In addition one is returned to absolute dependence on gas chromatography (GC) retention times for qualitation as is the case in pure gas chromatography experiments. The following spectra should indicate the thought processes behind the formulation of these experiments.
>
> We were interested in measuring a variety of biogenic amines as possible neurotransmitter substances in individual neurons. Similar experiments of neurotransmitters have been published by Costa's group [263], and by Narasimhachari and Vouros [264]. Figure [1.35] is the mass spectrum of the heptafluorobutyryl derivative of dopamine as used by Costa et al. The major fragmentation processes generate ions from the nonamine portion of the molecule. Narasimhachari and Vouros converted their primary amines to isothiocyanates with CS_2 and then trimethylsilylated. The spectrum of dopamine-NCS-TMS is shown in Figure [1.36]. Excellent structural data is present, but only compound-specific ions are important. We finally tried the TMS derivative whose spectrum is in Figure [1.37]. Nearly three-fourths of all the ion intensity is present in the m/e 174 peak representing the ion $CH_2=\overset{+}{N}-(TMS)_2$. It turns out that this ion is the base peak in all the primary biogenic amines, such as phenylethylamine, putrescine, tyramine, octopamine, norepinephrine, normetanephrine, 6-OH-dopamine, tryptamine, and serotonin. It is a major ion in Ω-amino acids possessing the $R-CH_2NH_2$ structure such as glycine, β-alanine, GABA, ornithine, and lysine. In fact, all these compounds can be separated by gas chromatography and detected in the same experiment at a single mass using a mass spectrometer detector. Figure [1.38] shows a standardization run of these

---

*Portions of text and selected figures reproduced with permission of the National Institute of General Medical Sciences (HEW).

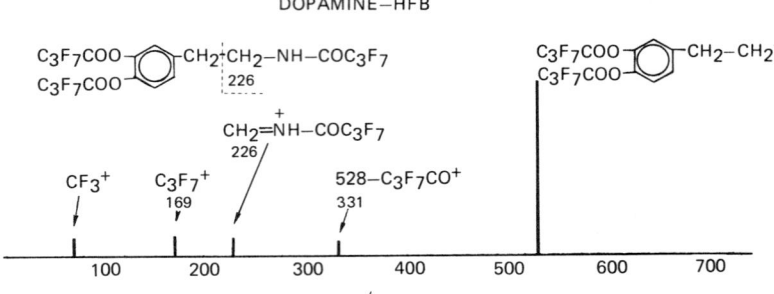

Figure 1.35. Mass spectrum of the heptafluorobutyryl derivative of dopamine. From Abramson [262], courtesy of National Institute of General Medical Sciences (HEW).

compounds at the approximate level of 4 pmoles. A 100-μg sample from an <u>Aplysia californica</u> ganglion is seen in Figure [1.39]. A number of individual neurons have been examined by this technique and some of the results have been validated by specific chemical assays.

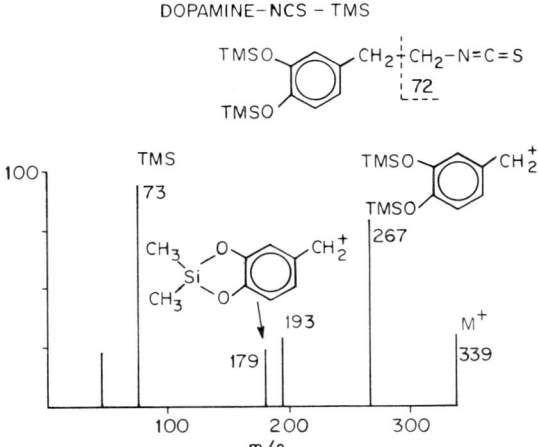

Figure 1.36. Mass spectrum of the isothiocyanate-TMS derivative of dopamine. 70 eV. From Abramson [262], courtesy of National Institute of General Medical Sciences (HEW).

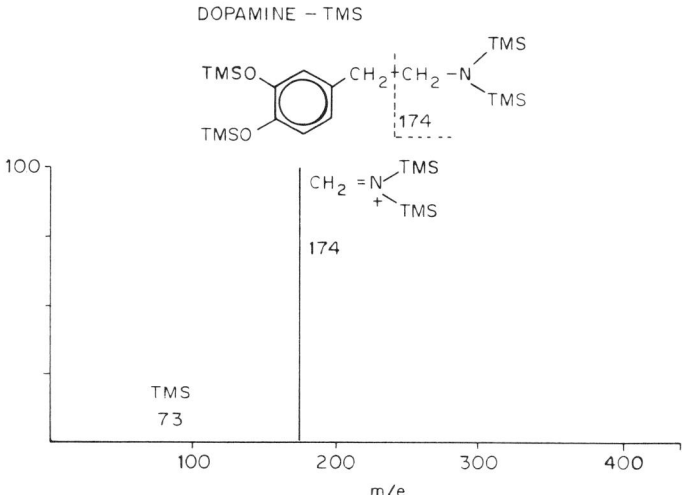

Figure 1.37. Mass spectrum of the poly-TMS derivative of dopamine. 70 eV. From Abramson [262], courtesy of National Institute of General Medical Sciences (HEW).

This technique was also applied to α-amino acids with the ability to quantify another eight amino acids using the ion m/e 218 $(CH_3)_3Si-\overset{+}{N}H=CH-COO-TMS$ which is important for many amino acids possessing the R-HC(NH$_2$)-COOH structure. In addition, α-methyl amines and α-amino acids may be specifically detected at their appropriate masses; m/e 188 and 232, respectively.

A rational extention of the functional group concept might be in the measurement of a drug and its metabolites. The metabolism of a drug often changes only one area of a molecule, allowing for the detection of those metabolites which keep unchanged the portion of the molecule being used as the functional group. My colleagues and I have begun a study of the clinical pharmacology of propranolol. This β-adrenergic blocking agent [I, Fig. 1.40] is extensively metabolized and among its many metabolites as studied by GC-MS are two more β-blocking compounds, 4-OH-propranolol (II) and N-deisopropyl-propranolol (III) [251]. Part of the fragmentation of the heptafluoro-butyryl derivative of these compounds is a fragment ion at m/e 252 containing the amino nitrogen, the propyl chain, and the N-hepta-fluorobutyryl group. Because the N-isopropyl group is lost in the course of this fragmentation anyway, III gives nearly an equal fragment at m/e 252 as I or II. ICI 45763 (IV) is used as an internal

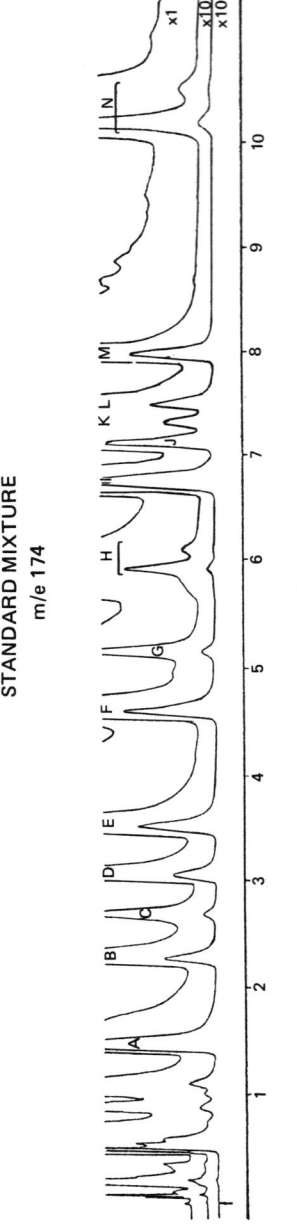

Figure 1.38. Mass chromatogram (m/e 174) of a standard mixture of amines and Ω-amino acids. At arrow, 1 μl of the TMS derivatives was injected. The peaks are identified as: A, glycine (21 pmole); B, β-alanine (6 pmoles); C, reagent blank; D, GABA (6.7 pmoles); E, phenylethylamine (5.4 pmoles); F, putrescine (3.4 pmoles); G, ornithine (4.2 pmoles); H, lysine (3.8 pmoles); I, octopamine (3.4 pmoles); J, DA (3.4 pmoles); K, normetanephrine (2.9 pmoles); L, norepinephrine (3.8 pmoles); M, 6-OH-DA (4.5 pmoles); and N, 5-HT (4.0 pmoles). From Abramson [262], courtesy of National Institute of General Medical Sciences (HEW).

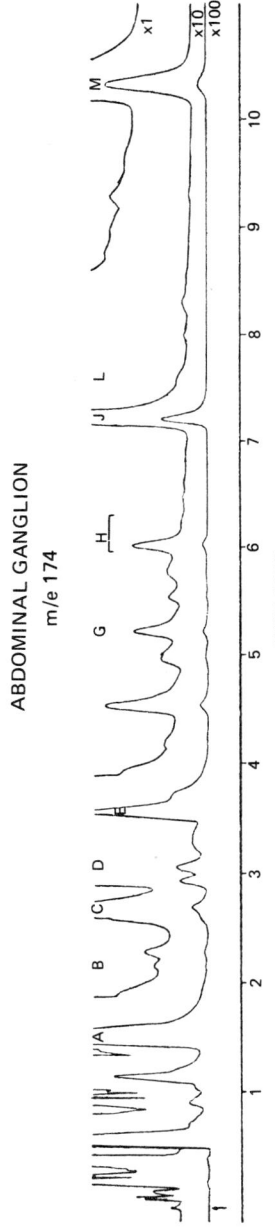

Figure 1.39. Mass chromatograph (m/e 174) of an extract of the abdominal ganglion from A. californica. One microliter of this solution (equivalent to 0.1 mg of tissue) was injected into the GC at arrow. Amino compounds were identified by comparison of retention times with those of the standard mixture (Fig. 1.38). From Abramson [262], courtesy of National Institute of General Medical Sciences (HEW).

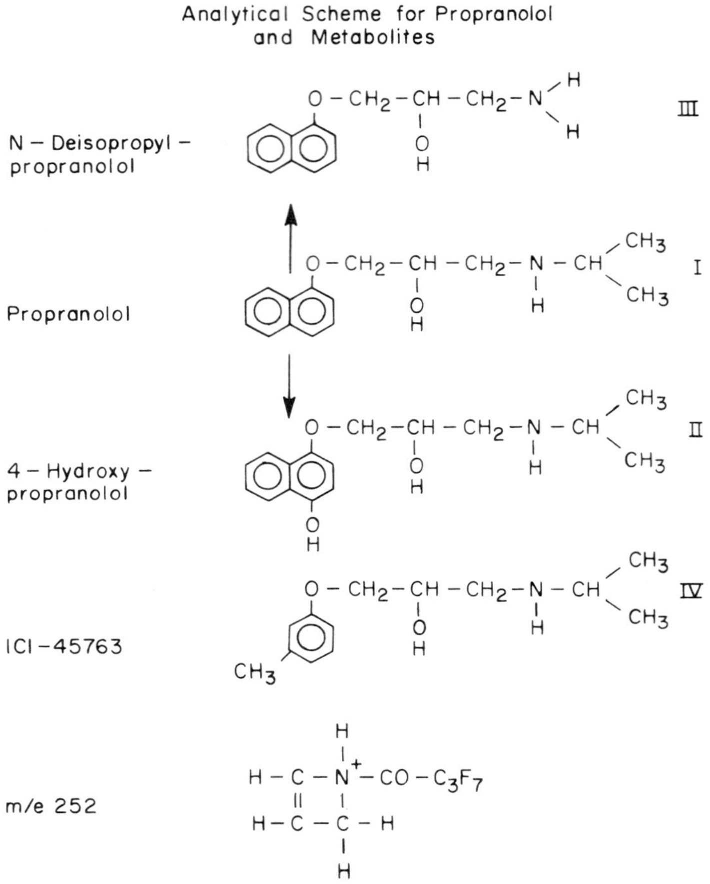

Analytical Scheme for Propranolol and Metabolites

N – Deisopropyl – propranolol — Structure III: naphthyl–O–CH$_2$–CH(OH)–CH$_2$–NH$_2$ (shown as N with two H)

Propranolol — Structure I: naphthyl–O–CH$_2$–CH(OH)–CH$_2$–NH–CH(CH$_3$)$_2$

4 – Hydroxy – propranolol — Structure II: 4-hydroxy-naphthyl–O–CH$_2$–CH(OH)–CH$_2$–NH–CH(CH$_3$)$_2$

ICI–45763 — Structure IV: (methylphenyl)–O–CH$_2$–CH(OH)–CH$_2$–NH–CH(CH$_3$)$_2$

m/e 252 — rearrangement ion: H–C(=CH–C(H)(H)–)–N$^+$(H)–CO–C$_3$F$_7$

Figure 1.40. The structure of propranolol in relationship to its two β-blocking metabolites and the internal standard. The ion structure shown at the bottom is a common ion formed from rearrangement of the heptafluorobutyryl derivative. From Abramson [262], courtesy of National Institute of General Medical Sciences (HEW).

standard for quantitation. Thus, by monitoring the chromatography at m/e 252, we can detect the parent drug, the active metabolites, and the internal standard in a very straightforward experiment. The nature of this fragmentation suggests that it will be a general one for other β-blocking drugs [265], such as bunalol, practolol, oxprenolol, and alprenolol as shown in Figure [1.41].

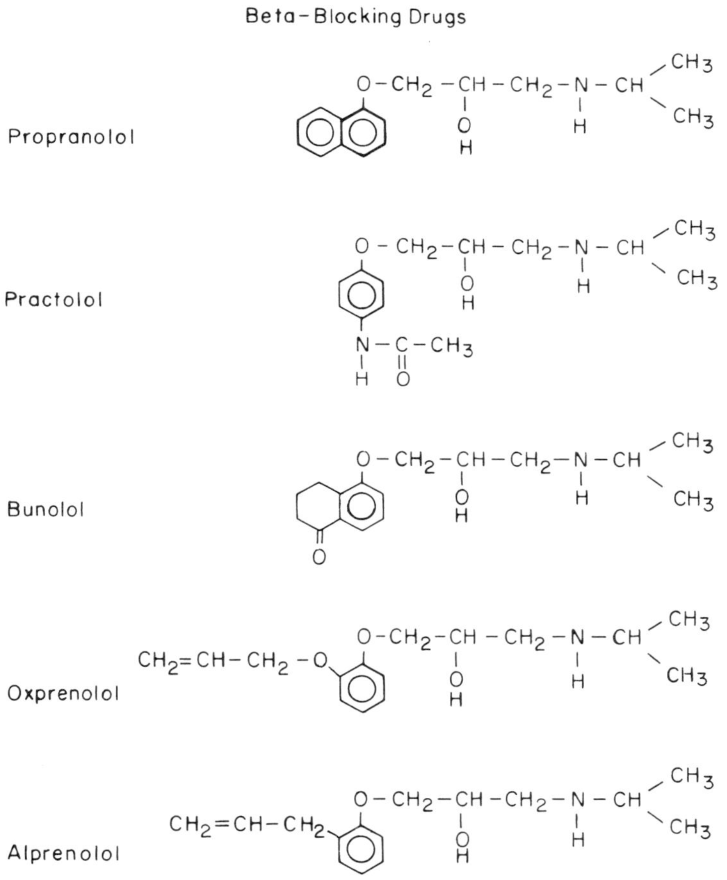

ANTIARRHYTHMIC AGENTS

Beta-Blocking Drugs

Figure 1.41. Some structures of representative β-blocking drugs. The commonality of the structural features leading to the m/e 252 fragment (see Fig. 1.40) suggests that any of them would be detectable in this manner. From Abramson [262], courtesy of National Institute of General Medical Sciences (HEW).

In 1976, Salens, Walle, and Privitera [266] described a method for the quantitative determination of propranolol and two of its active metabolites, 3-(α-napthoxy)-1,2-propanediol (propranolol glycol) and N-desisopropylpropranolol, in brain tissue of mice. In their procedure, tissues are homogenized in perchloric acid-acetonitrile. Propranolol and its metabolites are isolated from the supernatant by solvent extraction and

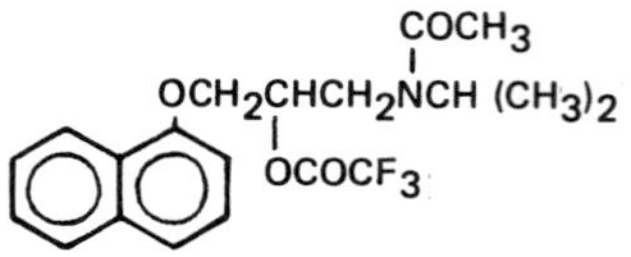

Propranolol

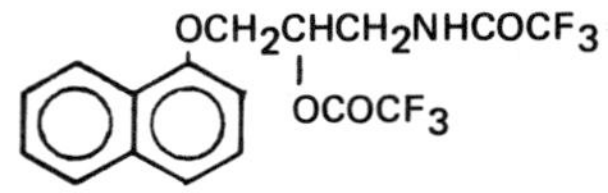

OCH$_2$CHCH$_2$N(CH$_3$)(COCH$_3$)
    |
    OCOCF$_3$
(naphthalene ring)

Propranolol

N-Desisopropylpropranolol

OCH$_2$CHCH$_2$NHCOCF$_3$
    |
    OCOCF$_3$
(naphthalene ring)

N-Desisopropylpropranolol

Propranolol Glycol

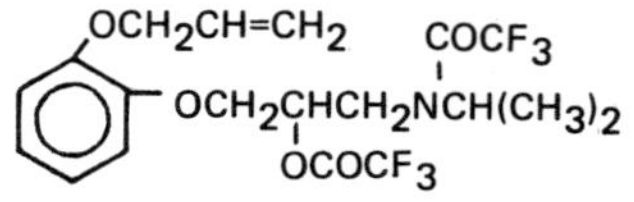

OCH$_2$CHCH$_2$OCOCF$_3$
    |
    OCOCF$_3$
(naphthalene ring)

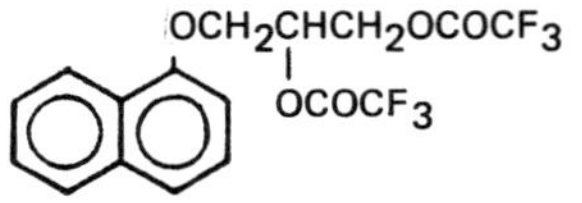

Propranolol Glycol

Oxprenolol

OCH$_2$CH=CH$_2$
OCH$_2$CHCH$_2$N(CH(CH$_3$)$_2$)(COCF$_3$)
    |
    OCOCF$_3$
(benzene ring)

Oxprenolol

separated and detected as their trifluoroacetyl derivatives by electron capture gas chromatography.

Using oxprenolol as internal standard, sample preparation for GC analysis consisted of the following:

To each sample of fresh mouse brain tissue (about 500 mg wet weight) were added 1.5 ml acetonitrile, 1.5 ml 0.8 N perchloric acid, and the internal standard oxprenolol (400 ng/mg). The sample was homogenized in ice with a Potter-Elvehjem homogenizer using a PTFE pestle. After centrifugation the supernatant was transferred to a conical centrifuge tube, made alkaline (pH 12) with 5 N NaOH, and extracted with 5 ml benzene.

The benzene was extracted with 2 ml of 1 N H$_2$SO$_4$, leaving the neutral metabolite, propranolol glycol, in the benzene phase (neutral fraction). The acidic aqueous phase containing the basic compounds, propranolol, N-deisopropylpropranolol, and oxprenolol, was then made alkaline (pH 12) with 5 N NaOH and extracted with 5 ml benzene (basic fraction).

Both 5-ml benzene extracts were evaporated to 500 µl at 50 to 60°C with a gentle stream of nitrogen. Twenty-five microliters of trimethylamine in benzene (1 M) and 25 µl of trifluoroacetic anhydride were added to each extract and the reaction mixtures were heated for 5 min at 50-60°C. The derivatized samples (di-TFA derivatives) were washed with 3 ml distilled water and centrifuged before analysis.

An aliquot of the aqueous solution containing the derivatives was injected into a Varian model 1440 gas chromatograph equipped with a ^{63}Ni electron capture detector and 180-cm by 2-mm-i.d. glass columns packed with 1% OV-17 and 2% OV-1 on 80-100 mesh Chromosorb W. With the specified GC conditions [injector temperature, 265°C; column temperature, 170°C (neutral fraction) or 195°C (basic fraction); detector temperature, 280°C; nitrogen carrier-gas flow rate, 30 ml/min], the retention times of the di-TFA derivatives of propranolol glycol, oxprenolol, N-desisopropylpropranolol, and propranolol were 2.49, 3.90, 6.28, and 9.80 min, respectively. On the other hand, the minimum detectable quantity for each compound (expressed in picograms and determined at a retention time of 3 min on a column with 3800 theoretical plates) was propranolol glycol, 0.2; oxprenolol, 1.1; N-desisopropylpropranolol, 0.4; and propranolol, 0.5. The recovery of propranolol and its two metabolites from brain tissue through homogenization in perchloric acid-acetonitrile followed by solvent extraction (as compared to water, from which recoveries were 90%) was propranolol, 58 ± 3%; propranolol glycol, 63 ± 4%; N-desisopropylpropranolol, 64 ± 3%; oxprenolol, 59 ± 6%. As noted by Saelens et al., brain levels of 10 to 250 ng/g can be detected of all three compounds with high specificity and good precision (at the 100-ng/g level, ±5% for propranolol and ±10% for desisopropylpropranolol).

Isoproterenol is a β-adrenergic stimulant that dilates blood vessels while it stimulates the heart. When used in the treatment of bronchial asthma, it may cause tachycardia, arrhythmias, and hypotension. It is used primarily in the treatment of bronchial asthma, atrioventricular block, and cardiac arrest [1].

Its analysis has been discussed in Chapter 2 of Volume 4 [28,59,267-273], but more recently, Watson and Lawrence [274] presented a simple, specific GC analytical procedure for the quantitative determination of isoproterenol, epinephrine, and phenylephrine in commercial tablets, powders, inhalation solutions, ophthalmic and nasal drops, and injectable preparations.

Following prescribed methods for sample preparation to which dibenzyl succinate was added as internal standard, each isoproterenol sample solution was treated with N-trimethylsilylimidazole (1 ml) and allowed to stand for 30 min in the dark at ambient temperature with occasional shaking.

Each epinephrine and phenylephrine sample solution containing the internal standard was treated with N,O-bis(trimethylsilyl)acetamide (1 ml) and allowed to stand for 30 min in the dark at ambient temperature with occasional shaking.

From either silylated solution, a 2-μl aliquot was injected into a Bendix series 2500 gas chromatograph equipped with flame ionization detectors and a 1.82-m by 6-mm-o.d. U-shaped glass column packed with 5% OV-101 on 100-120 mesh Chromosorb 750. With the specified GC conditions [injector temperature, 225°C; detector temperature, 225°C; column temperature, 170°C (10 min) and then programmed to 245°C at 2°C/min;

nitrogen carrier-gas flow rate, 70 ml/min], the retention times of the internal standard and the silyl derivatives of isoproterenol and epinephrine were approximately 23.62, 10.38, and 13.75 min, respectively.

The results obtained by applying the method to the analysis of each of the three drugs in several simulated decomposed mixtures were in good agreement with theoretical values, even at impurity levels of up to 80% by weight. When applied to commercial formulations, the procedure was feasible for tablets, powders, and solutions at drug concentrations of 0.2% or greater. The commonly incorporated buffering and antioxidant excipients (glycerin, lactic acid, ascorbic acid, citric acid, lactose, chlorobutanol, saccharin sodium, sodium bisulfite, sodium citrate, edetate sodium, phenol, and benzalkonium chloride) did not interfere.

F. Disopyramide

Disopyramide is a new antiarrhythmic agent that seems to possess a greater therapeutic index than quinidine. Pharmacokinetic studies in man have indicated that its plasma half-life is about 7 hr, almost 60% of the parent compound is excreted unchanged in the urine within 48 hr [275], and its primary metabolic product is mono-dealkylated disopyramide.

The determination of the parent compound and its metabolite by gas chromatography was first reported by Hutsell and Stachelski [276], who described their analysis in blood serum and urine. Their method involved extraction of the drugs from a basic aqueous medium into chloroform, derivatization of the metabolite with acetic anhydride, purification of the extract by use of Florisil to separate the drugs from interfering materials, and subsequent analysis by gas chromatography using a Packard GC system equipped with flame ionization detection and a 0.61-m by 2-mm-i.d. U-shaped column packed with 2.6% OV-17 on 80-100 mesh Chromosorb W-HP. Using p-chlorodisopyramide [4-diisopropylamino-2-(p-chlorophenyl)-2-(2-pyridyl)butyramide] as internal standard and the GC parameters listed in Table 1.26 for the assay of DIP and DIDIP in

Disopyramide
[4-Diisopropylamino-2-phenyl-2-(2-pyridyl) butyramide]
(DIP)

$$H_2N-\overset{O}{\overset{\|}{C}}-\underset{\underset{C_6H_5}{|}}{C}-(CH_2)_2-\overset{H}{\overset{|}{N}}-\underset{\underset{CH_3}{|}}{\overset{H}{\overset{|}{C}}}-CH_3$$

Monodealkylated Disopyramide
[4-Isopropylamino-2-phenyl-2-(2-pyridyl) butyramide]
(DIDIP)

biological specimens, the recoveries of DIP and DIDIP added to serum or urine were approximately 80% when compared with unextracted standards and essentially quantitative recoveries (>95%) when compared with standards that were carried through the assay procedure. On the other hand, the effective limits of detection (corrected for sample volume and dilution during analysis) relative to serum or urine were 85 ng DIP/ml and 170 ng DIDIP-acetate/ml or 65 ng DIP/ml and 125 ng DIDIP/ml, respectively.

Duchateau et al. [277] developed a rapid GC procedure for the determination of DIP in serum using a Pye Unicam G.C.V. gas chromatograph

TABLE 1.26

GC Operating Parameters for DIP and DIDIP Analysis[a]

Parameter	Assay system	
	DIP	DIDIP
Injector temperature (°C)	230	250
Column temperature (°C)	210	230
Detector temperature (°C)	260	260
Helium carrier-gas flow rate (ml/min)	60	60
Retention times (min)		
DIP	6.25	2.50
Internal standard	11.88	4.69
DIDIP-acetate	21.88	8.43

[a]Adapted from Hutsell and Stachelski [276].

equipped with a nitrogen detector and a 3-ft by 2-mm-i.d. glass coiled column packed with 3% OV-17 coated on 100-120 mesh Gas Chrom Q. To obtain retention times of 4.48 and 7.25 min for DIP and p-chlorodisopyramide (internal standard), respectively, the following GC conditions were used: injector temperature, 275°C; column temperature, 255°C; detector temperature, 275°C; nitrogen carrier-gas flow rate, 30 ml/min; hydrogen flow rate, 30 ml/min; air flow rate, 300 ml/min.

The procedure used for sample preparation for GC analysis was as follows:

Pipette into a glass-stoppered separating funnel 1.0 ml of serum, 2.0 ml of 0.1 N NaOH, 100 µl of internal standard solution (p-chlorodisopyramide, 100 µg per ml of solution in ethanol), and 10 ml of chloroform. Shake well for 30 sec, dry the chloroform layer with 1 g of anhydrous sodium sulfate, and filter. Extract the aqueous layer with 10 ml of chloroform for 15 sec, dry and filter off the chloroform phase. Evaporate the pooled chloroform extracts to dryness on a water bath at 50°C under a stream of nitrogen. Transfer the dried residue with small portions of chloroform into a 3-ml glass tube, evaporate the chloroform under a stream of nitrogen, and dissolve the residue in 25 µl of ethanol. Inject 1 µl of the final solution into the gas chromatograph.

Using a standard calibration curve (plot of the ratio of peak area of disopyramide to that of the internal standard versus DIP concentration), the recovery of DIP from serum was 102.5% with a standard deviation of 2.0% (n = 5).

Using the GC procedure developed by Hutsell and Stachelski [276] for the determination of DIP and DIDIP in biological media, Hinderling and Garrett [278] investigated the pharmacokinetics of DIP and its monodealkylated metabolite (DIDIP) in seven volunteers after intravenous (1 and 2 mg/kg) and oral (3 and 6 mg/kg) administration. As noted by these investigators, "the lower levels of sensitivity were 0.085 µg/ml and 0.065 µg/ml for the parent drug (DIP) and 0.17 µg/ml and 0.125 µg/ml for the metabolite (DIDIP) in plasma and urine, respectively. Mean and standard deviation of repetitively determined known serum concentration of DIP of 1.18 and 0.3 µg/ml were, respectively, 1.14 ± 0.11 µg/ml (n = 42), and 0.29 µg/ml (n = 44). In urine spiked with DIP to give concentrations of 7.50 and 1.50 µg/ml, the respective values of the mean and standard deviation were 7.51 ± 0.46 µg/ml (n = 26) and 1.42 ± 0.19 µg/ml (n = 26)."

Summarizing their findings, Hinderling and Garrett noted that:

Unchanged drug (52%) and the monodealkylated metabolite (25%) were renally excreted on intravenous administration. The pharmacokinetics of disopyramide were first order and dose dependent only when referenced to the drug not bound to plasma proteins since this binding was dose dependent. The apparent half-lives of the alpha and beta phases of intravenous administration were 2 min and 4.5 hr, respectively. The apparent volumes of distribution of the central and peripheral compartments, referenced to unbound DIP in the plasma, were 9 and 80 liters, respectively. The half-life of adsorption of oral aqueous disopyramide phosphate was 30 min with a lag time of 16 min and an apparent first-pass metabolism of 16% of the adsorbed dose, consistent with the hepatic efficiency of 14%. The renal and metabolic clearances were 125 and 111 ml/min, respectively. Graphical and computer analysis of the plasma and urine showed dose-independent first-order pharmacokinetics of plasma unbound in a two-compartment-body model to give two metabolites and a first-pass transformation of a fraction of the oral dose. The absorption efficiency of unchanged drug was 83%.

With regard to the plasma pharmacokinetics of the monodealkylated metabolite (DIDIP) after DIP administration, the data indicated that metabolite peak plasma levels of $0.23 \pm 0.02\%$ of the dose/liter of plasma (n = 3) occurred at 6.3 ± 1.3 hr (n = 3) after oral administration of 6 mg/kg DIP. Based on a semilogarithmic plot of time versus plasma concentrations of unbound DIDIP, an apparent half-life of 9.11 ± 0.68 and 9.21 ± 0.51 hr (n = 3) after intravenous administration of 1 and 2 mg/kg of DIP, respectively, was obtained.

On the other hand, they noted that:

The average renal clearance for the unbound DIDIP metabolite was 151 ± 10 ml/min (n = 3). The renal clearance values of the metabolite appeared to be independent of urine flow between 0.6 and 5.5 ml/min and of urinary pH between 5.2 and 7.7.

The endogenous creatinine clearances were within the normal range and were 119 ± 4.5 ml/min corrected for a body surface of 1.73 m^2 at urine flows of 1.04 ± 0.03 ml/min. The ratios of the renal clearances of DIP and DIDIP to creatinine were 1.01 ± 0.08 and 1.25 ± 0.07, respectively. The ratios of the mean renal clearances of DIP to DIDIP were 0.84 ± 0.17. This implies glomerular filtration for DIP and DIDIP since the values are not significantly different from unity.

In a subsequent report, Hinderling and Garrett [279] studied "the effects of heart rate, R-T' interval, and mean arterial blood pressure in seven healthy male volunteers after intravenous (1 and 2 mg/kg) and oral (3 and 6 mg/kg) administration of DIP. The left ventricular ejection time was measured after intravenous administration of 2 mg/kg of drug.

Simultaneously the plasma concentrations and urinary excretion of the parent drug and its monodealkylated metabolite were monitored as a function of time. Heart rate increases of 20% were observed at 2 mg/kg i.v. and 6 mg/kg p.o. and peaked at 0 to 4 min and 2 hr after administration, respectively. R-T' interval increases of 40% and 9% were observed at 2 mg/kg and 1 mg/kg i.v., respectively, and peaked at 0 to 2 min after administration. R-T' interval increases of 12% and 4% were observed at 6 mg/kg and 3 mg/kg p.o., respectively, and peaked at 2.5 hr. The ejection time index was unchanged, and although a 5 to 10% increase in the mean arterial blood pressure was observed in the 11 hr after administration, there was no pattern consistent with size or mode of administration of the four dosages."

G. α,α-Dimethyl-4-($\alpha,\alpha,\beta,\beta$-tetrafluorophenethyl)benzylamine

Zacchei and Weidner [280] developed a GC method for the analysis of a new orally active arrhythmic agent, α,α-dimethyl-4-($\alpha,\alpha,\beta,\beta$-tetrafluorophenethyl)benzylamine, for the treatment of ventricular arrhythmias resulting from myocardial infarction. The procedure involves the addition of an internal standard [4-($\alpha,\alpha,\beta,\beta$-tetrafluorophenethyl)benzylamine] to a plasma or urine sample followed by extraction of the drugs into benzene at pH 8.0. The extracted amines are converted to the trifluoroacetyl derivatives with trifluoroacetic anhydride as reagent and are analyzed with a Packard model 7400 gas chromatograph equipped with a ^{63}Ni electron detector and a 183-cm by 6-mm glass column containing 2% PPE-20 (polyphenyl ether) on 80-100 mesh Chromosorb W. The retention times of 4.0 and 6.6 min of DMTFPB and TPB as the trifluoroacetyl derivatives, respectively, were obtained using the following conditions: injector temperature, 230°C; column temperature, 200°C; detector temperature, 230°C; nitrogen carrier-gas flow rate, 50 ml/min. A summary of the

α,α-Dimethyl-4-($\alpha,\alpha,\beta,\beta$-tetrafluorophenethyl) benzylamine (DMTFPB)

4-($\alpha,\alpha,\beta,\beta$-Tetrafluorophenethyl) benzylamine (TPB)

recovery results of DMTFPB from water, dog plasma, and human urine over a 5- to 400-ng concentration range is given in Table 1.27, where one notes that DMTFPB recoveries added to dog plasma in amounts of 5 to 100 ng ranged from about 88 to 118.5% for analyses performed over several months; the mean recovery being 102.5 ± 13.5% over the entire concentration range. Based on human urine studies, recoveries of DMTFPB ranged from 64.5 to 103.5% over a 12- to 400-ng concentration range; the mean recovery being 93.7 ± 14.7%.

The TFA derivatives were characterized by GC-MS; specifically, a LKB 9000S GC-MS instrument equipped with two columns: a 183-cm by 5-mm glass column packed with 1% OV-17 on 80-100 mesh Supelcoport; the other a 183-cm by 5-mm glass column containing 2% PPE-20 on 80-100 mesh Chromosorb W. Using the specified conditions (column temperature, 190°C; helium carrier-gas flow rate, 30 ml/min; ionizing potential, 70 eV; accelerating potential, 3.5 kV; source temperature, 270°C; separator temperature, 260°C; injector temperature, 255°C), the retention times for DMTFPB and its TFA derivative were approximately 3.3 and 4.0 min, respectively.

H. Aprindine

Administered both orally and intravenously, aprindine [N,N-diethyl-N'-(2-indanyl)-N'-phenyl-1,3-propanediamine] was chromatographed by Rutherford and Bishara [281] in 1976 using a procedure in which the raw material of the new potent antiarrhythmic agent, supplied as the hydrochloride salt, is dissolved in deionized water (50 mg/5 ml), and the base is liberated by 25 ml of a 10% aqueous solution of sodium carbonate. Aprindine is extracted with three 10-ml portions of chloroform, filtered through anhydrous sodium sulfate into a 50-ml volumetric flask, and diluted to volume with chloroform. After the sample has been diluted 1:1 with the internal standard solution (60 mg of 5 α-cholestane/500 ml of chloroform), a 2-μl aliquot is withdrawn and injected into a Hewlett-Packard model 402 gas chromatograph equipped with a flame ionization

Aprindine

TABLE 1.27

Recovery of DMTFPB From Water, Dog Plasma, and Human Urine[a]

Water			Dog plasma			Human urine		
Added (ng)	Found (ng)	Recovery (%)	Added (ng)	Found (ng)	Recovery (%)	Added (ng)	Found (ng)	Recovery (%)
100	87.0	87.0	100	101.5	101.5	400	383	95.8
80	72.9	91.2	80	81.4	101.8	200	207	103.5
60	60.1	100.0	60	68.5	114.3	100	96	96.0
50	50.3	100.6	50	50.8	101.5	50	50	100.0
30	30.6	102.0	30	35.3	118.5	25	19	76.0
25	28.1	112.7	25	25.2	101.0	12.5	11	87.9
15	16.6	110.5	15	15.3	102.0	6.2	4	64.5
10	11.6	116.0	10	9.9	99.0			
5			5	4.4	88.0			

[a]Adapted from Zacchei and Weidner [280].

detector and a 122-cm by 3-mm-i.d. U-shaped glass column packed with 3.8% W-98 (methyl·vinyl silicone gum) on 80-100 mesh Chromosorb W-HP. To obtain retention times of approximately 2.0 and 5.8 min for aprindine and cholestane, respectively, the following GC conditions were maintained: injector temperature, 255°C; column temperature, 230°C; detector temperature, 255°C; helium carrier-gas flow rate, 60 ml/min.

Since previous GC studies [282-284] which assayed the drug in biological media did not validate their procedures with regard to precision, accuracy, and specificity, Rutherford and Bishara established the precision of their method as follows:

> Duplicate injections of five 50-mg raw material samples, extracted by a single analyst, gave a standard deviation (SD) of 0.01 and a relative standard deviation [RSD = (SD X 100)/mean] of 1.48%. Duplicate injections of five capsule samples containing 25 mg/capsule gave a relative standard deviation of 1.04%. The relative error calculated for this formulation was +0.2%. Duplicate injections of five solution samples (1 mg/ml) gave a relative standard deviation of 0.79%.

Whereas GC-MS spectral analysis indicated that the observed GC peak was that of aprindine, with a molecular ion at m/e 322, all synthetic precursors yielded shorter retention times than aprindine when chromatographed at a column temperature of 200°C. This GC study is summarized in Table 1.28. On the other hand, the percent recovery of aprindine by GC analysis for investigations conducted to measure the stability of aprindine to acid, base, dry heat, refluxing, and UV light, and to pH variations, is shown in Table 1.29.

I. Mexiletine

A recently introduced new antiarrhythmic agent, mexiletine, has been found to be effective in controlling serious ventricular arrhythmias in patients after acute infarction and has a potency comparable to that of lidocaine or procainamide.

Mexiletine
[1-(2',6'-Dimethyl)-phenoxy-2-aminopropane]

TABLE 1.28

Relative Retention Times (RRT) of Compounds
Related to Aprindine[a]

Identity[b]	Chemical name	RRT[c]
P	Indene	N.D.
P	2-Indonone	N.D.
P	2-Indanol	N.D.
P	2-Indanol methanesulfonate	0.07
P	N-Phenyl-2-indanamine	0.17
Aprindine	N,N-Diethyl-N'-(2-indanyl)-N'-phenyl-1,3-propanediamine	1.00
PDP	N,N-Diethyl-N'-phenyl-1,3-propanediamine	0.07
PDP	N-Ethyl-N'-(2-indanyl)-N'-phenyl-1,3-propanediamine	0.81
PDP	N-2-Indanyl-N-phenyl-1,3-propanediamine	0.66

[a]From Rutherford and Bishara [281], courtesy of the Journal of Pharmaceutical Sciences.
[b]P = synthetic precursor, and PDP = possible degradation product.
[c]Retention times were measured relative to aprindine (RRT = 1.00).
N.D. = compound not detected at the conditions used.

In recent years, several GC studies have been reported in the literature [285-289]. In 1973, Kelly et al. [285] developed methods for the estimation of mexiletine in plasma and urine based on spectrophotofluorometry and gas chromatography. Both methods involve extraction of the drug from alkaline plasma with ether. In the spectrophotofluorometric method the compound is reextracted into 0.05 N HCl and emission intensity determined at 300 nm with activation at 228 nm.

In the chromatographic procedure, sample preparation for GC analysis consisted of the following:

To plasma or urine (2.0 ml) in round-bottomed stoppered glass tubes are added 2 N NaOH (0.5 ml) and 0.5 ml of an aqueous solution containing about 2.5 µg/ml of the 2,4-methyl analog of mexiletine as the internal standard. Redistilled ether (5 ml) is added, the tubes are

TABLE 1.29

Degradation Studies: Percent Recovery of Aprindine Determined by GLC[a]

Treatment	Hours							
	0	2	6	12	24	48	72	144
Reflux in 1 N methanolic hydrochloric acid	100.6				100.4		99.5	99.0
Reflux in 1 N methanolic potassium hydroxide	102.0				102.5		101.1	101.5
Reflux in methanol	101.1		101.4	100.3	99.2			
Irradiation with UV light	99.7	57.4	27.0	21.0	15.6	7.6		
Heat at 110°C	100.0		100.5	100.5	99.7			
Solution in 5% dextrose in water at 50°C	100.5		100.9	100.4	99.8			
pH Profile at 50°C								
pH 1.0	101.0		100.5	99.4	100.4			
pH 4.0	101.7		101.5	101.5	100.9			
pH 7.0	101.5		102.0	101.2	100.5			

[a]From Rutherford and Bishara [281], courtesy of the Journal of Pharmaceutical Sciences.

shaken mechanically for 10 min and then centrifuged. The tubes are frozen, the ether decanted into tapered centrifuge tubes and butyric anhydride (3 μl) added to the ether. The organic solvent is evaporated to approximately 0.5 ml on a rotary vacuum evaporator at room temperature and the tubes are placed on a water bath at 60°C for 10 min. The residue is dissolved in 15 μl of ethanol using a Vortex mixer and 1- to 3-μl aliquots are taken for injection into the gas chromatograph.

In this study, Kelly et al. used a Hewlett-Packard model 5750 gas chromatograph equipped with a nitrogen-sensitive flame ionization detector (rubidium bromide as the alkali metal salt) and 4-ft by 1/4-in.-o.d. glass columns packed with 3% cyclohexane dimethanol succinate (HI-EFF 8BP) coated on 100-120 mesh Gas Chrom Q. With the specified GC conditions (helium carrier-gas flow rate, 70 ml/min; injector temperature, 240°C; column temperature, 220°C; detector temperature, 240°C), the retention times of the butyryl derivatives of mexiletine and the internal standard were 3.1 and 4.1 min, respectively. Capable of being estimated simultaneously, lidocaine had a retention time of 2.4 min, whereas the peak with a retention time of 5.5 min was postulated to be caffeine since it was observed to be much larger when blood samples were taken after consumption of coffee.

Using a calibration curve based on the ratio of the peak heights of mexiletine to internal standard plotted against concentration in the range 0.25 to 2.5 μg/ml, it was reported that the limit of detection was less than 10 ng/ml and that the recovery of drug from alkaline plasma was 85 to 90% of that obtained from corresponding aqueous standard solutions. It was further noted that routine analysis by spectrophotofluorometry and gas chromatography of duplicate plasma and urine samples containing mexiletine gave good agreement, with a correlation coefficient $r = 0.99$.

Willox and Singh [288] described a GC method for the determination of mexiletine in which a Hewlett-Packard model 5710A gas chromatograph equipped with an electron capture detector and 3-m by 4-mm glass columns packed with 1% cyclohexane dimethanol succinate on 100-120 mesh Gas Chrom Q was used.

Sample preparation consisted of adding 50 μl of 1 M KOH solution, 2 ml of diethyl ether, and 50 μl of the aqueous internal standard solution (alprenolol, 10 μg/ml) to 1 ml of plasma contained in a 15-ml glass-stoppered centrifuge tube. After a 2-min mixing period on a Vortex mixer, the tube was centrifuged and the diethyl ether layer aspirated; this aspirated ether phase was subsequently mixed for 2 min with 0.5 ml of 1 M HCl and then discarded. After washing the acid phase with 1 ml of fresh ether, 0.5 ml of 1.1 M KOH was added and the resulting basic aqueous phase was again extracted with 1.5 ml of diethyl ether. After drying the ether over potassium carbonate (20-30 mg) for 1 hr, the ether was transferred to a 1-ml "Reacti-vial," a boiling chip was added, and the ether boiled off using a heating block. To the residue, 25 µl each of benzene and heptafluorobutyric anhydride were added; the solvent and HFBA were removed with a stream of nitrogen after incubation at 90°C for 30 min. The final dry derivatives were dissolved in 30 to 50 µl of diethyl ether and 1 µl was injected into the GC column.

With the carrier-gas flow rate (5% methane in argon) set at 45 ml/min and the injector, column, and detector temperatures maintained at 250, 180, and 250°C, respectively, the retention times of the HFB derivatives of mexiletine and alprenolol were 3.3 and 5.2 min, respectively. Based on GC data, their data confirmed previous observations that mexiletine has a longer plasma half-life after oral ingestion than currently available antiarrhythmic drugs.

In 1977, Beckett and Chidomere [289] developed sensitive and specific GC methods for the analysis of mexiletine and its metabolites (see Table 1.30) in urine of man. In the identification and analysis of mexiletine and its metabolic products in man, Beckett and Chidomere noted that "the identity of the GC peaks was established by mass spectrometry. The hydroxylamine (V-1) was qualitatively identified and determined quantitatively after conversion to the more stable oxime (V-2). Selective extraction procedures, thin-layer chromatography, and derivatization with hexamethyldisilazane (HMDS) and trifluoroacetic anhydride (TFA) were used in the qualitative identification of the major metabolites (VI-IX), particularly in distinguishing the basic products VI and VII from their corresponding alcoholic products VIII and IX. The limit of detection of the GC method was 6 to 12 ng/ml for compounds I-IV, and 40 to 50 ng/ml for compounds V-2 to IX."

GC and mass spectral studies were performed with a Perkin-Elmer equipped with a flame ionization detector and a VG 12F Micromass spectrometer or an A.E.I. MS-9 mass spectrometer, respectively. All mass spectra with the GC-MS system were obtained at an ionization potential of 70 eV; the columns and conditions for GC and GC-MS investigations were as follows:

1. GC-MS study: column A, 1 m by 0.64 cm o.d., glass, with 3% OV-17 on 80-100 mesh Chromosorb W; temperature 150 to 160°C; helium carrier-gas flow rate 60 ml/min; column B, 1 m by 0.64 cm o.d., glass, with 7.5% Carbowax 20M on 80-100 mesh Chromosorb W; temperature 175 to 190°C; helium flow rate 100 ml/min.

2. GC study: column A, 2 m by 0.64 cm, glass, with 3% OV-17 on 80-100 mesh Gas Chrom Q; column temperature 160°C; nitrogen

TABLE 1.30
Structures of Mexiletine and Its Metabolites[a]

$$\text{R}_1 - \overset{\text{CH}_2\text{R}_2}{\underset{\text{CH}_3}{\bigcirc}} - \text{O} - \text{CH}_2 - \overset{\text{CH}_3}{\underset{|}{\text{C}}} - \text{R}_3$$

Ident no.	Substituents			Compound
	R_1	R_2	R_3	
I	H	H	HNH_2	Mexiletine
II	H	H	$HNHCH_3$	N-Methyl mexiletine
III	H	H	(=O)	1-(2',6'-Dimethyl)-phenoxypropan-2-one
IV	H	H	HOH	1-(2',6'-Dimethyl)-phenoxypropan-2-ol
V-1	H	H	HNHOH	N-Hydroxymexiletine
V-2	H	H	(=NOH)	1-(2',6'-Dimethyl)phenoxypropan-2-one oxime
VI	OH	H	HNH_2	1-(4'-Hydroxy,2',6'-dimethyl)-phenoxy-2-aminopropane
VII	H	OH	HNH_2	1-(2'-Hydroxymethyl,6'-methyl)-phenoxy-2-aminopropane
VIII	OH	H	HOH	1-(4'-Hydroxy,2',6'-dimethyl)-phenoxypropan-2-ol
IX	H	OH	HOH	1-(2'-Hydroxymethyl,6'-methyl)-phenoxypropan-2-ol

[a] Adapted from Beckett and Chidomere [289].

carrier-gas flow rate 60 ml/min; column B, 1 m by 0.64-cm, glass, with 7.5% Carbowax 20 M on 80-100 mesh Chromosorb W; this column was operated at two different temperatures: B_1, 175 to 185°C; B_2, 125 to 135°C; nitrogen carrier gas flow rate (same at both column temperatures) 100 ml/min.

Using the various derivatives and GC conditions discussed above, the retention times of mexiletine and its derivatives as well as recoveries from water and urine specimens (following prescribed extraction procedures) are listed in Table 1.31.

III. CORONARY VASODILATORS

In this section will be discussed organonitro and nonorganonitro vasodilators as well as several drugs that have relaxing effects on smooth muscle.

A. Organonitro Compounds

The predominant organonitro vasodilators are shown structurally in Figure 1.42. Some of these compounds have been examined by GC [28, 290-301] as early as 1964 and as recently as 1977. Because of their relaxing effect on various smooth muscles, the coronary blood vessels are so susceptible to this action that minute doses can cause an increase in coronary blood flow [1].

In 1964, Camera and Pravisani [290] separated by GC monoethylene glycol dinitrate, glycerol trinitrate, diethylene glycol dinitrate, triethylene glycol dinitrate, 1,2-dinitropropanediol, and 1,5-dinitropentanediol. In their investigation, the analyses were performed with an Erba Fractovap model C, equipped with a hot-wire thermal conductivity detector (250 mA current) and two stainless steel columns (35 and 50 cm long), both packed with 10% ethylene glycol succinate (EGS) on 40-60 mesh, acid-washed Celite C-22. As noted by the authors, operational conditions were as follows:

> The 35-cm column was operated at 145°C at a pressure of 0.3 kg/cm^2. The 50-cm column was operated at 150°C at a pressure of 0.44 kg/cm^2. Evaporator temperature was 160°C, flow rate (measured by soap bubble) was 50 ml/12 sec, and chart speed was 1 in./3 min. Helium was used as the carrier gas and kept at the highest velocity that did not cause turbulence. Sample size was 10 µl.

Whereas a column temperature of 145°C was employed for the separation of components with short retention times, such as EGDN and 1,2-dinitropropanediol, a column temperature of 150°C was preferred in

TABLE 1.31

Mexiletine and Its Metabolites: Retention Times and Recoveries from Water and Urine[a]

Compound	Retention times (mins)					Percent recovery	
	Column A			Column B$_1$	Column B$_2$	Conc. (μg/ml)	Found (mean)
	Normal	TFA	TMSi				
I	3.5	6.8		2.0	10.0	5–200	97.1 (U, W)
II	4.0	12.6		1.8	8.0	0.1–1.0	98–100 (U, W)
III	3.5			2.2	12.0	1.0–10	98–100 (U, W)
IV	3.5	2.2		3.0	18.0	1.0–10	98–100 (U, W)
V-1	9.0	decomp.	7.4	11.8			
V-2	9.0	decomp.	7.2	17.0 (anti)		10	100.8 (W)
						8	102.0 (W)

CORONARY VASODILATORS

			15.0 (syn)	2	99.1 (W)
				2-10	100.0 (U)
VI	18.0	11.4	14.0	25	90.0 (W)
				20	94.0 (U, W)
				5	90.0 (U)
				5	93.6 (W)
VII	14.0	10.0	12.0	21.0	100.0	40	87.5 (W)
				32	90.0 (U, W)
				8	88.0 (U)
				8	89.2 (W)
VIII	16.0	3.6	14.0		
IX	14.0	3.6	12.0	34.0	

[a] Adapted from Beckett and Chidomere [289].

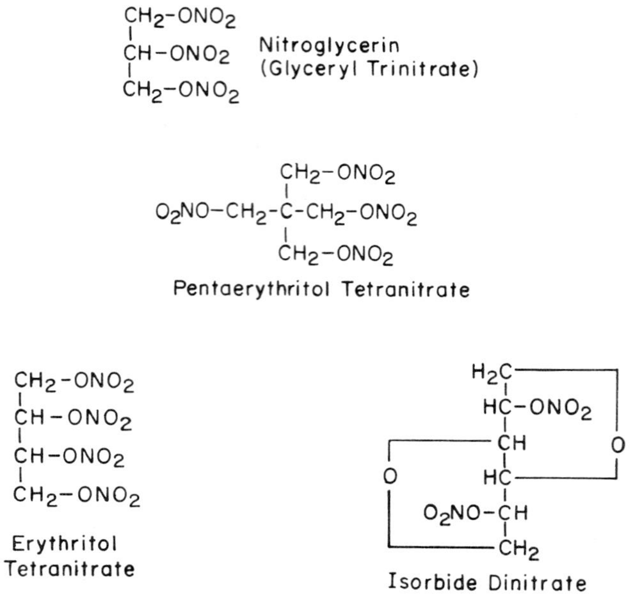

```
        CH2-ONO2
        |
        CH-ONO2    Nitroglycerin
        |          (Glyceryl Trinitrate)
        CH2-ONO2


                  CH2-ONO2
                  |
        O2NO-CH2-C-CH2-ONO2
                  |
                  CH2-ONO2
             Pentaerythritol Tetranitrate
```

```
    CH2-ONO2                      H2C────────┐
    |                             |          │
    CH-ONO2                       HC-ONO2    │
    |                      ┌──────CH         O
    CH-ONO2                │      |          │
    |                      O      HC─────────┘
    CH2-ONO2               │      |
                           │  O2NO-CH
      Erythritol           │      |
      Tetranitrate         └──────CH2
                              Isorbide Dinitrate
```

Figure 1.42. Structures of common organonitro vasodilators.

order to elute TEGN in a more reasonable retention time, as shown in Figure 1.43. In Table 1.32, calibration data (relative to DEGN) are shown, where CF of DEGN is calculated versus 1,5-dinitropentanediol (P5). Furthermore, based on the DEGN peak, the number of theoretical plates determined for the 35-cm and 50-cm columns were 166 and 237, respectively.

Fossel [291] resolved and determined quantitatively glycerol trinitrate and chloroglycerol dinitrate in pharmaceutical preparations from ethanol solution using an Aerograph A-90P gas chromatograph equipped with a thermal conductivity detector and a 7.5-ft by 1/4-in. aluminum column packed with 3% SE-30 coated on 50-60 mesh Anakrom AB. Using the specified GC conditions (column temperature, 100 and 130°C for glycerol trinitrate and chloroglycerol dinitrate, respectively; detector temperature, 192°C; injector temperature, 148°C; filament current, 230 mA; helium carrier-gas flow rate, 37.5 ml/min), sample preparation was as follows: "Tablets totalling 60 mg of active ingredient were pulverized and suspended in 20 ml of absolute ethanol. The tightly stoppered mixtures were shaken intermittently for 3 hr, then filtered through rapid-flow filter paper. The concentration was determined by comparison of the signal from a 40-μl

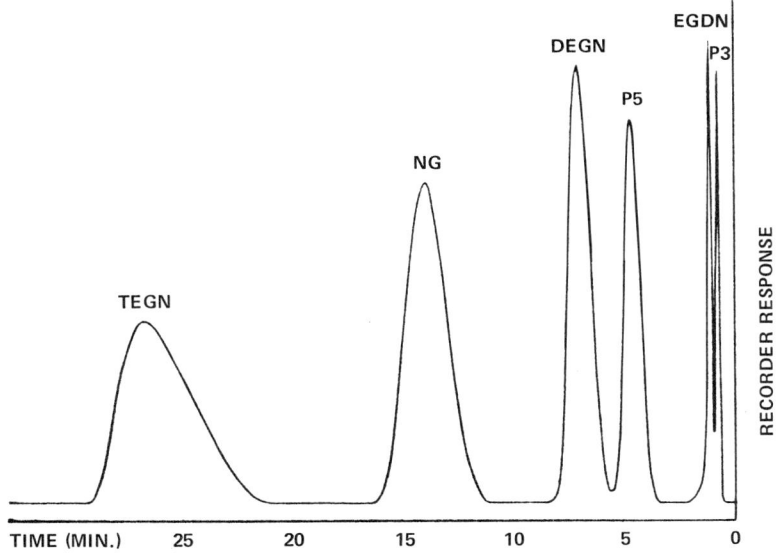

Figure 1.43. Chromatogram of nitric esters at 150°C. P3 = 1,2-dinitropropanediol, EGDN = ethylene glycol dinitrate, P5 = 1,5-dinitropentanediol, DEGN = diethylene glycol dinitrate, NG = glycerol trinitrate, TEGN = triethylene glycol dinitrate. From Camera and Pravisani [290], courtesy of Analytical Chemistry.

sample with the calibration curve." This calibration curve was prepared from the response of the detector to 30, 40, and 50 μl of a standard solution containing 0.50 g of a 10% nitroglycerine in lactose mixture dissolved in 16.66 ml of absolute ethanol.

In 1966, Williams et al. [292] determined by GC traces of ethylene glycol dinitrate and glycerol trinitrate in blood and urine, devising a procedure using the electron capture detector which could easily detect less than 0.04 ng of EGDN and 1.0 ng of glycerol trinitrate.

Sample preparation for the determination of EGDN in heparinized blood or in urine consisted of transferring a measured volume (about 0.5 ml) of the sample to a 10-ml stoppered glass tube followed by the addition of 1 ml of water and 0.3 g of sodium chloride, which was dissolved by shaking the tube. As noted by Williams et al., the solution so obtained was thoroughly shaken with 2 ml of n-hexane and the organic extract was then used directly for chromatography after centrifuging. The GC separation was carried out with an instrument equipped with an electron capture detector (tritium

TABLE 1.32

Calibration Data for Nitric Esters[a]

Compound	RRT[b]		CF[c]	
	145°C	150°C	145°C	150°C
EGDN	0.17	0.18	0.914	0.915
NG	1.95	1.96	1.319	1.476
P3	0.12	0.12	0.935	0.944
P5	0.66	0.66	0.931	0.926
DEGN	1.00	1.00	1.000	1.000
TEGN	3.98	3.78	1.083	1.115

[a] Adapted from Camera and Pravisani [290].
[b] RRT = relative retention time.
[c] CF = calibration factor (weight percent basis).

source) and a 2-ft by 1/4-in. metal column packed with 10% E-301 (silicone elastomer) coated on Embacel as solid stationary phase. For the elution and detection of EGDN, the GC instrument was operated in the following manner: detector potential, 30 V; nitrogen carrier-gas flow rate, 150 ml/min; column temperature, 140°C; injector temperature, 160°C; detector temperature, about 140°C. Analyses of blood and urine samples obtained from five plant operators yielded the following results: (1) blood specimens: 0.04, 0.01, 0.07, 0.06, and 0.05 ppm EGDN; (2) corresponding urine samples contained 0.02, 0.03, 0.02, 0.04, and 0.08 ppm EGDN, respectively. Whereas these samples were taken from a peripheral vein within a few minutes of the operator leaving his work (all samples were examined within 30 min after being taken), when the same operators were reexamined after 16 hr away from explosives manufacture, EGDN was no longer detectable in either their blood or their urine.

Sherber et al. [293] summarized their initial studies of the analysis of isosorbide dinitrate as follows:

> Isosorbide dinitrate (ISDN) administered to man and animals presents special difficulties in determination of blood levels because of the low dosage required for pharmacological effectiveness. The sensitivity of flame ionization or electron capture detection after GC partition is uniquely suitable to investigation of the metabolism of the stated compound.

Whole blood is extracted with ethyl acetate in the ratio of 1:10. The organic solvent is dried over anhydrous sodium sulfate and reduced to dryness at 40°C in vacuo. The residue after extraction of 10 ml of blood is redissolved in 0.5 ml ethyl acetate and 4 μl injected into the GC column under either of the following conditions:

Six-foot column packing of 3% XE-60 on Gas Chrom Q; oven temperature, 150°C; flash heater, 160°C; detector, 180°C; nitrogen carrier, 55 ml/min; or 4-ft column packing of 3.8% SE-30 on Gas Chrom P; oven temperature, 110°C; flash heater, 130°C; detector, 190°C; nitrogen carrier, 55 ml/min.

Meta-dinitrobenzene was used as internal standard.

As little as 1×10^{-2} μg of ISDN in blood may be determined in this manner.

Preliminary studies with electron capture detection have shown that with this method (same conditions) it is possible to detect as little as 1×10^{-6} μg of ISDN standard solutions. Detector overload with contaminants in biological extracts, however, precludes this form of detection without extensive purification.

ISDN levels 90 sec after intravenous administration has been found by this manner to average 14%, thus suggesting extremely rapid clearing of this compound from the systemic circulation.

In 1970, Trowell [294] analyzed by GC nitrated derivatives of glycerol in aged double-base propellants using a F&M model 5754B gas chromatograph equipped with dual flame ionization detectors and dual columns, 6 ft by 1/8 in., packed with a 2.5% OV-17/2.5% QF-1 liquid stationary phase mixture coated on 60-80 mesh Gas Chrom Q. The conditions maintained, which yielded retention times of approximately 7.61, 11.67, 13.12, 14.57, 16.12, 17.00, 17.80, 19.50, and 25.15 min for disilylated mononitroglycerol, monosilylated 1,2-dinitroglycerol, disilylated resorcinol, monosilylated 1,3-dinitroglycerol, triacetin, nitroglycerine (glycerol trinitrate), dimethylphthalate, dimethylsebacate, and 2-nitrophenylamine, respectively, were column temperature, programmed from 70 to 230°C at 10°C/min; injector temperature, 250°C; detector temperature, 250°C; helium carrier-gas flow rate, 65 ml/min; hydrogen flow rate, 28 ml/min; air flow rate, 500 ml/min; sample size, 0.004 ml.

For this particular analysis of double-base propellants, samples of propellant extracts were obtained by extracting 1 to 2 g of propellant with methylene chloride or diethyl ether. The extract volume was then reduced to approximately 2 ml and reacted with 1 ml of bis-(trimethylsilyl)-acetamide (BSA) catalyzed with 1% trimethylchlorosilane (TMCS). Reaction of the BSA with the resorcinol and nitroglycerine derivatives was essentially instantaneous at room temperature. To the reacted sample sufficient internal standard (dimethyl phthalate) was added to yield a final concentration of 1 mg/ml when diluted to 25 ml with dichloroethane.

Sherber et al. [295] studied by GC the rapid clearance of ISDN from rabbit blood, using the instrument and conditions previously described in 1969 [293]. With the 3% XE-60 column, the retention times of meta-dinitrobenzene (internal standard) and ISDN were approximately 6.57 and 17.45 min, respectively. Their GC data for ISDN demonstrated that 86% of this drug, administered intravenously, is cleared from rabbit blood within 90 sec.

Davidson et al. [297] presented a GC method for the separation and quantitation of submicrograms of pentaerythritol tetranitrate and other organic nitrate esters of common therapeutic use. As described, the procedure for PETN provides a routine method for general analytical use with detection of micro- and submicrogram quantities with the flame ionization detector and with the electron capture detector to determine nano- and subnanogram quantities, adequate sensitivity for application to detection of PETN simultaneously with the lesser nitrate esters and their alkyl alcohol as trifluoroacetyl derivatives in biological samples. Separation of these compounds was accomplished using a Varian Aerograph model 2100-20 gas chromatograph equipped with a hydrogen flame ionization (FID) and a tritium (250 mCi) electron capture (ECD) detector and two U-shaped glass columns: column A, 5.5 ft by 2 mm i.d., packed with 1% SE-30 coated on 100-120 mesh Chromosorb P; column B, 6 ft by 2 mm i.d., packed with 1% Dexsil 300 on 100-120 mesh Chromosorb W. The GC conditions found most suitable for the separation of these compounds were as follows:

1. Flame ionization detector
    a. Injector temperature, 200°C
    b. Detector temperature, 200°C
    c. Column temperature, programmed from 65 at 10°C/min
    d. Nitrogen carrier-gas flow rate, 20 ml/min
    e. Hydrogen flow rate, 20 ml/min
    f. Air flow rate, 300 ml/min
2. Electron capture detector
    a. Nitrogen carrier-gas flow rate, 75 ml/min
    b. Other conditions as noted above for FID detection

With the flame ionization detector, the retention times, elution temperatures, and response values of the nitrate esters are shown in Table 1.33 using both column systems.

TABLE 1.33

Retention Times, Elution Temperatures, and Response Values of Nitrate Esters[a]

Compound	Ret. time (min)		Elution temp. (°C)		Response value[c]	
	SE-30	Dexsil	SE-30	Dexsil	SE-30	Dexsil
PE tetra-TFA[b]	1.6	2.5	83	90	1305	1265
PE mononitrate, tri-TFA	2.8	4.0	96	106	855	835
PE dinitrate, di-TFA	4.4	5.7	111	124	395	395
PE trinitrate, mono-TFA	6.1	7.6	128	144	275	235
PE tetranitrate	7.8	9.6	146	165	185	195
Isosorbide dinitrate	6.0	7.8	126	146		
Erythritol tetranitrate	6.3	8.2	130	150		
Mannitol hexanitrate	10.1	11.6	170	185		

[a] Adapted from Davidson et al. [297].
[b] PE = pentaerythritol.
[c] Calculated as underivatized compound, $mm^2/\mu g$.

On the other hand, the retention times and response values (peak area/ng) using both columns and the electron capture detector at the column temperatures indicated are given in Table 1.34. From the chromatographic data obtained, it was estimated that the minimal detectable quantities by the procedure for PE (tetra-TFA) and PE tetranitrate were 250 pg and 2 ng, respectively.

In 1972, Rosseel and Bogaert [298] developed a GC procedure for assay of mixtures of glycerol trinitrate with its nitrated metabolites, and of mixtures of isosorbide dinitrate and its two mononitrates as well as isomannide dinitrate (a stereoisomer of ISDN) and its mononitrate. Using a Packard series 7400 gas chromatograph equipped with a flame ionization detector, a tritium (150-mCi) electron capture detector, and 6-ft by 2-mm-i.d. glass columns packed with either 3% XE-60 or 3.5% QF-1 on 60-80 mesh Gas Chrom Q, the separation were achieved with the following conditions: injector temperature, 160°C; detector temperature, 200°C; column temperature, the QF-1 at 110°C and the XE-60 at 150°C for FID, and the QF-1 at 120°C and the XE-60 at 150°C for ECD; nitrogen carrier-gas flow rate, 25 ml/min; for FID, the hydrogen and air flow rates maintained at 18 and 370 ml/min, respectively.

Using the above GC operating conditions, Table 1.35 lists the relative retention times obtained with the flame ionization detector for both columns and compares the minimum amounts of different nitrates that can be determined with each detector.

In a subsequent study, Rosseel and Bogaert [299] described a procedure for the identification and quantitative determination of nitroglycerin and isosorbide dinitrate in plasma after administration of therapeutic doses in man. Prior to GC analysis, the extraction procedure used to remove the drugs from plasma consisted of the following:

Five milliliters of plasma and 5 ml of ethyl acetate were shaken for 5 min in glass-stoppered tubes; after centrifugation for 10 min at 4000 rpm, the organic phase was transferred over an activated charcoal filter to a conical tube by means of a Pasteur pipette, avoiding the lipoprotein interface. The filter was rinsed before use with ethyl acetate and covered with sodium sulfate; afterward it was rinsed with 0.5 ml of ethyl acetate. The organic phase was then evaporated under nitrogen to near dryness at room temperature. The plasma was extracted two more times. The yellow evaporation residue from the three extractions was dissolved in 0.5 ml of ethyl acetate, filtered again through a filter, reevaporated to dryness, and immediately dissolved in 10 μl of benzene to prevent evaporation of nitroglycerin. The benzene solution (1.6 μl) was injected into the gas chromatograph. The injection was done as soon as possible after the extraction procedure; in between the stoppered samples were stored at 180°C to minimize evaporation of the benzene.

TABLE 1.34

Retention Times and Response Values of PE Nitrates with ECD[a]

Compound	Ret. time (min)					Response value[b]			
	SE-30		Dexsil			SE-30		Dexsil	
	75°C	110°C	100°C	125°C		75°C	110°C	100°C	125°C
PE tetra-TFA	0.47	0.16	0.47	0.12		66.0		26.3	
PE mononitrate, tri-TFA	0.71	0.24	1.24	0.35		54.0		24.3	
PE dinitrate, di-TFA	4.71	0.63	3.76	0.94		28.5	18.0	13.0	6.5
PE trinitrate, mono-TFA		0.94		2.82			41.5		15.5
PE tetranitrate		4.55		8.82			24.5		8.5

[a] Adapted from Davidson et al. [297].
[b] Calculated as undervatized compound, mm^2/ng.

TABLE 1.35

Relative Retention Times and Minimum Detection Limits of Different Nitrates Using Both Columns and Detectors[a]

Nitrate	Rel. ret. time (FID)		Detection limits	
	QF-1	XE-60	FID (μg)	ECD (ng)
Glyceryl trinitrate	0.415	0.548	5	1
Glyceryl 1,3-dinitrate	0.198	0.641	1	10
Glyceryl 1,2-dinitrate	0.184	0.560	1	10
Glyceryl 1-mononitrate	0.075	0.237	1	10
Isosorbide dinitrate	1.000[b]	1.000	0.5	8
Isosorbide 5-mononitrate	0.420	1.024	1	2
Isosorbide 2-mononitrate	0.208	0.269	0.5	2
Isomannide dinitrate	1.420	1.580	1	10
Isomannide mononitrate	0.360	0.500	0.5	10

[a] Adapted from Rosseel and Bogaert [298].
[b] RT at 110°C on QF-1 column = 31.7 min.

To determine NG quantitatively, ISDN was added to the plasma as internal standard prior to solvent extraction. On the other hand, isoidide dinitrate was used as internal standard when assaying isosorbide dinitrate. Using calibration curves based on peak area measurements, extracts were analyzed with a Packard series 7400 gas chromatograph equipped with a tritium electron capture detector (150 mCi) and 1.83-m by 2-mm-i.d. glass columns packed with 3.5% QF-1 on 60-80 mesh Gas Chrom Q and operated isothermally at 117 and 120°C for ISDN and NG determinations, respectively; the other operating parameters being injector temperature, 160°C; detector temperature, 180°C; nitrogen carrier-gas flow rate, 30 ml/min; pulse voltage, 25 V.

As noted by Rosseel and Bogaert, the recoveries for 25 ng of NG and 15 ng of ISDN added to blank plasma were 97.3 ± 6.1% and 96.8 ± 3.2%, respectively, using this extraction technique.

Using the GC conditions listed above, the lower limit of detection was about 0.5 ng/ml for NG and somewhat lower for ISDN. The relative retention time for NG as compared to ISDN was 0.443 (see Fig. 1.44A), whereas the retention times of 2-isosorbide mononitrate, 5-isosorbide

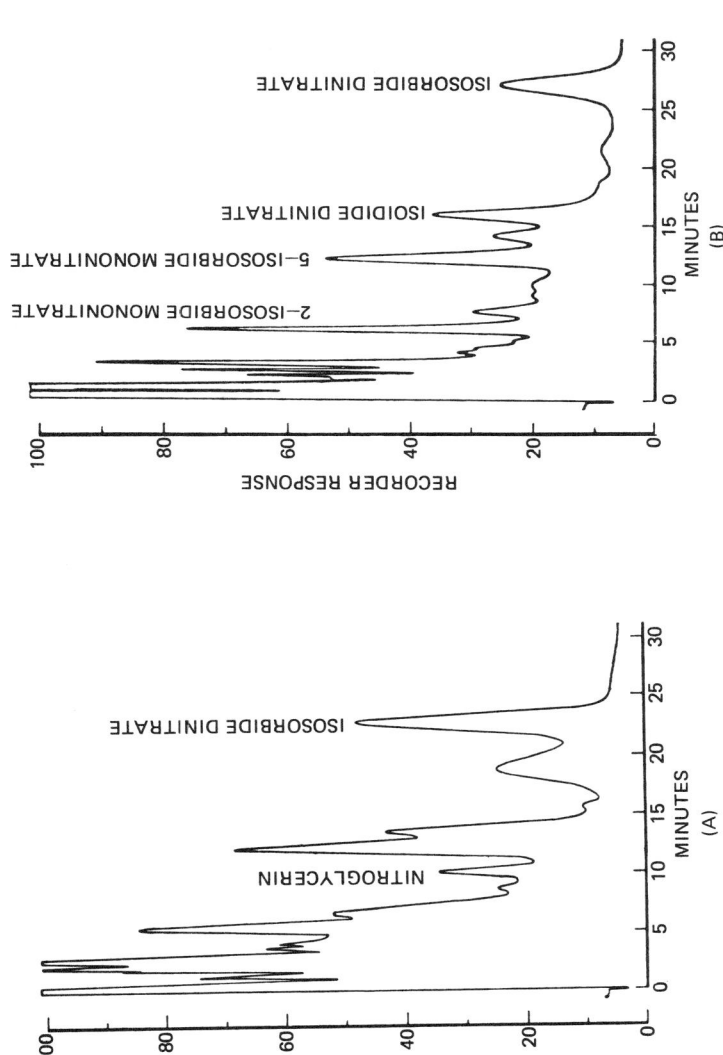

Figure 1.44. Gas chromatograms of extracted human plasma. A. isosorbide (15 ng) added to 5 ml of plasma after sublingual administration of NG, 800 μg. B. isoidide dinitrate (5 ng) added to 5 ml of plasma after oral administration of 5 mg of ISDN. Adapted from Rosseel and Bogaert [299].

mononitrate, and isosorbide dinitrate relative to isoidide dinitrate (internal standard) were 0.374, 0.760, and 1.705, respectively (see Fig. 1.44B).

Malbica et al. [300] described a GC method for the determination of ISDN using electron capture detection that was expedient, sensitive, and reproducible for routinely handling large number of samples. ISDN was extracted from plasma prior to GC analysis as indicated below:

> Five-milliliter aliquots of benzene were added to a 15-ml graduated conical centrifuge tube containing 1.0 ml of plasma spiked with 10 ng of isoidide dinitrate as an internal standard. The tube was mixed on a Vortex for 1 min and centrifuged at 2000 rpm to separate the phases. Then the benzene phase was carefully removed to another 15-ml centrifuge tube. A 0.5-g portion of benzene-washed sodium sulfate and three benzene-washed charcoal-treated paper disks were added to the benzene extract.
>
> The tube and its contents were again vortexed for 15 sec and centrifuged as previously described. As much of the benzene layer as possible was carefully removed to another centrifuge tube and dried completely under a nitrogen stream (using an in-line activated silica gel dessicant filter). To each residue was added 100 μl of ethyl acetate just prior to injection.

The residues from the benzene extracts were analyzed with a Hewlett-Packard HP 7620A gas chromatograph equipped with a ^{63}Ni electron capture detector and a 120-cm by 4-mm-i.d. glass column packed with 3% QF-1 on 100-120 mesh Gas Chrom Q. To obtain retention times of 2.0 and 3.0 min for isoidide dinitrate and ISDN, respectively, the following GC conditions were maintained: injector temperature, 210°C; column temperature, 150°C; detector temperature, 175°C; detector pulse interval, 150 μsec; argon with 5% methane carrier-gas flow rate, 95 ml/min.

Having a reported lower limit of detection of 0.5 ng/ml, Malbica et al. noted that:

1. The overall coefficient of variation of the procedure in the 1- to 75-ng/ml range was less than 20% except in the 1- to 10-ng/ml range where, as expected, it sometimes increased with decreasing concentration.

2. A plot of the response ratio versus concentration showed that the described procedure was reproducible from day to day and that linearity was established throughout the 0- to 75-ng/ml range.

3. The ISDN human plasma levels following a 5-mg dose of chewable ISDN were highest after 15 min after administration in all four subjects who participated in the program. No ISDN levels were

detectable at 120 min or more after administration. The average human plasma levels of ISDN after administration of a 5-mg chewable tablet at sampling times of 15, 30, and 60 min were 4.3 ± 1.3, 2.1 ± 0.6, and 0.7 ± 0.4 ng/ml, respectively.

4. The overall recovery of ^{14}C-ISDN in the 2.2- to 90-ng/ml concentration range was independent of concentration; the average recovery at the 2.2, 4.5, and 90.0 levels (ng/ml) being $80.1 \pm 1.2\%$, $75.0 \pm 1.3\%$, and $75.8 \pm 0.3\%$, respectively.

In 1977, Chin et al. [301] developed a GC assay method for the determination of ISDN and two of its metabolites (ISDN 2-mononitrate and ISDN 5-mononitrate) in plasma. The extraction procedure used for this investigation consisted of the following steps:

To a 3-ml sample of dog plasma or to 4 ml of human plasma in a 50-ml centrifuge tube, equipped with a polypropylene stopper, was added 2 ml of 1 N NaOH or 1 ml of 2 N NaOH, respectively. Then 30 ml of ether was added, and the tube was stoppered and shaken mechanically at low speed for 20 min. It was centrifuged at 1500 rpm for 5 min, and the aqueous layer was discarded. Then 0.5 g of anhydrous magnesium sulfate was added, and the mixture was shaken and centrifuged.

A 25-ml aliquot of the ether layer was transferred to a 30-ml centrifuge tube and evaporated to dryness under a gentle stream of nitrogen with the water bath held below 30°C. The residue was redissolved in 1.0 ml of ethyl acetate. An aliquot (1 to 3 μl) of this solution was injected and compared with the calibration curve.

The separation of ISDN and its two metabolites was performed with a Microtek MT-220 or a Varian model 2100-20 gas chromatograph equipped with a ^{63}Ni electron capture detector and a 1.83-m by 2-mm-i.d. silanized glass column packed with 30% SE-30 on 60-80 mesh Gas Chrom Q. The unusually heavy liquid-phase loading was necessary to eliminate irreversible adsorption on the solid support. Maintaining recommended GC conditions (injector temperature, 190°C; column temperature, 165°C; detector temperature, 250°C; carrier-gas (not specified) flow rate, about 60 ml/min; detector operation, pulse mode with a width of 5 μsec at 44 V and a pulse interval of 220 μsec), the retention times of ISDN 2-mononitrate, ISDN 5-mononitrate, and ISDN were approximately 1.79, 2.74, and 4.00 min, respectively.

With the response of the EC detector to ISDN and its two metabolites being linear with concentration over the 50- to 1000-ng/ml range, the recoveries of ISDN, ISDN 2-MN, and ISDN 5-MN from spiked dog plasma were 83, 59, and 71%, respectively; from human plasma their respective values were 67, 65, and 59%.

With regard to in vivo studies, Chin et al. summarized their findings as follows:

> The average plasma (ISDN, ISDN 2-MN, ISDN 5-MN) levels in four dogs are shown in Figure [1.45A]. The results are in qualitative agreement with the data obtained in a ^{14}C-labeled study [302]. There were very low and erratic blood levels of ISDN, consistently higher levels of ISDN 2-MN, and much higher and prevalent levels of ISDN 5-MN. Very rapid absorption of ISDN took place, since ISDN levels were detected at 5 min postadministration.
> The average plasma levels of ISDN, ISDN 2-MN, and ISDN 5-MN in two human volunteers are shown in Figure [1.45B]. Significant ISDN levels were detected at 10, 20, and 30 min and up to 1 hr postadministration. The two metabolites reached a maximum at 30 min, and the ISDN 5-MN levels were approximately twice the ISDN 2-MN levels.

B. Nonorganonitro Compounds

In addition to papaverine (see Chapter 1, Volume 5), whose main pharmacologic effect is smooth muscle relaxation (its vasodilator properties being well documented), the xanthines, particularly theophylline, which tend to dilate smooth muscles and cause increased coronary blood flow (see Chapter 1, Volume 4), ethyl alcohol, which has the undeserved reputation of being a coronary vasodilator [1] (see Chapter 2, Volume 1), MAO inhibitors, which have been advocated by some investigators for the management of angina [1] (see Chapter 2, Volume 3), dipyridamole [28], adrenergic vasodilators such as isoproterenol and nylidrin [28,339], prenylamine [59], cyclandelate [28,58,59], as well as other muscle relaxants such as orphenadrine [59], phenyramidol [59], chlorzoxazone [59], and those discussed in Chapter 2, Volume 2, more recent compounds possessing similar therapeutic properties have appeared in the literature and are amenable to GC analysis.

Fanelli and Frigerio [303] described a sensitive and specific method for the quantitative determination of piribedil in brain tissue and plasma.

Piribedil
[1-(3,4-Methylenedioxybenzyl)-4-(2-pyrimidinyl)piperazine]

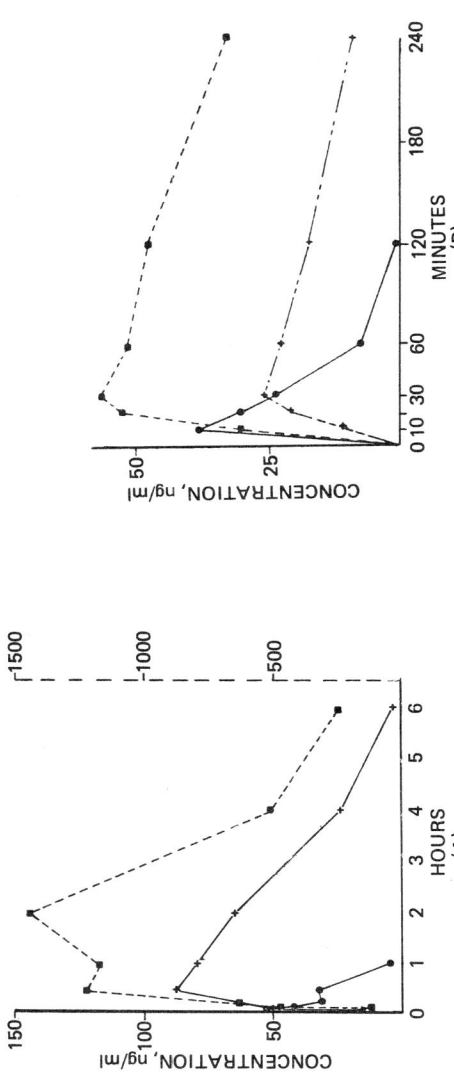

Figure 1.45. Plasma levels of ISDN, ISDN 2-MN, and ISDN 5-MN versus time. A. Average plasma levels of ISDN (●), ISDN 2-MN (+), and ISDN 5-MN (■, right-hand scale) in four beagle dogs after an oral administration of 40 mg of ISDN. B. Average plasma levels of ISDN (●), ISDN 2-MN (+), and ISDN 5-MN (■) in two human volunteers after sublingual administration of 10 mg of ISDN. Adapted from Chin et al. [301].

Piribedil, in addition to its known vasodilator activity [304, 305] has been shown to possess the capacity to stimulate dopaminergic receptors [306-308].

Following prescribed procedures for the extraction of piribedil from plasma and brain tissue, piribedil is detected by GC using a flame ionization detector or GC-MS (mass fragmentography); the limits of detection being 250 (GC) and 10 (GC-MS) ng/ml or ng/g of piribedil present in biological samples.

For GC studies, separations were performed with a Carlo Erba Fractovap model G1 equipped with a flame ionization detector and a 2-m glass column packed with 3% OV-17 coated on 60-80 mesh Gas Chrom Q. Other GC conditions were nitrogen carrier-gas flow rate, 30 ml/min; injector temperature, 270°C; column temperature, 240°C.

For GC-MS studies, a LKB model 9000 equipped with an alternating voltage alternator was used. As noted, the GC conditions were as given above, except that helium at a flow rate of 25 ml/min was used as the carrier gas. The MS was operated as follows: molecular separator temperature, 280°C; ion source temperature, 290°C; trap current, 60 μA; electron energy, 30 eV; accelerating voltage, 3.5 kV; filters, 20 Hz; AVA focused alternately on the ions at m/e 298 for piribedil and at m/e 321 for 2-N-benzylamino-5-chlorobenzophenone (BACB) (internal standard).

Using the above chromatographic conditions, the retention time of piribedil relative to the internal standard was 0.64. On the other hand, the recovery of piribedil obtained by adding varying amounts (0.01 to 50.0 μg/ml or μg/g) to rat plasma and brain tissue and by utilizing the flame ionization detector or the mass fragmentographic technique is given below:

	Recovery (%)	
	FID	GC-MS-MF
Plasma	97.1 ± 0.7	95.6 ± 1.3
Brain tissue	80.4 ± 3.1	79.6 ± 1.4
Range, μg/ml or μg/g	1 to 50	0.01 to 0.10

Higuchi et al. [309] developed a highly sensitive method for the quantitative determination of 2,6-dimethyl-4-(3-nitrophenyl)-1,4-dihydropyridine-3,5-dicarboxylic acid 3-[2-(N-benzyl-N-methylamino)]-ethyl ester 5-methyl ester (YC-93) in plasma by electron capture gas chromatography. Introduced as a new potent vasodilator with preferential effect on the cerebral circulation, after extraction, YC-93 was oxidized to a pyridine analog with nitrous acid prior to its GC analysis. Sensitive to

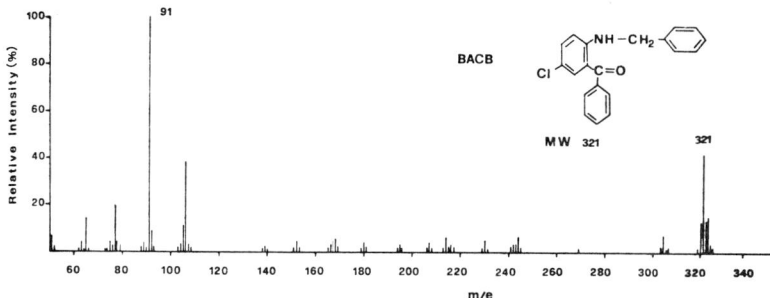

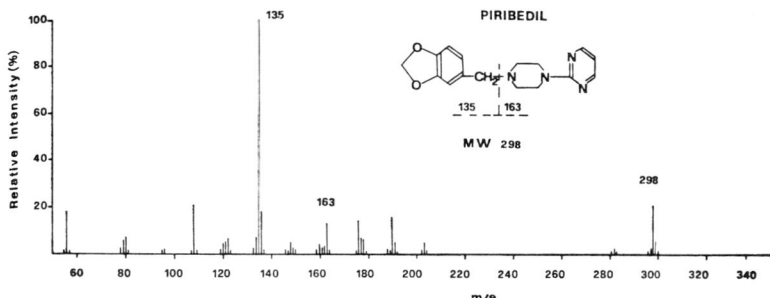

YC-93

{2,6-Dimethyl-4-(3-nitrophenyl)-1,4-dihydropyridine-3,5-dicarboxylic acid 3-[2-(N-benzyl-N-methylamino)]-ethyl ester 5-methyl ester}

YC-93 →[HNO₂, 45°C, 1hr]→ Pyridine Analog

2 to 3 ng/ml, which is sufficient to determine plasma concentrations of YC-93 after oral administration of clinical doses to humans, and using 2,6-dimethyl-4-dihydropyridine-3,5-dicarboxylic acid 3-[3-(N-benzyl-N-methylamino)]-propyl ester 5-isopropyl ester as internal standard which, in turn, undergoes oxidation with nitrous acid to its pyridine analog, qualitative and quantitative results were obtained with a Hewlett-Packard model 5700A gas chromatograph equipped with a ^{63}Ni electron capture detector and a 90-cm by 1.8-mm-i.d. glass column packed with 3% OV-1 on 80-100 mesh Chromosorb W. To obtain retention times of 1.4, 2.2, 3.3, and 4.4 min, respectively, for YC-93, internal standard, and the corresponding pyridine analogs, the following conditions were used: injector temperature, 300°C; column temperature, 260°C; detector temperature, 300°C; argon-methane (95:5) carrier-gas flow rate, 40 ml/min. Based on a standard curve prepared by plotting peak height ratios of the pyridine analogs of YC-93 and internal standard against YC-93 concentration, the average recoveries of ^{14}C-labeled YC-93 added to plasma at two concentration levels, 10 and 50 ng/ml, were 78.8 ± 1.3% and 89.7 ± 2.1%, respectively.

In their investigation, the effects of $NaNO_2$ concentration, HCl concentration, reaction time, and reaction temperature on the oxidation of dihydropyridines to pyridines were studied. Their data revealed that oxidation was effected most satisfactorily by incubating the sample with 0.3 ml of a 1% $NaNO_2$ solution at 45°C for 1 hr in 4 ml of 0.05 N HCl. Using a Hitachi RMU-7 mass spectrometer and direct-probe insertion of the samples, it was shown that the YC-93 pyridine analog had a parent peak at m/e 477, which is two mass units less than the parent compound, indicating the oxidation of the 1,4-dihydropyridine ring to the pyridine ring. In like manner, the same situation was observed with the similarly structured internal standard.

Li and Cervoni [339] described a method in 1976 for the detection of nanograms of nylidrin in human urine. Used in the treatment of some peripheral vascular disorders, sample preparation for GC analysis consisted of the following:

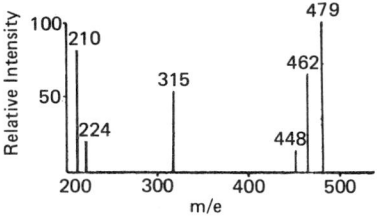

Mass Spectrum of YC-93

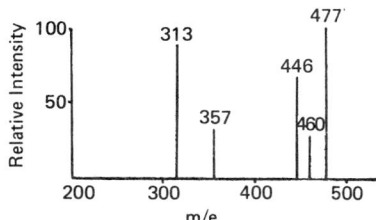

Mass Spectrum of YC-93
Pyridine Analog

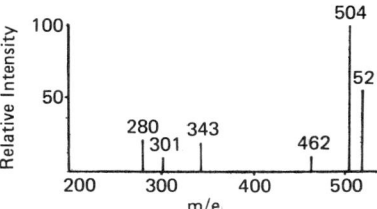

Mass Spectrum of Internal Standard

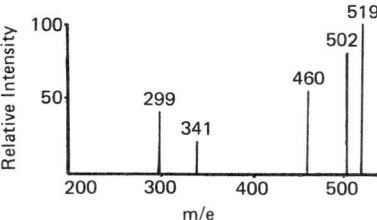

Mass Spectrum of Internal Standard
Pyridine Analog

After adjustment of the urine to pH 5.0 with acetic acid, the volume was measured. A 5.0-ml aliquot was then pipetted into a 100-ml glass-stoppered bottle, and 5 ml of 0.1 M acetate buffer solution (pH 5.0) containing 5000 units of β-glucuronase was added. The samples were then kept in a Dubnoff metabolic shaking incubator at 37°C for 18 hr in the presence of air.

The hydrolyzed urine mixture was saturated with sodium bicarbonate and extracted three times with 25 ml of spectral-grade chloroform. The chloroform extracts were pooled and dried over anhydrous sodium sulfate and condensed to a small volume. The drug was then back-extracted two times with 2.5 ml of 0.1 N HCl.

A 4.0-ml aliquot of the pooled acid extract was transferred to a glass-stoppered conical tube, and the acid was evaporated to dryness in a freeze-drying unit. The side of the tube was washed with a small volume of methanol, and the methanol solution was evaporated to complete dryness under a stream of dry nitrogen for derivatization.

The trimethylsilyl (TMSi) derivative of nylidrin was prepared by adding 30 μl of bis(trimethylsilyl)trifluoroacetamide and 20 μl of a

0.2% chloroform solution of docosane (internal standard) into conical tubes containing the dried acid extracts. The reactants were then thoroughly mixed using a vortex agitator. Silylation was carried out in an oil bath at 55 to 60°C for 1 hr. Five microliters of the reaction mixture was injected directly into the chromatograph for analysis.

Li and Cervoni performed their separations with a Perkin-Elmer model 900 gas chromatograph equipped with a flame ionization detector and a 1.8-m by 0.63-cm-o.d. glass column packed with 0.2% OV-1 coated on

Nylidrin

[1-(p-Hydroxyphenyl)-2-(1'-methyl-3'-phenylpropylamino)-1-propanol]

80-100 mesh, DMCS-treated Corning GLC-110 glass beads. To obtain retention times of approximately 4.7 and 11.7 min for docosane and the di-TMSi derivative of nylidrin, respectively, the following operating conditions were maintained: injector temperature, 230°C; column temperature, initially 170°C and then programmed at a rate of 0.5°C/min; detector tempreature, 230°C; helium carrier-gas flow rate, 50 ml/min. Using integrated CG-MS in the chemical ionization mode, the peak at m/e 444 was postulated to be the M+1 ion of di-TMSi nylidrin, the molecular weight of which is 443, with silylation taking place at the phenolic and β-hydroxyl groups (the sterically hindered nitrogen remaining underivatized).

Using standard curves prepared by plotting the relative area of the TMSi peaks versus nylidrin concentration, the lower limit of detection of urinary nylidrin as determined by eight experiments was about 68 ng/ml of urine whereas the average recovery (n = 6) of nylidrin added to urine over the 178- to 1068-ng/ml concentration range was 67 ± 4%.

In 1975, Mardente and De Marchi [310] described a specific, rapid, and sensitive GC method for purity control of hexadiphane (a papaverine-like compound with weak anticholinergic effects that is employed as an antispasmodic) and its determination in pharmaceutical preparations. Using solvent extraction and diphenylpyraline as internal standard, the

Hexadiphane
(1,1-Diphenyl-3-hexamethyleneiminopropane)

preparations examined included a liquid form for oral use, a combination with oxazepam hemisuccinate in hard gelatin capsules, and a combination with digestive enzymes and dimethylpolysiloxane.

The analyses were performed with a Carlo Erba Fractovap model D equipped with a flame ionization detector and a 2-m by 2-mm-i.d. stainless steel column packed with 0.5% OV-17 on 80-100 mesh Gas Chrom Q; the operating conditions were injector temperature, 300°C; column temperature, held isothermally at 190°C for 6 min and then programmed to 250°C at a rate of 22°C/min; nitrogen carrier-gas flow rate, 35 ml/min. With these operating parameters, the retention times of the internal standard, hexadiphane, and 1,1-diphenyl-3-hexamethyleneiminobutyronitrile were approximately 2.91, 5.03, and 9.40 min, respectively. The assay results of the hexadiphene-oxazepam hemisuccinate combination, liquid commercial preparation of hexadiphane hydrochloride, and hexadiphane-digestive enzymes-dimethylpolysiloxane combination are summarized in Table 1.36.

Hucker and Stauffer [311] developed a GC procedure for the determination of cyclobenzaprine (a unique, centrally acting, skeletal muscle relaxant currently in clinical trial) in plasma and urine.

Cyclobenzaprine
(N,N-Dimethyl-5H-dibenzo[a,d]cycloheptene-Δ^5,γ-propylamine)

Their recommended procedure for the extraction of cyclobenzaprine from plasma or urine was as follows:

TABLE 1.36

GC Analyses of Various Hexadiphane Pharmaceutical Preparations[a]

Analysis number	Sample A[b]		Sample B[c]		Sample C[d]	
	Found (mg)	Recovered (%)	Found (mg)	Recovered (%)	Found (mg)	Recovered (%)
1	3.24	101.9	2.03	101.5	2.03	101.5
2	3.12	97.5	1.98	99.0	1.94	97.0
3	3.20	100.0	1.98	99.0	1.97	98.5
4	3.16	98.7	1.99	99.5	1.98	99.0
5	3.26	101.9	2.03	101.5	2.01	100.5
6	3.19	99.7	2.04	102.0	2.02	101.0

[a] Adapted from Mardente and De Marchi [310].
[b] Hexadiphane–oxazepam hemisuccinate combination (hexadiphane maleate, 3.2 mg/capsule).
[c] Liquid commercial preparation of hexadiphane hydrochloride (label claim, 2 mg/10 ml).
[d] Hexadiphane–digestive enzymes–dimethylpolysiloxane combination (hexadiphane hydrochloride, 2 mg/tablet).

Two milliliters of plasma or urine, 200 ng of internal standard
[N,N-dimethyl-5H-dibenzo(a,d)cycloheptene-Δ^5, α-ethylamine (in
0.1 ml of water)], 1 ml of 0.5 N NaOH, and 25 ml of n-heptane-
isopentyl alcohol (97:3) were shaken for 20 min in a 45-ml glass-
stoppered centrifuge tube. The tube was centrifuged, and as much of
the organic phase as possible was transferred to a similar tube containing 5 ml of 0.1 N HCl. The tube was shaken for 10 min and
centrifuged, and the organic (upper) phase was discarded by
aspiration.

The aqueous phase was washed three times with n-heptane (25 ml
each) to remove any residual isopentyl alcohol, the washings being
discarded each time by aspiration. Then the aqueous phase was
transferred to a clean 13-ml glass-stoppered centrifuge tube. Five
milliliters of freshly distilled ether and 1.5 ml of 0.5 N NaOH were
added, and the tube was shaken for 10 min. After centrifuging, the
ether layer was transferred with a Pasteur pipette to a glass tube
with a constricted tip.

The solvent was removed in a warm water bath (40°C), with
periodic chilling in ice water to rinse down the sides. The residue
was dissolved in 25 μl of ethyl acetate, and a 5-μl aliquot was
injected into the chromatograph.

Quantitative results were obtained using a Hewlett-Packard model 810
gas chromatograph equipped with a hydrogen flame ionization detector and
a 1.8-m by 4-mm-i.d. glass column packed with 1.5% OV-17 on 80-100
mesh Gas Chrom Q. All determinations were performed under the following conditions: injector temperature, 260°C; column temperature, 218°C;
detector temperature, 285°C; helium carrier-gas flow rate, 100 ml/min.
Under these conditions, the retention times of the internal standard, cyclobenzaprine, desdimethyl cyclobenzaprine, and desmethyl cyclobenzaprine
were 2.2, 2.8, 3.1, and 3.2 min, respectively.

With a limit of detection of approximately 4 ng/ml, Hucker and Stauffer
noted that the plasma levels and urinary excretion of the drug in two
human subjects after oral and intravenous administration of a 40-mg dose
suggested that the drug is somewhat slowly absorbed, since peak plasma
levels of 29.6 ng/ml were observed after 4- to 6 hr whereas intravenous
drug administration gave plasma levels that were somewhat unusual in that
the sample taken after 15 min was no higher than the samples taken over
the following 2 hr.

Summarizing their findings, they concluded that:

> This finding suggests, as does an estimate of the apparent volume of
> distribution, that cyclobenzaprine is rapidly taken up by tissues from
> which sites the drug is slowly and relatively constantly released into

the blood. Levels after the intravenous dose were considerably higher during the first 4 hr than those attained following the oral dose, suggesting also that first-pass hepatic metabolism is important and that this phenomenon may be involved in the pharmacokinetics of cyclobenzaprine absorption in humans.

The presence of only a relatively small amount of unchanged drug in the urine (0.2 to 1.5% of the administered doses) would suggest that the drug was virtually completely metabolized in humans. The extent of metabolism may not be quite this complete since, after administration of ^{14}C-labeled drug, only 6.3% of a 10-mg p.o. dose and 7.1% of a 10-mg i.v. dose were excreted in the 24-hr urine.

GC analysis of urine samples showed the desmethyl metabolite to be most predominant in the 8- to 24-hr urine samples and appeared to be present in equal or higher concentrations compared to unchanged cyclobenzaprine. When treated with trifluoroactic anhydride, the TFA derivative of the desmethyl metabolite had a retention time of 5.0 min (the same retention time as the TFA derivative of authentic N-desmethylcyclobenzaprine), whereas the TFA derivative of N-desdimethylcyclobenzaprine was eluted in 4.0 min under the same GC conditions.

Miyazaki et al. [312] developed a method for the mass fragmentographic determination of 1-piperidino-2,4'-dimethylpropiophenone (Mydocalm), an effective central-acting muscle relaxant.

$$CH_3-\langle\bigcirc\rangle-\underset{\underset{O}{\overset{\|}{C}}}{}-\underset{\underset{CH_3}{|}}{CH}-CH_2-N\langle\bigcirc\rangle$$

Mydocalm
(1-Piperidino-2,4'-dimethylpropiophenone)

The instrumentation used to perform quantitative determinations of Mydocalm consisted of a LKB 9000 GC-MS system equipped with multiple ion detectors, a data processing system, and a 2-m by 2.5-mm glass coiled column packed with 3% OV-3 coated on 80-100 mesh Chromosorb W-HP. The GC-MS operating conditions used were column temperature, 190°C; helium carrier-gas flow rate, 30 ml/min; injector temperature, 230°C; GC-MS separator temperature, 230°C; ionization source temperature, 250°C; accelerating voltage, 3.5 kV; ionization energy, 20 eV; trap current, 60 µA.

In their multiple-ion detection system, volunteers were given a single 100-mg oral dose of a mixture (1:1) of nonlabeled Mydocalm and Mydocalm-^{15}N. As noted by Miyazaki et al., "the synthesis of

$^{15}NH_2OH \cdot HCl \rightarrow$ [cyclopentanone oxime with ^{15}N-OH] $\rightarrow$ [δ-valerolactam with ^{15}N] $\rightarrow$ [piperidine with ^{15}N] $\rightarrow$

A   B   C   D

$CH_3-\langle\text{phenyl}\rangle-\underset{\underset{O}{\|}}{C}-\underset{\underset{CH_3}{|}}{CH}-CH_2-^{15}N\langle\text{piperidine}\rangle$

E

1-piperidino ^{15}N-2,4'-dimethylpropiophenone (summarized above) consisted of converting hydroxylamine (A) to cyclopentanone oxime (B) which, in turn, was converted to δ-valerolactam-^{15}N (C, followed by Beckmann rearrangement). δ-Valerolactam-^{15}N was reduced to piperidine-^{15}N hydrochloride with LiAlH$_4$ (D). Mydocalm-^{15}N (E) was synthesized by Mannich reaction using 4'-methyl-propiophenone, paraformaldehyde, and piperidine-^{15}N hydrochloride."

The internal standard, 1-piperidino [d_{10}]-2,4'-dimethylpropiophenone (Mydocalm-d_{10}), was also prepared by his procedure, using decadeutero-piperidine hydrochloride which was obtained by catalytic hydrogenation of perdeuteropyridine with deuterium gas.

The procedure used for sample preparation for subsequent GC-MS analysis involved the following steps:

> The volunteers were given a single oral dose of 100 mg of the mixture of Mydocalm and Mydocalm-^{15}N. Blood specimens were taken at 30 min after administration, and 1, 2, 3, 4, and 7 hr.
> To 1.0 ml of serum in a 50-ml centrifuge tube, 1.0 ml of internal standard solution (1.0 μg of Mydocalm-d_{10}/ml), 1 ml of water, and 0.1 ml of concentrated ammonia water were added and mixed. Then, 30 ml of ethanol was added. The tube was shaken well by hand and allowed to stand for 30 min, and then centrifuged for 10 min at 3000 rpm. The supernatant was evaporated to dryness below 25°C under reduced pressure. The residue was dissolved with 5 ml of benzene and 5 ml of saturated potassium carbonate solution, shaken well, and transferred into a separatory funnel. This extration procedure was repeated twice. The benzene layer was separated and washed with water until the washing did not color a litmus paper blue. The benzene layer was shaken well with 5 ml of 0.01 N HCl. The acid layer was transferred into a 10-ml glass-stoppered tube, and

to this was added 0.5 ml of saturated potassium carbonate solution and 1 ml of n-hexane. The tube was shaken for 2 min and then centrifuged for 10 min at 3000 rpm. The n-hexane layer was subjected to a gas chromatograph-mass spectrometer.

Using the GC-MS operating conditions previously cited, the retention times of Mydocalm, decadeuterium-labeled Mydocalm, and Mydocalm-^{15}N were approximately 4.5, 4.4, and 4.5 min, respectively (all appearing as a single peak in the gas chromatogram). However, by monitoring m/e 245 (molecular ion of Mydocalm), 255 (molecular ion of Mydocalm-d_{10}), and 246 (molecular ion of Mydocalm-^{15}N), each component is recorded as a single peak via the mass fragmentographic technique.

With the limit of detection by this technique reported to be 0.01 µg/ml of serum (0.05 µg of Mydocalm/ml of serum detectable with a S/N ratio of 3:1), the absolute recovery via their extraction/clean-up procedure was nearly 85% for 0.1 µg of Mydocalm/ml of serum.

The accuracy of the mass fragmentographic technique was determined by adding 100 ng of Mydocalm and a tenfold amount of internal standard to 1 ml of serum. In this study, the recovery was found to be (n = 5) 98.6 ± 7.8%.

Of 13 known metabolites reported [313], most of the parent drug was excreted in the form of two major metabolites: 3-piperidino-2-methyl-1-(4'-carboxyphenyl)-1-propanone and 3-piperidino-2-methyl-1-(4'-carboxyphenyl)-1-propanol.

Crombez, Van Den Bossche, and De Moerloose [314] in 1976 described a GC method for the quantitative determination of camylofine, a spasmolytic agent which is often combined with other spasmolytics and analgesics such as papaverine hydrochloride, codeine phosphate, novalgin (dipyrone), and aninopyrine. By determining the 3-methyl-1-butanol formed after an alkaline hydrolysis of the drug (n-butanol added as internal standard), the method has been applied to the quantitative determination of the drug in two galenical forms, tablets and suppositories.

Following prescribed procedures for the extraction of camylofine from tablets and suppositories (lipophilic base) and its subsequent hydrolysis in

Camylofine
{N-[2-(Diethylamino)ethyl]-2-phenylglycinate}

the presence of the internal standard, the final hydrolyzate was analyzed with a Packard series 7400 all-glass gas chromatograph equipped with a flame ionization detector and a 5-ft by 4-mm-i.d. glass-spiraled column packed with Porapak Q. Using the specified GC conditions (injector temperature, 200°C; column temperature, 180°C; detector temperature, 210°C; nitrogen carrier-gas flow rate, 30 ml/min), the retention times of n-butanol and 3-methyl-1-butanol were approximately 11.32 and 21.80 min, respectively.

Using this method, the recovery of camylofine in a powder mixture of composition camylofine dihydrochloride (402.4 mg), codeine phosphate (406.5 mg), papaverine hydrochloride (804.8 mg), novalgin (2.992 g), and aminopyrine (5.007 g), based on the amount of 3-methyl-1-butanol formed after extraction and hydrolysis of the drug, was 100.9 ± 1.7% (n = 6). For the recovery of known amounts of drug in tablets and suppositories, the following data were obtained: tablets, 95.4%; suppositories, 92.5%.

IV. COUMARIN-TYPE ANTICOAGULANTS

During the past 15 years, many GC and/or GC-MS studies have been reported for coumarin-type anticoagulants [28,59,102,315-333]. As noted by Goth [1], the various coumarin anticoagulants act by the same basic mechanism: They inhibit the formation of prothrombin, factor VII (proconvertin), factor IX (Christmas), and factor X (Stuart-Power factor).

In 1962, studies by Brown and Shyluk [315] on the biosynthesis of certain coumarins had been handicapped by the lack of satisfactory purification techniques for the isolation of pure compounds. An extension of their previous successful GC investigations for the separation and purification of coumarin and herniarin (7-methoxycoumarin) [316] was undertaken to include other neutral (nonphenolic) coumarins and several phenolic coumarins as acetate derivatives.

For their investigations, a gas chromatograph equipped with a thermal conductivity cell operated with a filament current of 200 mA was used. Three different liquid stationary phases were examined: (1) two columns of succinate-ethylene glycol polyester on 60-80 mesh Chromosorb, the first (SEG 1) having a liquid phase/support ratio of 1:20, whereas the second (SEG 2) was 1:6; (2) a phthalate-ethylene glycol polyester (PhEG) on 60-80 mesh Gas Chrom P in a ratio of 1:10; and (3) high-vacuum silicone grease on 40-60 mesh Celite 545. The dimensions of the copper columns used with these various coated solid supports were 2.4 m by 5 mm o.d., 0.61 m by 5 mm o.d., 1.2 m by 5 mm o.d., and 0.61 m by 5 mm o.d. for SEG 1, SEG 2, phthalate-ethylene glycol, and silicone grease, respectively. The column and injector temperatures for the SEG 1, SEG 2, and phthalate-ethylene glycol coated supports were approximately 208 and 245°C, respectively, and a column temperature of 178°C and an injector temperature of 210°C were used with the silicone grease-packed column.

In addition to the above GC conditions, the helium carrier-gas flow rate used with each column was SEG 1, 40 ml/min; SEG 2, 100 ml/min; PhEG, 100 ml/min; silicone grease, 100 ml/min.

The SEG 2 column had the most general application for neutral coumarins (see Table 1.37) and was the only one examined which resolved pimpinellin, bergapten, and sphondin, as shown in Figure 1.46. Osthol and psoralen, which were not separated by this packed column, were readily resolved on the phthalate-ethylene glycol polyester coated Gas Chrom P support. The relative retention times for 13 neutral coumarins investigated are listed in Table 1.37, as are the retention time data for the phenolic coumarins with the silicone grease column. The phenolic coumarins were chromatographed as their acetates and, presumably because of decomposition even at low column temperatures, coumarins of the isoprenoid ether type, imperatorin and umbelliprenin, were not eluted from the columns.

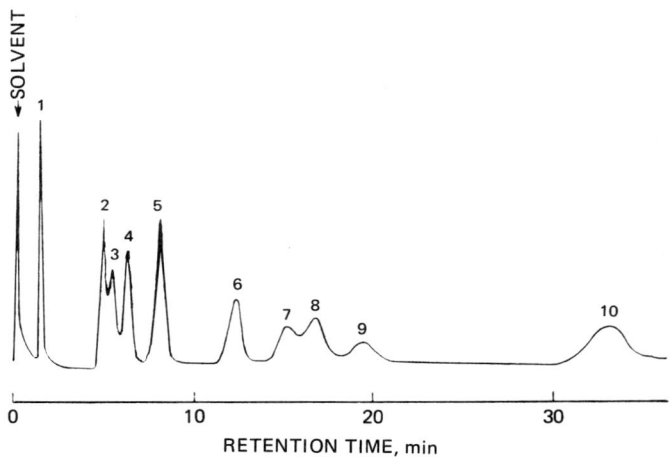

Figure 1.46. Chromatogram of synthetic mixture of neutral coumarins (SEG 2 column). 1, Coumarin; 2, herniarin; 3, angelicin; 4, seselin; 5, osthol + psoralen; 6, isobergapten; 7, pimpinellin; 8, bergapten; 9, sphondin; and 10, isopimpinellin. From Brown and Shyluk [315], courtesy of Analytical Chemistry.

TABLE 1.37
Relative Retention Times of Coumarins[a,b]

		Column		
Neutral coumarins		SEG 1	SEG 2	PhEG
1. Coumarin		0.21	0.29	
2. Herniarin		1.00	1.00	1.00
3. Angelicin			1.10	1.30
4. Seselin			1.25	
5. Osthol			1.65	6.50
6. Psoralen			1.65	1.75
7. Isobergapten			2.50	
8. Pimpinellin			3.10	
9. Aesculetin dimethyl ether			3.15	

TABLE 1.37 (continued)

Neutral coumarins		Column		
		SEG 1	SEG 2	PhEG
10. Bergapten	(structure)			3.40
11. Xanthotoxin	(structure)			3.60
12. Sphondin	(structure)			3.90
13. Isopimpinellin	(structure)			6.70

Phenolic coumarins[c]		Silicone grease
1. Umbelliferone	(structure)	1.00
2. 7-Hydroxy-8-methoxy coumarin	(structure)	1.35

Phenolic coumarins[c]		Column		
		SEG 1	SEG 2	PhEG
3. Daphenetin	(structure)			2.25
4. Scopoletin	(structure)			2.25

TABLE 1.37 (continued)

Phenolic coumarins[c]	Column		
	SEG 1	SEG 2	PhEG
5. Aesculetin			2.95

[a] From Brown and Shyluk [315], courtesy of Analytical Chemistry.
[b] Based on herniarin = 1.00 for neutral coumarins and umbelliferone = 1.00 for phenolic coumarins.
[c] Chromatographed as the acetates.

With the SEG columns, the neutral coumarins exhibited marked correlation between their retention times and the number of ether linkages in their respective molecules. For example, Brown and Shyluk showed that coumarin, with no ether linkage, had the shortest retention time, whereas this compound was followed by the monoethers (herniarin, angelicin, seselin, osthol, and psoralen), the diethers (isobergapten, bergapten, aesculetin dimethyl ether, sphondin, and xanthotoxin), and the triethers (pimpinellin and isopimpellin, with the former falling among the diethers).

The neutral coumarin fraction isolated from lavender (Lavandula officinalis Chaix) contained only herniarin and coumarin. The lactone fractions recovered from roots of Heracleum sibiricum and Angelica archangelica are shown in Figures 1.47 and 1.48, respectively. In Figure 1.48, only three peaks were identified; peak 1, angelicin; peak 2, osthol; and peak 5, bergapten. In contrast to the lactone fraction, seven of the eight peaks obtained from the H. sibiricum sample were identified; each peak was confirmed by paper chromatography when compared to authentic samples. With the exception of daphnetin and scopoletin, which could not be resolved, the phenolic coumarins investigated could be easily chromatographed, as shown in Figure 1.49.

In 1963, Kazyak and Knoblock [102] demonstrated the versatility of gas chromatography by its many applications to the separation and determination of barbiturates and many of the alkaloids and tranquilizers. Using U-shaped borosilicate glass columns, 6 ft by 4 mm i.d., packed with 1% SE-30 on 100-120 mesh Anakrom ABS and an argon ionization detector, the authors presented chromatographic data for compounds of general toxicological interest. For example, they reported that warfarin, an anticoagulant coumarin-type compound, could be easily eluted at column temperatures ranging from 165 to 200°C with retention times varying from 2.0 to 1.7 min, respectively.

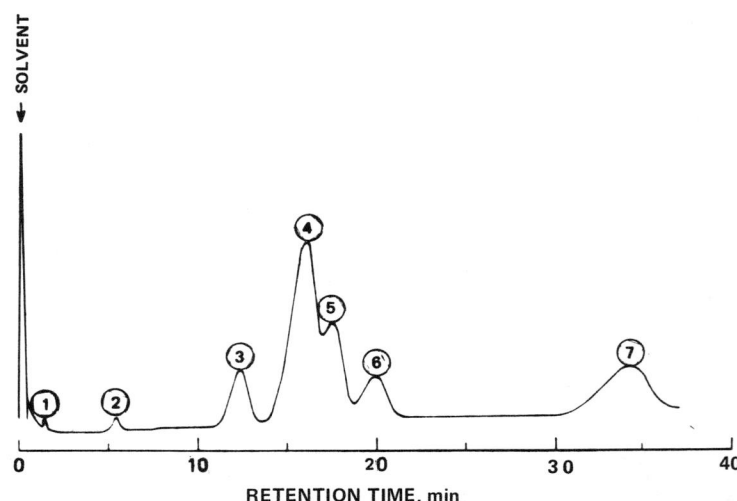

Figure 1.47. Chromatogram of neutral lactone fraction from H. sibiricum (SEG 2 column). 1, Unidentified; 2, angelicin; 3, isobergapten; 4, pimpinellin; 5, bergapten; 6, sphondin; and 7, isopimpinellin. From Brown and Shyluk [315], courtesy of Analytical Chemistry.

In addition to the initial GC studies of the separation of plant coumarins performed by Brown and Shyluk, other investigations of naturally occurring coumarins were undertaken by Furuya and Kojima [318], Steck and Bailey [319,320], Pellizzari et al. [321], and Hoque and Dutta [324]. In their studies, many other nautrally occurring coumarins were chromatographed; their structures are shown in Figure 1.50.

In 1967, Furuya and Kojima [318] studied the GC separation of 17 standard samples (coumarins, pyranocoumarins, and furanocoumarins), either in the free form or as their trimethylsilyl (TMSi) ethers, and several plant extracts using SE-30 and HI-EFF-BP (diethylene glycol succinate) as liquid stationary phases.

The separations were performed with a Shimadzu GC-1C gas chromatograph equipped with a flame ionization detector and two columns (dimensions not specified): column A, packed with 1.5% SE-30 on 60-80 mesh Chromosorb W and held isothermally at 180°C concurrently with an injector temperature, a detector temperature, and a nitrogen carrier-gas flow rate of 250°C, 230°C, and 70.4 ml/min, respectively; and column B, packed with 12% HI-EFF-BP on 80-100 mesh Gas Chrom P. The GC conditions used with column B were column temperature, 210°C; injector temperature,

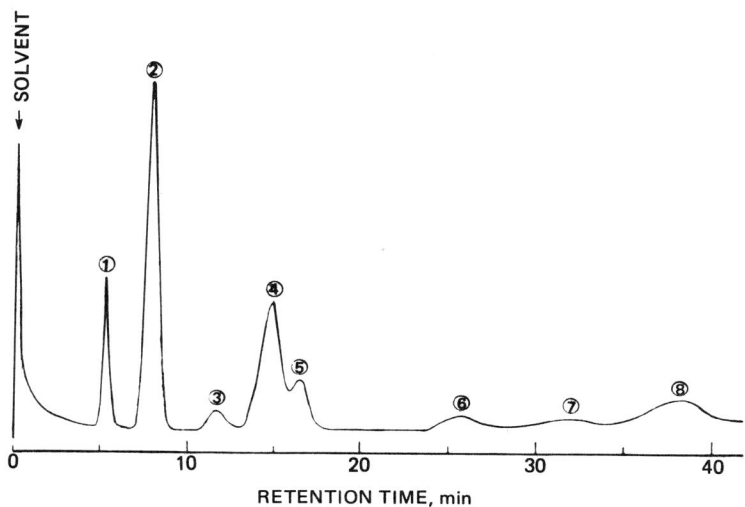

Figure 1.48. Chromatogram of neutral lactone fraction from A. archangelica (SEG 2 column). From Brown and Shyluk [315], courtesy of Analytical Chemistry.

250°C; detector temperature, 230°C; nitrogen carrier-gas flow rate, 69.1 ml/min. Samples in the free form or as their TMSi derivatives (hexamethyldisilazane and trimethylchlorosilane used as silylating reagents) were injected into the gas chromatograph as acetone solutions. The furanocoumarins were extracted according to the method of Svendsen and Ottestad [334]; their neutral fractions were also injected into the GC unit as acetone solutions. With the columns and GC conditions listed above, the retention times of various coumarins are given in Table 1.38.

With regard to possible correlations among carbon numbers, hydroxyl numbers, and retention times, Furuya and Kojima summarized their findings as follows:

> Especially aesculetin and its methyl ethers showed a good relationship between the hydroxyl numbers and retention times, the order being as follows: t_R = 23.4 min for aesculetin bistrimethylsilyl ether, 17.9 min for scopoletin trimethyl ether, 17.7 min for 7-methylaesculetin trimethylsilyl ether, and 13.1 min for dimethylaesculetin, using 1.5% SE-30.
> Daphnetin and aesculetin, each having two hydroxyl groups in the ortho position, gave lower retention times than 4,7-dihydroxycoumarin.

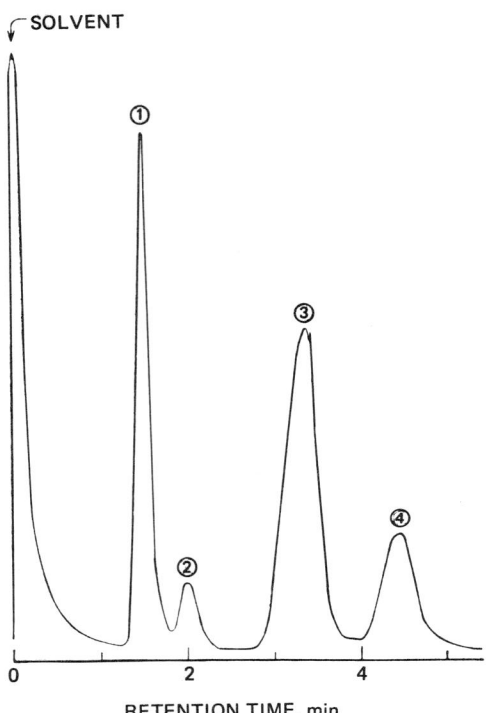

Figure 1.49. Chromatogram of synthetic mixture of phenolic coumarin acetates (silicone grease column). 1, Umbelliferone; 2, 7-hydroxy-8-methoxycoumarin; 3, daphnetin + scopoletin; 4, aesculetin. From Brown and Shyluk [315], courtesy of Analytical Chemistry.

Trihydroxycoumarin, such as 4,5,7-trihydroxycoumarin, after trimethylsilylation showed the longest retention time. Pyranocoumarins gave sharp peaks; angular types such as seselin (t_R = 15.1 min) had a lower retention time than linear ones such as xanthyletin (t_R = 19.4 min).

Furanocoumarins also gave good gas chromatograms.

Angular furanocoumarins had shorter retention times than linear ones, and the increase in the retention times with increasing number of methoxy groups was noticeable. In the methoxyfuranocoumarins, different positions of the methoxyl group gave different retention times, as illustrated by isobergapten and sphondin (angular) and bergapten and xanthotoxin (linear type).

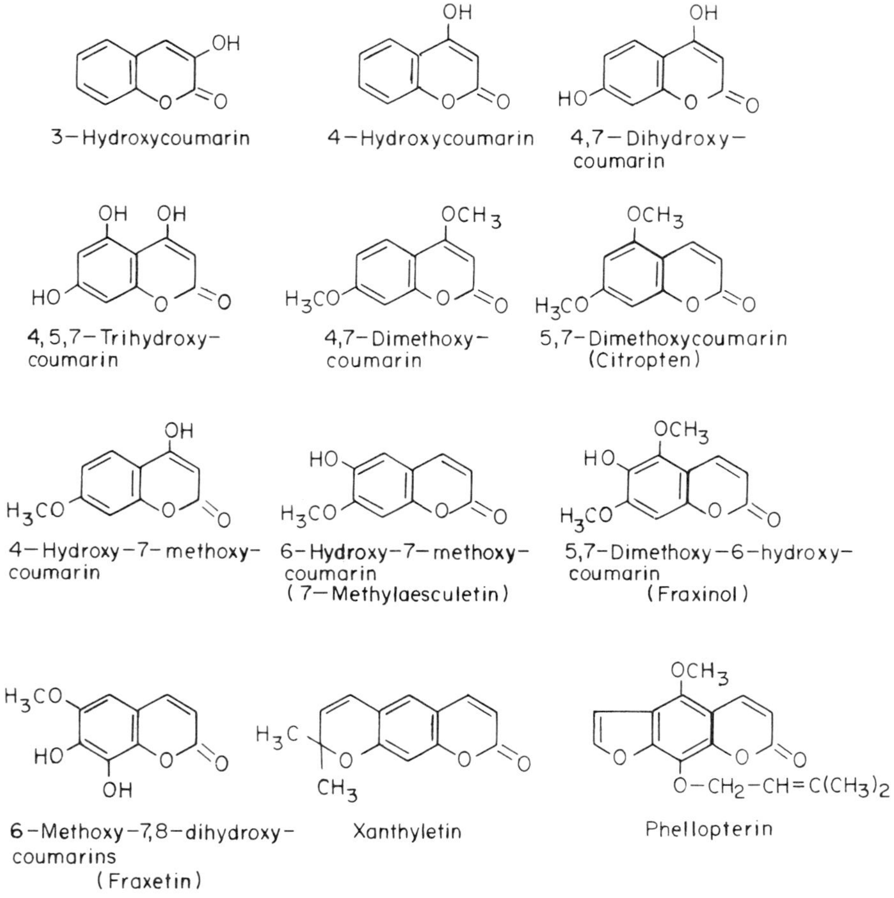

COUMARIN-TYPE ANTICOAGULANTS

3-Hydroxycoumarin

4-Hydroxycoumarin

4,7-Dihydroxy-coumarin

4,5,7-Trihydroxy-coumarin

4,7-Dimethoxy-coumarin

5,7-Dimethoxycoumarin (Citropten)

4-Hydroxy-7-methoxy-coumarin

6-Hydroxy-7-methoxy-coumarin (7-Methylaesculetin)

5,7-Dimethoxy-6-hydroxy-coumarin (Fraxinol)

6-Methoxy-7,8-dihydroxy-coumarins (Fraxetin)

Xanthyletin

Phellopterin

Figure 1.50. Structures of other plant coumarins.

Pimpinellin ran faster than sphondin using 1.5% SE-30, but was slower when 12% HI-EFF-BP was used. It would appear that the presence of the two vicinal methoxyl groups in pimpinellin makes the polarization of the molecule low, and consequently the absorption of the polar phase weak.

In 1969, Steck and Bailey [320] devised a submilligram method for the characterization of plant coumarins by combined gas chromatography, ultraviolet absorption spectroscopy, and nuclear magnetic resonance

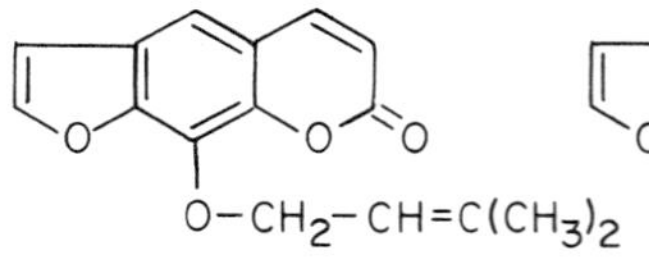

Imperatorin: O-CH₂-CH=C(CH₃)₂ furanocoumarin

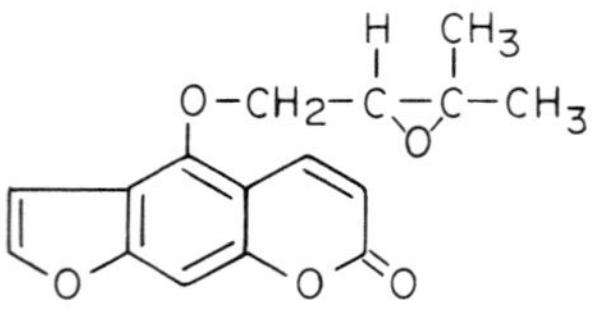

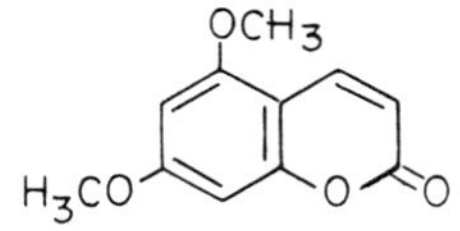

Oxypeucedanin: O-CH₂-CH(-)C(CH₃)₂ with epoxide, furanocoumarin

Limettin: 5,7-dimethoxycoumarin

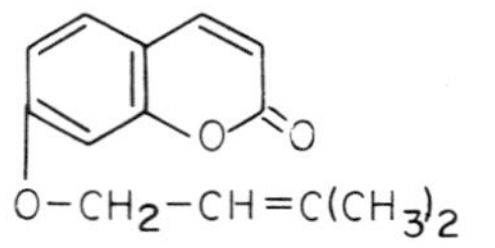

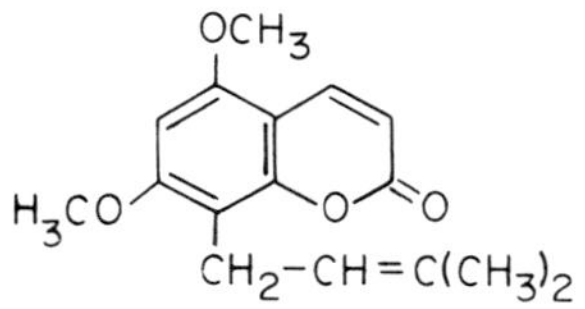

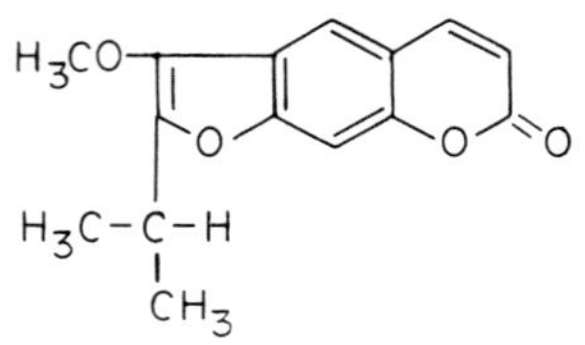

O-Prenylumbelliferone: O-CH₂-CH=C(CH₃)₂

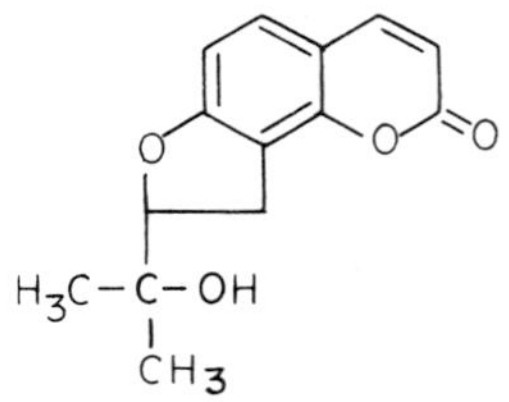

Columbianetin: dihydrofuranocoumarin with H₃C-C(OH)-CH₃

Coumurrayin: dimethoxy coumarin with CH₂-CH=C(CH₃)₂

Peucedanin: methoxyfuranocoumarin with H₃C-C(H)-CH₃

Figure 1.50. (continued)

analysis. With regard to their GC investigations, the separations were performed with an Aerograph model A-700 gas chromatograph equipped with a thermal conductivity detector and a 3.0-m by 4.7-mm-i.d. copper column packed with 5% SE-30 on 70-80 mesh Chromosorb W (DMCS-treated and acid-washed). Using the specified GC conditions (injector temperature, 252°C; column temperature, 205°C; detector temperature, 264°C; helium carrier-gas flow rate, 60 ml/min), the retention times in minutes of various coumarins were as follows: coumarin, 2.1; angelicin,

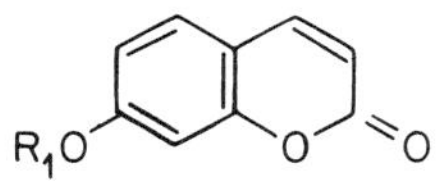

COUMARIN-TYPE ANTICOAGULANTS

Marmin

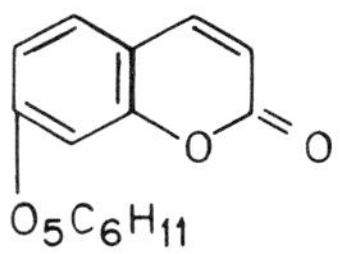

Scopolin

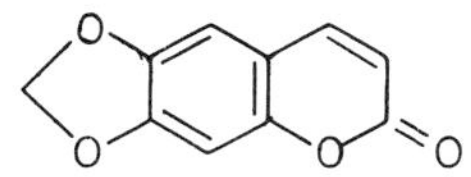

Ayapin

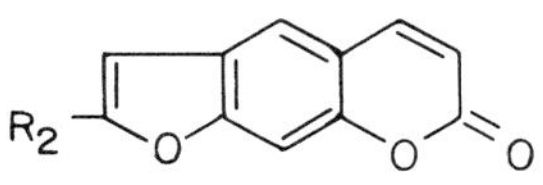

Marmesin

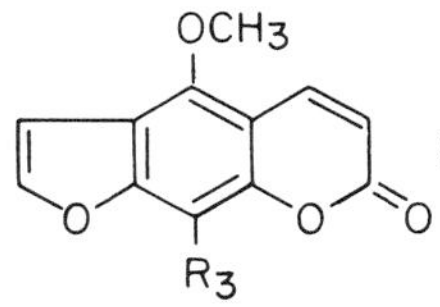

Byakangelicin

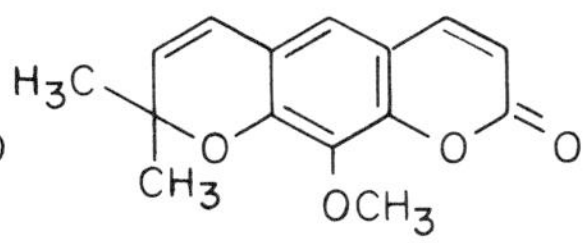

Luvangetin

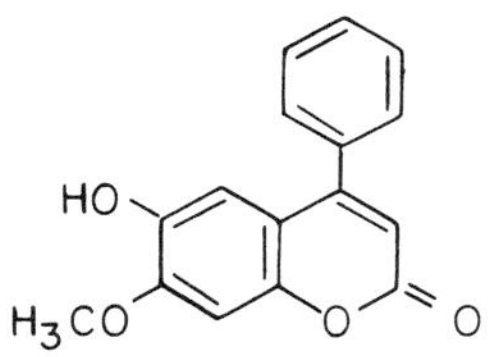

Dalbergin

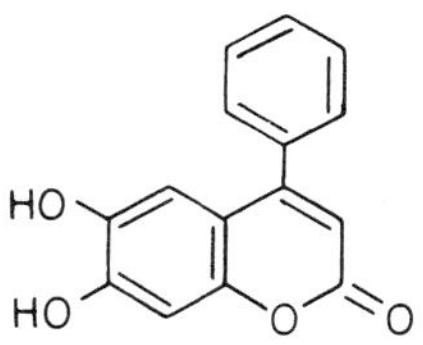

Nor-Dalbergin

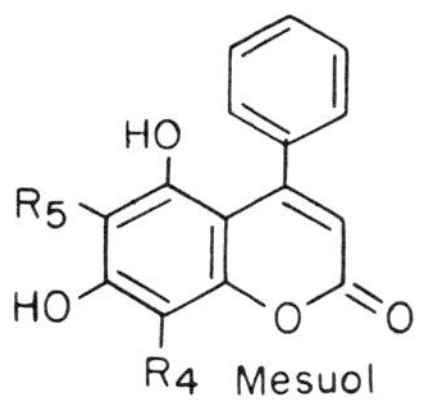

Mesuol

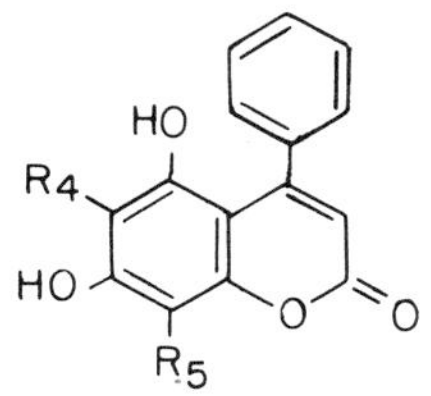

Iso-Mesuol

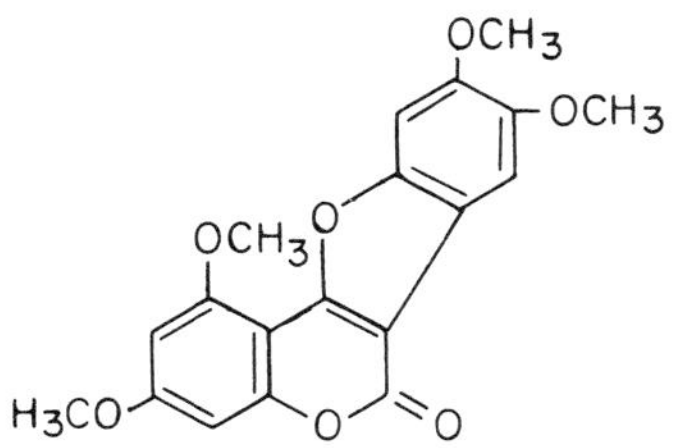

Tri-O-methyl-wedelo-lactone

where
$R_1 = -CH_2-CH=C(CH_3)-CH_2-CH_2-CH(OH)-C(CH_3)_2-OH$;
$R_2 = -CH(OH)-C(CH_3)_2-OH$
$R_3 = -O-CH_2-CH(OH)-C(CH_3)_2-OH$;
$R_4 = -CH_2-CH=C(CH_3)_2$
$R_5 = -CO-CH(CH_3)_2$

Figure 1.50 (continued)

TABLE 1.38
Retention Times of Some Naturally Occurring Coumarins[a]

	Compound	Retention time (min)		
		Column A		Column B
		Free	TMSi	Free
1	Coumarin	2.6		6.0
2	3-Hydroxycoumarin		5.5	
3	4-Hydroxycoumarin		9.0	
4	Umbelliferone (7-Hydroxycoumarin)		8.9	
5	4,7-Dihydroxycoumarin		34.5	
6	Aesculetin (6,7-Dihydroxycoumarin)		23.4	
7	Daphnetin (7,8-Dihydroxycoumarin)		15.5	
8	4,5,7-Trihydroxycoumarin		49.5	
9	Herniarin (7-Methoxycoumarin)	6.2		21.6
10	4,7-Dimethoxycoumarin	17.1		74.4
11	Citropten (5,7-Dimethoxycoumarin)	14.3		50.3
12	Dimethylaesculetin (6,7-Dimethoxycoumarin)	13.1		55.1
13	Osthol	8.8		37.6
14	4-Hydroxy-7-methoxycoumarin		23.3	
15	7-Methylaesculetin (6-Hydroxy-7-methoxycoumarin)		17.7	
16	Scopoletin (6-Methoxy-7-hydroxycoumarin)		17.9	
17	Fraxinol (5,7-Dimethoxy-6-hydroxycoumarin)		25.5	
18	Fraxetin (6-Methoxy-7,8-dihydroxycoumarin)		29.0	
19	Seselin	15.1		28.0
20	Xanthyletin	19.4		47.2
21	Angelicin	7.0		24.0

TABLE 1.38 (continued)

	Compound	Column A Free	Column A TMSi	Column B Free
22	Isobergapten	15.6		54.4
23	Sphondin	17.0		86.9
24	Pimpinellin	22.3		69.0
25	Psoralen	8.4		35.4
26	Bergapten	17.4		74.8
27	Xanthotoxin	15.8		80.1
28	Isopimpinellin	32.2		151.1
29	Phellopterin	12.8		

a Adapted from Furuya and Kojima [318].

6.0; herniarin, 6.5; psoralen, 6.9; 6,7-dimethoxycoumarin, 10.2; umbelliferone, 10.2; limettin, 10.5; scopoletin, 11.1; isobergapten, 11.7; xanthotoxin, 12.0; sphondin, 12.6; O-prenylumbelliferone, 13.2; bergapten, 13.8; pimpinellin, 15.9; osthol, 15.9; columbianetin, 20.4; isopimpinellin, 21.6; phellopterin, 23.1; peucedanin, 23.1; coumurrayin, 26.0; and oxypeucedanin, 48.0 (double peak).

Pellizzari et al. [321] examined plant phenolics and related compounds by gas chromatography and mass spectrometry; coumarin being included among the compounds studied.

The GC analyses were performed with a Hewlett-Packard model 810 gas chromatograph equipped with dual flame ionization and dual thermal conductivity detectors and 4-ft by 4-mm-i.d. glass columns packed with 3% OV-1 on 60-80 mesh Chromosorb Q. The GC operating conditions used were helium carrier-gas flow rate, 50 ml/min; injector temperature, 310°C; FID temperature, 310°C; column temperature, its initial temperature and program rate dependent on the mixture to be analyzed. Chromatographed as TMSi ether derivatives, the retention times of various components of six mixtures, the programmed temperature rates used, and the parent m/e ions are listed in Tables 1.39 and 1.40.

Mass spectral data were obtained with a LKB 9000 GC-MS instrument; the TMSi ether derivatives being chromatographed as above except that thermal conductivity and 8-ft columns were used. The effluent of each

TABLE 1.39

Retention Times of TMSi Derivatives of Some Plant Phenolics and Related Compounds[a]

TMSi derivative	Parent ion (m/e)	Retention time (min)
Mixture A[b]		
Coumarin	146	4.33
Cinnamic acid	220	6.27
p-Hydroxyphenylacetic acid	296	8.20
p-Hydroxyphenylpropionic acid	310	10.30
o-Coumaric acid	308	11.05
3,4-Dihydroxyphenylacetic acid	384	11.65
m-Coumaric acid	308	12.10
p-Coumaric acid	308	13.13
Mixture B[c]		
Coumarin	146	4.33
Vanillin	224	6.35
p-Hydroxbenzoic acid	282	8.35
Vanillic acid	312	10.60
Umbelliferone	234	11.20
3,4-Dihydroxyphenylacetic acid	384	11.65
Quinic acid	552	13.30
Ferulic acid	338	16.00
Mixture C[d]		
Quinic acid	552	5.52
p-Hydroxyphenylpyruvic acid	324	6.86
Caffeic acid	396	7.60
Chlorogenic acid	786[e]	15.55

[a] Adapted from Pellizzari et al. [321].
[b] Column programmed from 100 to 196°C at 6°C/min.
[c] Column programmed from 100 to 202°C at 6°C/min.
[d] Column held isothermally at 146°C for 1 min, then programmed to 300°C at 10°C/min.
[e] Did not give parent ion.

TABLE 1.40

Retention Times of TMSi Derivatives of Some Plant Phenolics and Related Compounds[a]

TMSi derivative	Parent ion (m/e)	Retention time (min)
Mixture D[b]		
Scopoletin	264	6.27
Esculetin	322	7.02
Phloretin	562	12.70
Naringenin	488	13.30
Catechin	650	13.80
Quercitin	662	15.82
Myricetin	750	16.30
Mixture E[c]		
Arbutin	632	7.60
Esculin	700	9.70
Phloridzin	940	11.33
Mixture F[d]		
Chalcone	208	3.28
2-Hydroxychalcone	296	5.98
Phloretin	562	10.43
Phloridzin	940	15.70

[a] Adapted from Pellizzari et al. [321].
[b] Column held isothermally at 146°C for 1 min, then programmed to 300°C at 10°C/min.
[c] Column held isothermally at 144°C for 1 min, then programmed to 302°C at 20°C/min; the 302°C temperature was held isothermally for 7 min.
[d] Column held isothermally at 180°C for 1 min, then programmed to 320°C at 10°C/min.

component in a mixture entered directly into the mass spectrometer and mass spectra as well as the mass of the parent ion of each TMSi derivative were determined using the following conditions; electron energy, 20 eV;

accelerator voltage, 3.5 kV; ion source temperature, 280°C; molecular separator temperature, 275°C; scan rate, 100 m/e per second.

Hoque and Dutta [324] studied the chromatographic behavior of 22 natural coumarins on different polar and nonpolar columns, establishing the optimum conditions regarding column length, concentration of the liquid stationary phase, carrier-gas flow rate, and column temperature for the separation of these compounds on each type of column.

This study was performed with a F&M model 700 gas chromatograph equipped with a dual flame ionization detector and seven different column systems: column A, 2-ft by 4-mm-i.d. aluminum tubing (all columns used the same 4-mm-i.d. aluminum column material) packed with 10% SE-30 (solid substrate and its mesh size not specified); column B, 6 ft, packed with 10% SE-30; column C, 2 ft, packed with 10% diethylene glycol adipate polyester (DEGA); column D, 6 ft, packed with 10% DEGA; column E, 2 ft, packed with 10% Apiezon L; column E, 6 ft, packed with 10% Apiezon L; and column F, 2 ft, packed with 5% Apiezon L. Using a nitrogen carrier-gas flow rate of 45 ml/min with the injector and detector temperature maintained 30°C above column temperature, the 22 coumarins were divided into two groups prior to GC analysis: Group I contained coumarin, herniarin, angelicin, psoralen, ayapin, aesculetin dimethyl ether, seselin, xanthotoxin, bergapten, xanthyletin, pimpinellin and luvangetin; and group II included scopolin, marmin, dalbergin, nor-dalbergin, byakangelicin, marmesin, mesuol, isomesuol, dimethyl mesuol, and tri-O-methyl wedelolactone.

For the separation of group I components, columns B and D were found to be suitable for the complete separation of all coumarins at a column temperature of 200°C, as shown in Table 1.41. On the other hand, Group II compounds could be separated very well using column A at 280°C with a carrier-gas flow rate of 40 ml/min, as indicated in Table 1.41, where both t_R (retention time) and RRT (relative retention) data are listed.

With regard to GC and/or GC-MS analysis of coumarin anticoagulants such as those illustrated in Figure 1.51, Finkle et al. [28] reported relative retention data for almost 600 common poisons, drugs, and human metabolites using four columns and three liquid stationary phases (see Chapter 1 of Volume 2 for column, GC operating, extraction, and coding details); the data being tabulated in two indices. In their study, the relative retention times and the column system used for several anticoagulants were as follows: acenocoumarin, RRT = 0.20, column system II; anisindione, RRT = 0.75, column system II; diphenadione, RRT = 0.72, column system VII; warfarin, RRT=0.28, column system I; ethyl biscoumacetate, RRT = negative on column systems I, II, IV, and VII.

Moffat [59] suggested the use of SE-30 as a stationary phase for the identification of drugs based on retention indices alone. Included in the compiled retention index data for 480 drugs were the retention indices of several anticoagulants: acenocoumarin, 1900; anisindione, 2285; diphenadione, 2910; warfarin, 1460.

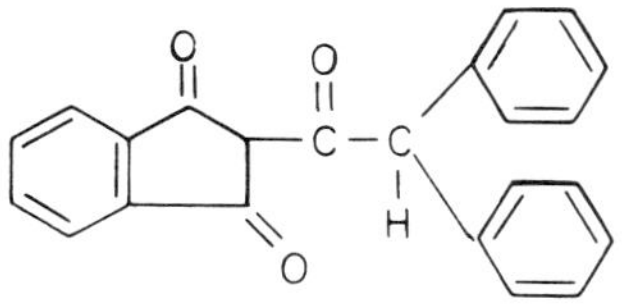

Diphenadione

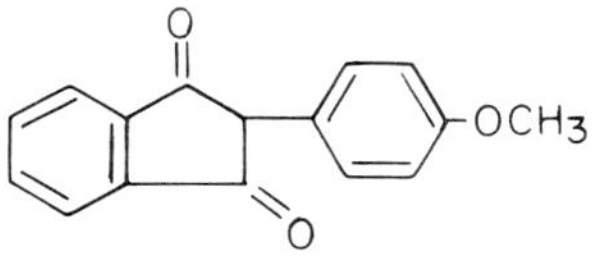

Anisindione

In 1972, Deckert [322] described GC results obtained with coumarin, 4-hydroxycoumarin, five anticoagulants derived from 4-hydroxycoumarin, and the TMSi ethers of some of these compounds. Silylation was performed with hexamethyldisilazane-trimethylchlorosilane (2:1 ratio) as

TABLE 1.41

Retention Time Data for 22 Coumarins on Various Columns[a]

1. Group I Compounds

Column	B	D
Column temperature (°C)	200	200
Carrier gas flow rate (ml/min)	42	45
	$t_R{}^b$	$t_R{}^b$
Coumarin	6.08	1.26
Herniarin	13.50	6.32
Angelicin	15.12	7.31
Psoralen	18.20	9.04
Ayapin	21.20	17.90
Aesculetin dimethyl ether	27.40	9.71
Seselin	29.60	7.95
Xanthotoxin	34.00	18.95
Bergapten	35.90	24.30
Xanthyletin	38.10	13.70
Pimpinellin	45.50	14.83
Luvangetin	58.10	24.60

TABLE 1.41 (continued)

2. Group II Compounds

Column	A	A	C	E
Column temperature (°C)	300	280	200	250
Carrier-gas flow rate (ml/min)	40	40	45	45
	RRT	t_R^b	RRT	RRT
Scopolin	0.78	1.07		0.60
Luvangetin	1.00	1.62	1.00	1.00
Marmesin	1.17	1.98	1.00	2.01
Byakangelicin	1.43	2.80	1.14	2.90
Marmin	2.60	3.24	1.14	3.96
Dalbergin	3.17	3.84	1.41	4.98
Nor-Dalbergin	5.07	4.55	1.77	7.21
Dimethylmesuol	6.07	7.29	2.36	9.02
Isomesuol		10.90	3.18	12.35
Mesuol		12.95	3.77	14.50
Tri-O-methyl wedelolactone		16.40	4.45	19.60

[a]Adapted from Hoque and Dutta [324].
[b]t_R = retention time (min).

silylating reagents, and all chromatographic retention data were obtained with a Varian Aerograph model 1200 gas chromatograph equipped with a flame ionization detector and a 5-ft by 1/8-in.-o.d. copper column packed with 5% SE-30 on 60-80 mesh Chromosorb W (DMCS-treated). Using a nitrogen carrier-gas flow rate of 30 ml/min and injector, column, and detector temperatures of 245, 205, and 270°C, respectively, the retention times of underivatized coumarin, 4-hydroxycoumarin, phenprocoumon, warfarin, acenocoumarin, bishydroxycoumarin, and ethyl biscoumacetate were 0.5, 1.0, 4.4, 8.8, 1.1, 32.0, and 56.0 min, respectively. The retention times of TMSi derivatives of 4-hydroxycoumarin, phenprocoumon, warfarin, and acenocoumarin were 1.2, 6.4, 9.7, and > 30 min, respectively.

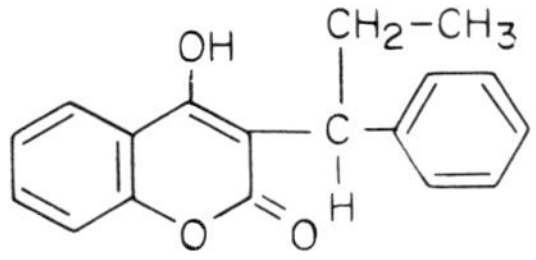

Phenprocoumon

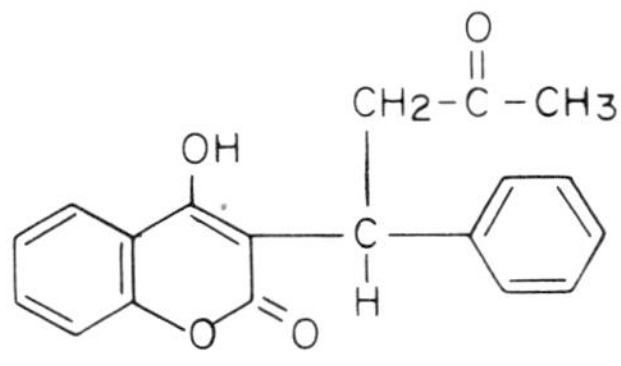

Warfarin

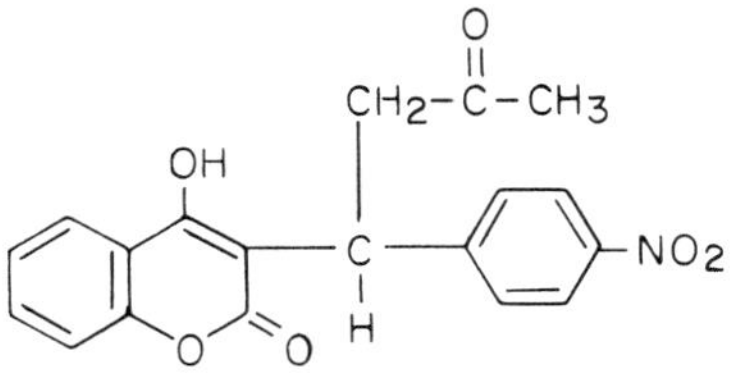

Acenocoumarin

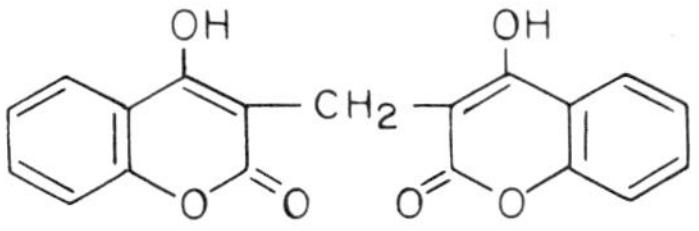

Bishydroxycoumarin

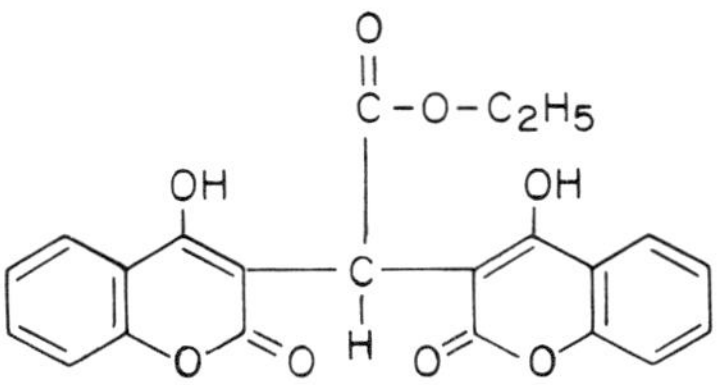

Ethyl biscoumacetate

Figure 1.51. Structures of coumarin-type anticoagulants. Structure of coumarin and 4-hydroxycoumarin given in Table 1.37 and Figure 1.50, respectively.

Soon thereafter, Deckert [323] reported results with 4-hydroxycoumarin, phenprocoumon, warfarin, and their TMSi ethers, acetates, trichloroacetates, and trifluoroacetates. In this study, Deckert used a Varian Aerograph model 1520 gas chromatograph equipped with a flame ionization detector and a 5-ft by 1/8-in.-o.d. aluminum column packed with 5% SE-30 on 60-80 mesh, DMCS-treated Chromosorb W. Using a nitrogen carrier-gas flow rate of 30 ml/min and injector, column, and detector temperatures of 240, 205, and 260°C, respectively, the retention times of the anticoagulants and their various derivatives are listed in Table 1.42.

In 1974, Kaiser and Martin [325] developed a GC method for the determination of warfarin in human plasma in order to evaluate the pharmacokinetics and potential drug interactions at relatively low doses (i.e., 7.5 mg). As developed, the method consisted of an ethylene chloride extraction of the acidified specimen, TLC of the ethylene chloride extract residue, formation of the pentafluorobenzyl derivatives of the materials

TABLE 1.42

Retention Time Data for Several Anticoagulants[a]

Derivative	Retention time (min)		
	4-Hydroxycoumarin	Phenprocoumon	Warfarin
Underivatized	1.0	6.2	13.0
TMSi ether	1.3	9.6	14.3
Acetyl	1.3	11.7	16.6
Trichloroacetyl	3.0	22.0	39.0
Trifluoroacetyl	0.6	3.5	9.0

[a] Adapted from Deckert [323].

eluted from the thin-layer chromatogram, and quantification of the pentafluorobenzyl derivatives by gas chromatography, utilizing electron capture detection.

With 3-(α-acetonyl-p-chlorobenzyl)-4-hydroxycoumarin selected as internal standard, separations of the PFB derivatives were accomplished with a Tracor model MT-220 gas chromatograph equipped with a ^{63}Ni electron capture detector and 0.61-m by 3-mm-i.d. U-shaped glass columns packed with 1% OV-17 on 80-100 mesh Gas Chrom Q. During analysis, the injector, column, and detector temperatures were maintained isothermally at 275, 240, and 285°C, respectively, with the nitrogen carrier-gas flow rates (used as carrier and purge) set a 75 and 30 ml/min, respectively. Under these conditions, the PFB derivatives of warfarin [3-(α-acetonylbenzyl)-4-hydroxycoumarin] and the internal standard were eluted from the OV-17 column in 3.6 and 6.1 min, respectively.

Having a lower limit of detection for measurement of intact warfarin in plasma of 0.02 μg/ml, the recoveries of known amounts of warfarin and internal standard added to plasma were 98.8 ± 10.9% and 95.6 ± 3.7%, respectively; these being essentially quantitative as compared to an unextracted standard of the derivatives.

With regard to plasma levels of warfarin in humans, Kaiser and Martin summarized the data from this study as follows:

Results from measurement of plasma warfarin concentrations in six normal human subjects, after single-dose oral administration of 7.5 mg of drug (as three 2.5-mg tablets), demonstrated the utility of the analytical methodology [Fig. 1.52]. A peak mean (± SEM) level

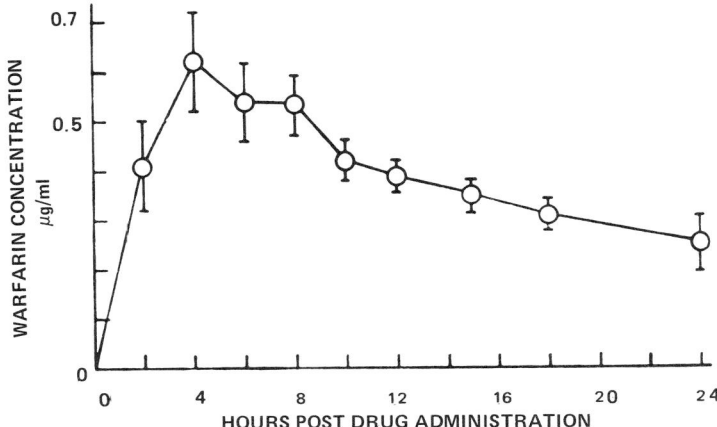

Figure 1.52. Mean (± SEM) plasma concentrations of warfarin versus time in humans (n = 6) after single-dose oral administration of 7.5 mg of drug as compressed tablets. From Kaiser and Martin [325], courtesy of the Journal of Pharmaceutical Sciences.

of warfarin (0.62 ± 0.10 µg/ml) was observed at 4 hr after drug administration. Substantial amounts of intact drug (0.25 ± 0.06 µg/ml) were found in the 24-hr plasma specimens, indicating slow drug disappearance from peripheral circulation.

Midha et al. [326] described a novel method for the quantitative determination of warfarin in plasma; in which a 2-ml sample of plasma containing warfarin to which a known amount of phenylbutazone (1 ml of 5 µg/ml aqueous solution) is added as internal standard is acidified and extracted with 20 ml of ethylene dichloride. The drug and the internal standard are then back-extracted into alkali which, in turn, is acidified and reextracted with ethylene dichloride. The organic extract, after washing with phosphate buffer (pH 7.2), is evaporated and the evaporated extract is reacted with an ethereal solution of diazomethane (100 µl). The reaction mixture is evaporated and then dissolved in 25 µl of carbon disulfide. A 2- to 3-µl aliquot is withdrawn and injected into a Perkin-Elmer model F-11 gas chromatograph equipped with a flame ionization detector and a 1.8-m by 0.25-cm glass spiral column packed with 5% OV-7 coated on 80-100 mesh Chromosorb W (acid-washed, DMCS-treated).

With the GC operated at prescribed conditions (injector temperature, 280°C; column temperature, 260°C; detector temperature, 270°C; nitrogen carrier-gas flow rate, 63 ml/min), the retention times of the methylated derivatives were warfarin, 9.8 min; phenylbutazone, 3.9 and 7.7 min (respective peak heights being in the ratio of 0.7:1.0), with the latter peak used for quantitative studies. Examined by mass spectrometry, the methylated derivative of warfarin, 3-(α-acetonylbenzyl)-4-methoxycoumarin, showed a molecular ion at m/e 322 and abundant ions at m/e 280, 279, 265, 263, 246, 235, 221, 219, 203, 202, 201, 145, and 131. For these ions, structures I-XIV were postulated.

The phenylbutazone peak at 7.7 min was shown to be consistent (molecular ion at m/e 322 and other diagnostic ions at m/e 77, 183, 266, and 279) with the structure 1,2-diphenyl-3-methoxy-4-n-butyl-5-oxopyrazaline.

With regard to warfarin metabolism, Midha et al. noted that "the metabolites of warfarin, namely, 3-[α-(2-hydroxypropyl)benzyl]-4-hydroxycoumarin (two diastereoisomers), 6-hydroxywarfarin, and 7-hydroxywarfarin, do not interfere with the assay since, on methylation with diazomethane, they gave retention times of 10.5, 12.5, 19.6, and 22.7 min, respectively. No metabolites were detected in plasma samples of dosed volunteers (n = 10) following single doses of 20 mg of sodium warfarin, an observation that confirms the findings of Welling et al. [335]."

The recoveries (average) of warfarin and phenylbutazone added to plasma using the above extraction-methylation-GC procedure were 94.47 ± 0.85 and 55.57 ± 1.30%, respectively.

In 1976, Yacobi et al. [329] studied the serum protein binding and elimination kinetics of warfarin in 31 patients with cardiovascular disease who were taking warfarin regularly. The warfarin levels in serum were determined with a Hewlett-Packard model 5830A gas chromatograph, using the GC method of Midha et al. [326], which was modified slightly as follows: a 2-ml serum sample was extracted into 11 ml of ethylene dichloride, of which 10 ml were used to extract into 2.5 ml of sodium hydroxide solution, of which 2 ml were acidified and extracted into 2.5 ml of ethylene dichloride. Two milliliters of the ethylene dichloride phase were evaporated at room temperature under nitrogen and, after phenylbutazone (2.5 μg in 0.05 ml of chloroform) was added, this solution was evaporated. The residue was methylated with an ethereal solution of diazomethane and, after the evaporation of the reaction mixture and dissolution of the methylated extract with carbon disulfide, a 2- to 3-μl aliquot was withdrawn and injected into the gas chromatograph. They noted that, relative to warfarin added directly to the final ethylene dichloride phase, the recovery by their modified procedure was 94.9 ± 3.0%, with no apparent dependence in the 0.5- to 4.0-μg/ml concentration range.

Their data indicated that "the free fraction of warfarin in the serum ranged from 0.00436 to 0.0189, indicating 98.11% to 99.56% protein binding. There was no apparent relationship between the extent of protein binding of warfarin and the concentration of albumin or total protein in the

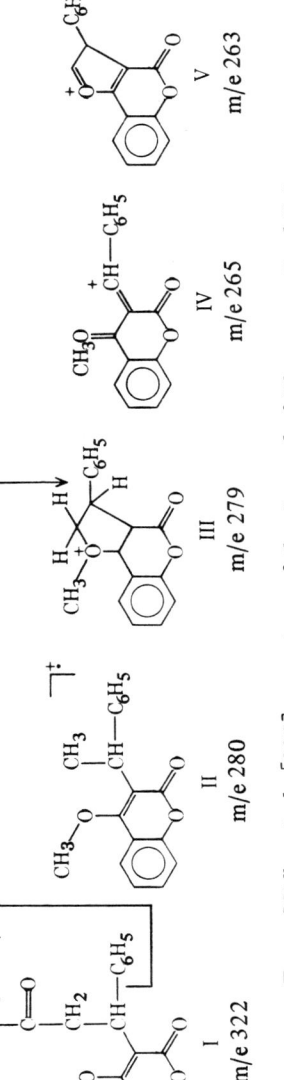

From Midha et al. [326], courtesy of the Journal of Pharmaceutical Sciences.

From Midha et al. [326], courtesy of the Journal of Pharmaceutical Sciences.

serum. The estimated total body clearance of warfarin in patients ranged from 1.16 to 4.35 ml/hr/kg of body weight and correlated significantly with the free fraction of warfarin in serum. This correlation has been predicted on theoretical grounds and shows that serum protein binding is a major determinant of the elimination kinetics of warfarin in man and an important cause of interindividual variations in its body clearance. The interindividual variation of free warfarin concentrations in the serum of patients with similar prothrombin times was somewhat smaller than the variations in total serum-warfarin concentrations and in the daily dose of warfarin. There was no correlation between prothrombin time and the concentration of free warfarin in serum, indicating that variables other than protein binding also affect the anticoagulant response of patients."

In 1976, Bianchetti et al. [328] developed a method for the determination of acenocoumarin in plasma based on solvent extraction, formation of its pentafluorobenzyl derivative with pentafluorobenzyl bromide as reagent, use of clonazepam as internal standard, and subsequent analysis by gas chromatography with electron capture detection.

For this study, a Carlo Erba Fractovap G-1 gas chromatograph was used, equipped with a ^{63}Ni electron capture detector and 60-cm by 4-mm-i.d. glass columns packed with 3% OV-17 on 100-120 mesh Chromosorb Q. The operating conditions were injector temperature, 290°C, column temperature, 285°C; detector temperature, 290°C; nitrogen carrier-gas flow rate, 20 ml/min; scavenger gas (nitrogen) flow rate, 60 ml/min; pulse voltage, 50 V; pulse interval, 30 μsec. With these operating conditions, the retention times of clonazepam and the PFB derivative of acenocoumarin were 4.5 and 1.5 min, respectively.

With the calibration curve exhibiting good linearity for concentrations from 100 to 400 ng/ml in plasma [curve obtained by plotting the ratios of the peak area of the PFB derivative to that of clonazepam (this compound did not react with pentafluorobenzyl bromide under the conditions used) versus known amounts of acenocoumarin added to the plasma], the limits of detection for acenocoumarin and the recovery of the extraction procedure were 500 pg and about 75%, respectively.

When applied to patient studies, they noted that administration of acenocoumarin (5 mg orally in two doses with a 12-hr interval) to two patients for 2 to 3 weeks gave steady-state levels varying between 20 and 70 ng/ml in plasma. Based on this observation, they postulated that the wide fluctuation of the plasma levels during the "steady state" might be explained either by a low compliance and an erratic absorption owing to the presence of food in the gastrointestinal tract, or by an inappropriate dosage interval that is inadequate compared with the apparent half-life of acenocoumarin. From preliminary results, drug levels appeared to be strictly correlated with prothrombin time, and plasma levels of 40 to 60 ng/ml seemed to be sufficient to maintain prothrombin activity of about 20%.

Midha and Cooper [333] also described in 1977 a quantitative method for the estimation of acenocoumarin plasma levels. In this procedure, plasma containing acenocoumarin, to which a known amount of γ-oxo derivative of phenylbutazone is added as an internal standard, is acidified and extracted with ethylene dichloride. The drug and internal standard are then back-extracted into alkali, which, in turn, is acidified and reextracted with ethylene dichloride. The organic extract is evaporated and treated with an ethereal solution of diazomethane (100 μl). The reacted mixture is evaporated, and the residue is dissolved in 25 μl of carbon disulfide.

γ—Oxo Derivative of Phenylbutazone

Aliquots (2 to 3 μl) of the CS_2 solution are injected into a Perkin-Elmer model 3920 gas chromatograph equipped with a flame ionization detector and a 180-cm by 0.25-cm-i.d. spiral glass column packed with 3% OV-11 coated on acid-washed, DMCS-treated 80-100 mesh Chromosorb W. Retention times for the methoxy derivatives of the γ-oxo derivative of phenylbutazne and acenocoumarin of 2.6 and 7.1 min, respectively, were obtained using the following GC operating conditions: injector temperature, 300°C; column temperature, 285°C; detector temperature, 310°C; nitrogen carrier-gas flow rate, 70 ml/min. When examined by integrated GC-MS, Midha et al. noted that the mass spectrum of the methylated derivative of acenocoumarin "showed a molecular ion at m/e 367 and abundant ions at m/e 351, 337, 324, 310, 308, 294, 280, 264, 236, 203, 201, 187, 176, and 43. Structures III-XVII (Scheme 1.1) are postulated for these ions. These fragmentations are in agreement with those reported for warfarin [326,336] and phenprocoumon [330,337,338] and suggest that the methylated derivative of acenocoumarin has the structure 3-(α-acetonyl-p-nitrobenzyl)-4-methoxycoumarin. Combined GC-mass spectral evidence for the structure of the internal standard indicated it to be 1,2-diphenyl-4-methyl-4-(2-butanone)-3,5-dioxopyrazoline (molecular ion at m/e 336

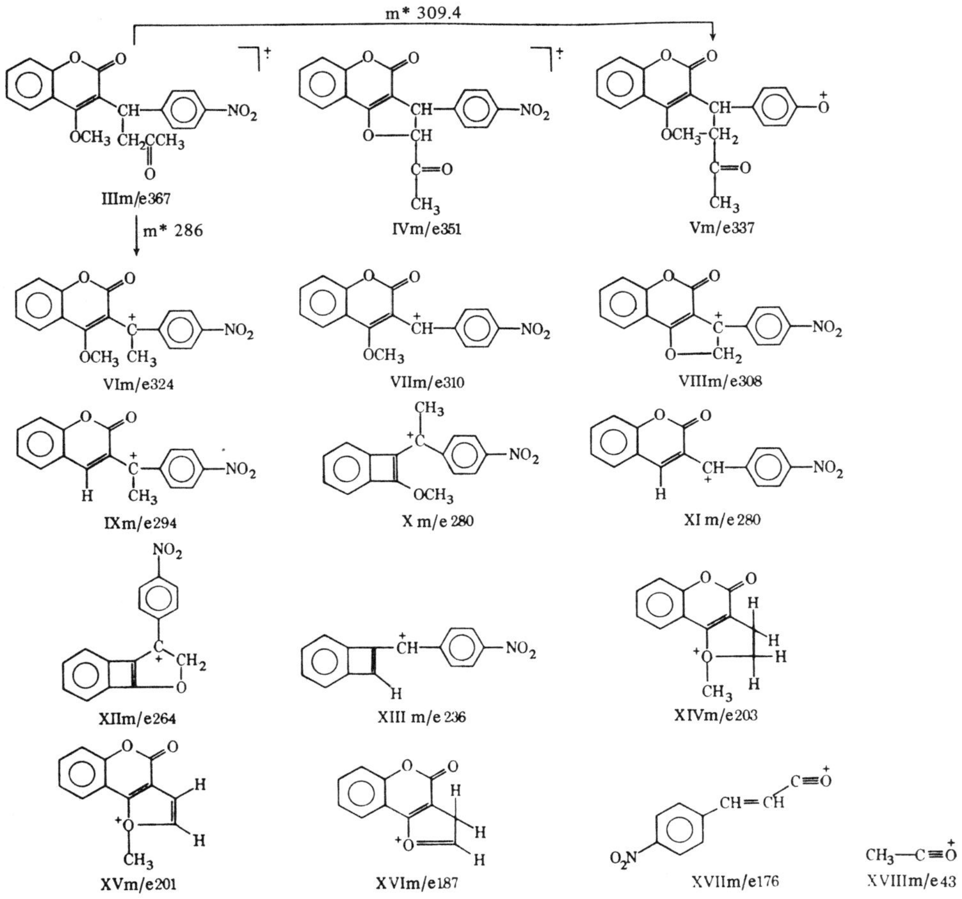

COUMARIN-TYPE ANTICOAGULANTS

Scheme 1.1. From Midha and Cooper [333], courtesy of the _Journal of Pharmaceutical Sciences._

and other diagnostic ions at m/e 321, 308, 293, 279, 264, 202, 177, 160, 119, 77, 51, and 43).

The recoveries (average) of acenocoumarin and the internal standard added to plasma using the above extraction-methylation-GC procedure were 99.90 ± 1.73 and $47.42 \pm 1.64\%$, respectively, whereas the method had sufficient sensitivity to determine 0.25 µg/ml of the drug in plasma with a relative standard deviation of 4%.

With regard to the GC analysis of phenprocoumon in plasma, Midha et al. [330] developed a GC method in which plasma containing phenprocoumon, to which a known amount of diphenylhydantoin is added as the internal standard, is acidified and extracted with ethylene dichloride. The drug and internal standard are then back-extracted into alkali, which is acidified and reextracted with ethylene dichloride. The organic extract is evaporated, and the evaporated residue is mixed with 50 µl of trimethylanilinium hydroxide in methanol.

Aliquots (1 to 2 µl) are then withdrawn and injected into a Perkin-Elmer model F-11 gas chromatograph equipped with a flame ionization detector and a 1.8-m by 0.3-cm-o.d. coiled stainless steel column packed with 5% OV-25 coated on 80-100 mesh Chromosorb W. Using injector, column, and detector temperatures of 325, 260, and 300°C, respectively, with a nitrogen carrier-gas flow rate of 60 ml/min, the retention times of the methoxy derivatives of diphenylhydantoin and phenprocoumon were 5.70 and 9.36 min, respectively.

Examining both methylated compounds by mass spectrometry, the mass spectrum of phenprocoumon showed a molecular ion of m/e 294 and a base peak at m/e 265. Other abundant ions were observed at m/e 279, 249, 247, 221, 203, 121, and 91. Structures III-XI have been postulated for these ions.

Capable of detecting 0.125 µg/ml of the drug in plasma with a coefficient of variation of 7%, the overall recoveries of phenprocoumon and diphenylhydantoin from plasma were of the order of 86.70 ± 1.38 and 90.23 ± 1.16%, respectively.

In 1977, Schmitt and Jahnchen [332] described a rapid GC method for the determination of underivatized phenprocoumon in plasma of patients treated with this drug. The preparation of samples for GC analysis consisted of the following:

Internal standard solution (0.1 ml of human plasma containing 6 µg of p-chlorophenprocoumon) and 2.0 ml of distilled water were added to plasma samples of 0.5 to 2.0 ml. The samples were acidified with 0.5 ml of 3 N HCl and extracted into 10 ml of ethylene dichloride. After centrifugation, 8 ml of the organic phase were removed and evaporated to dryness on a rotary evaporator. The residue was dissolved in 1.0 ml of acetone and transferred into 1.5-ml custom-made vials. The acetone solution was concentrated in an air bath (about 60°C) with slight vibration to a volume of about 5 µl. One to two microliters were then injected into a gas chromatograph.

In this investigation, Schmitt and Jahnchen performed all analyses with a Carlo Erba Fractovap G-1 gas chromatograph equipped with a flame ionization detector and 6-ft by 2-mm-i.d. glass columns packed with 3% OV-17 coated on 100-120 mesh Chromosorb W-HP. Retention times for

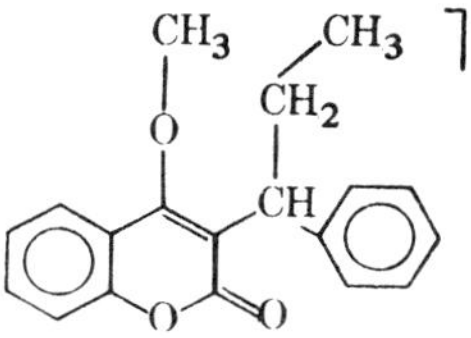

III m/e 294

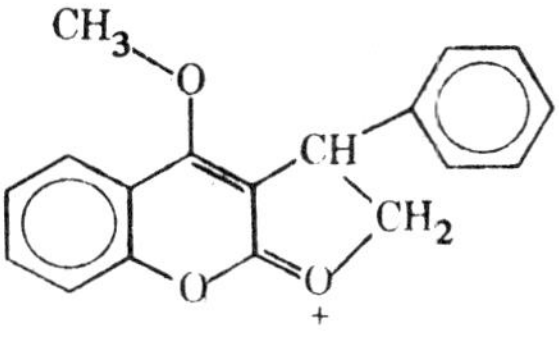

IV m/e 279

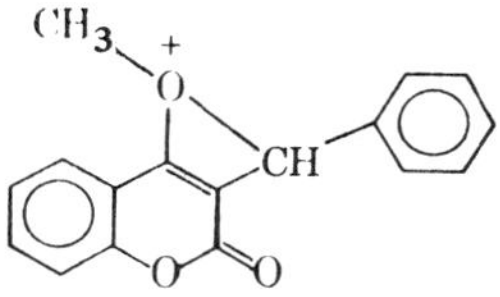

V m/e 265

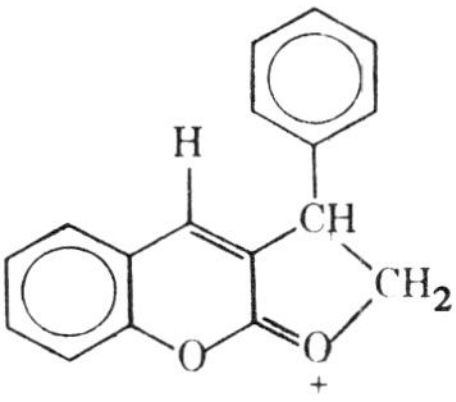

VI m/e 249

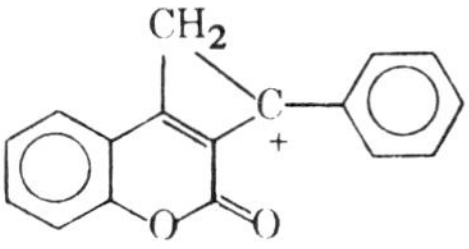

VII m/e 247

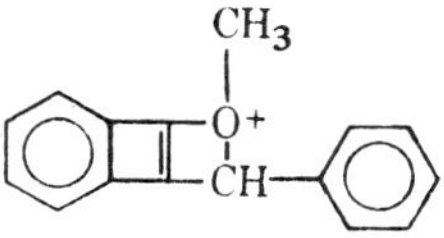

VIII m/e 221

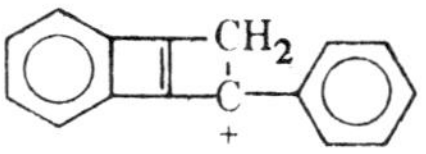

IX m/e 203

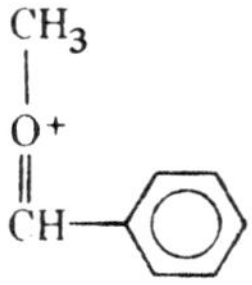

X m/e 121

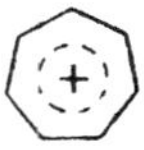

XI m/e 91

From Midha et al. [330], courtesy of Journal of Pharmaceutical Sciences.

phenprocoumon and p-chlorophenprocoumon of approximately 6.5 and 12.0 min, respectively, were obtained using the following GC conditions: injector temperature, 300°C; column temperature, 265°C; detector temperature, 300°C; nitrogen carrier-gas flow rate, 50 ml/min. The recoveries of phenprocoumon and p-chlorophenprocoumon from spiked plasma samples were 83 ± 10% and 88 ± 11%, respectively. With regard to detection limits of phenprocoumon, it was noted that concentrations of 0.2 μg/ml could be readily determined in 1-ml plasma samples; lower levels could be detected by increasing the volume of the plasma sample.

V. DIURETICS

With regard to general concepts pertaining to diuretics, Goth [1] notes that:

> Diuretics are drugs that increase the net renal excretion of solute and water. The renal tubule utilizes numerous transport processes for the reabsorption of most of the glomerular filtrate. Diuretics inhibit some of these transport processes, and their site of action within the nephron determines the quantitative and qualitative influence they exert on water and solute excretion.
>
> Although the mercurial diuretics are looked on by many as having mainly historical interest, they still have important clinical uses. They produce predictable diuresis without excessive potassium loss and are given by intramuscular injection.
>
> The carbonic anhydrase inhibitors (acetazolamide, sulfanilamide, ethoxzolamide) are somewhat ineffective in edematous states but are used in other conditions, such as glaucoma and as adjuncts in conditions in which alkaline urine may be of benefit.
>
> The thiazide diuretics (hydrochlorothiazide, chlorothiazide, methylclothiazide) are administered orally and are especially useful in hypertensive patients with congestive failure. They have disadvantages such as the induction of hypokalemic alkalosis, occasional hyperglycemia, and hyperuricemia.
>
> Furosemide and ethacrynic acid are powerful diuretics, and their potent action requires close supervision of the patient.
>
> Spironolactone and triamterene conserve potassium. They are not potent when used alone but may increase the degree of diuresis obtained by other drugs.

In addition to the above compounds, the structures of other diuretics are illustrated in Figure 1.53, including chlorthalidone and bumetanide. On the other hand, the xanthines—theophylline, theobromide, and caffeine (see Chapter 1, Volume 4)—have a combined effect on renal hemodynamics and tubular reabsorptive capacity, but the overall potency of these compounds is very much less than that of the mercurials or chlorothiazide.

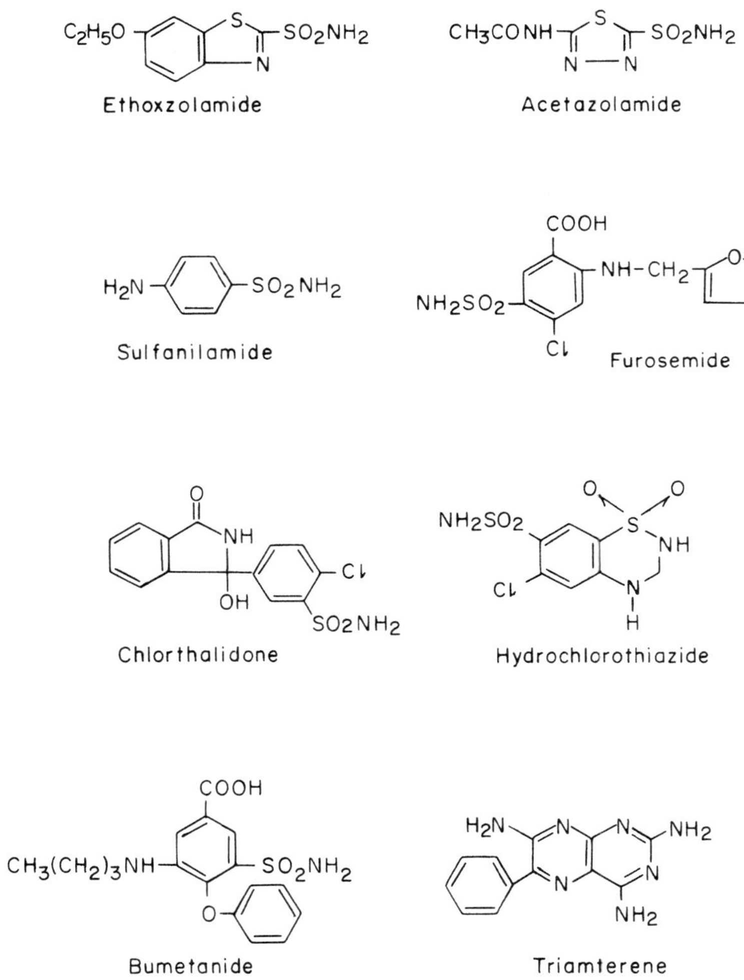

DIURETICS

Figure 1.53. Structures of Common Diuretics

As a consequence, the xanthines are occasionally useful as adjuncts to mercurial diuretics [1].

Within the past decade, many of these and other compounds exhibiting favorable diuretic properties have been examined by GC or integrated

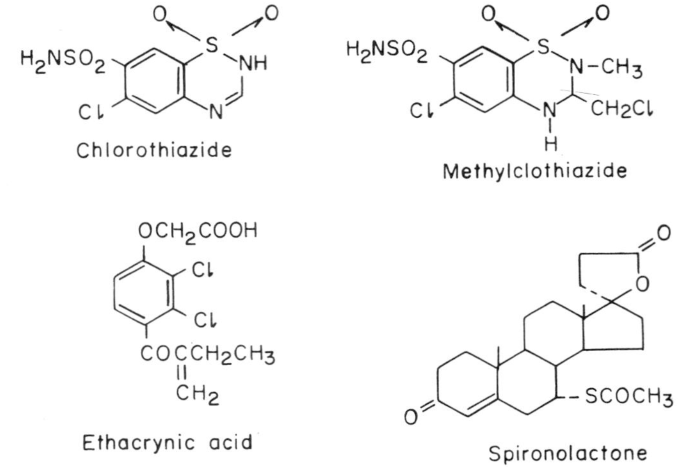

Chlorothiazide

Methylclothiazide

Ethacrynic acid

Spironolactone

Figure 1.53. (continued)

GC-MS [28,58,59,62,167,236,340-353]. Studies of a more qualitative nature were those performed by Finkle and co-workers [28,58], Foltz et al. [62], Moffat [59], Law et al. [236], and Milne et al. [340].

In 1971, the simple GC system developed by Finkle et al. [28] (see Chapter 1, Volume 2, for column, GC operating, extraction, and coding details) reported the following relative retention times and column systems used for several diuretic compounds: aldactone (spironolactone), RRT = 1.73, column system VII; amisometradine, RRT = 0.32, column system II; ethoxzolamide, RRT = 1.92, column system II; mercumallylic acid, RRT = 0.35 and 0.41, column system II; chlorthalidone, negative response using column systems I, II, IV, and VII; dichlorphenamide, negative response using column systems I, II, IV, and VII; ethacrynic acid, negative response using column systems I, II, IV, and VII; hydrochlorothiazide, negative response using column systems I, II, IV, and VII; trichloromethiazide, negative response using column systems I, II, IV, and VII.

Law et al. [236] described GC-MS techniques which could be used to obtain mass spectra of toxicological materials in biological media such as gastric lavage, serum, or urine. Following chloroform extractions at acidic and basic pH's, the organic layers were dried and evaporated to dryness or near dryness (as is the case with the more volatile drugs ethchlorvynol and the amphetamines). Taking up the residue in a suitable solvent, mass spectra were measured on a LKB-9000 GC-MS instrument with an electron-beam voltage of 70 eV and a source temperature of 250°C. Whereas the standard drugs were admitted to the mass spectrometer by

DIURETICS

means of a direct-insertion probe, extracts from biological specimens could be introduced by either of two inlets: the direct-insertion probe or the gas chromatograph. Using a helium carrier-gas flow rate of 20 to 40 ml/min, a 1% OV-17 column, and temperature programming up from 80°C at 5°C/min, the low-resolution mass spectra of 58 commonly used drugs were extracted with a DEC PDP-8I computer with a memory of 4096 12-bit words and 65536 words of disk storage. Each entry in Table 1.14 (Chapter 1, Volume 2) consisted of the five largest m/e peaks in the mass spectrum, listed in order of decreasing abundance. Excluding all ions less than m/e 40, the entire spectrum was normalized to the most intense ion above m/e 40, and if two ions were of equal abundance, they were listed in order of decreasing m/e value.

In order to search the drug list, which includes drugs whose spectra fall into seven main categories with respect to their biological activity (classified as sedatives, tranqualizers, narcotics, stimulants, analgesics, antihistaminics, or alkaloids), a computer program was written which compared experimental data with the entries on the list. As noted by the authors, the computer retrieves the disk-stored master file and checks each entry on it against the input data. Any entry that consists of the same five numbers as the input data is considered to be a solution and is displayed as such, but if no such "five-peak fit" is found, the analyst is notified and asked if a four-peak fit will suffice.

Included in the master file of drug mass spectra giving the five largest peaks, Law et al. recorded the following information for two diuretics: chlorothiazide (Diuril), m/e 295, 268, 297, 97, and 57; triamterene, m/e 253, 252, 43, 254, and 104.

In 1971, Milne et al. [340] dispensed with the gas chromatographic step and analyzed gastric extracts by direct insertion of the sample into a chemical ionization-source mass spectrometer system. They measured the isobutane chemical ionization spectra of 48 commonly used drugs (Table 1.16 in Chapter 1, Volume 2), the majority of which gave only an MH^+ ion which can be used to identify the compound. In a few cases, the fragmentation of the MH^+ ion was observed and could be rationalized in terms of simple acid-catalyzed reactions. In the isobutane CI mass spectra of drugs were included caffeine, theophylline, and triamterene; the peaks in descending order of intensity for these compounds were caffeine, 195, 194 (30), 196 (10), 110 (3); theophylline, 181, 182 (9), 180 (6); triamterene, 254, 255 (16), 250 (6), 240 (2), 256 (1), 252 (1).

Finkle et al. [58] included mannitol, acetazolamide, chlorothiazide, sulfanilamide, and triamterene in a supplement to an earlier 1972 report, which gives revised GC-MS reference data for toxicological and biomedical purposes including chemical ionization data and the facility of an interactive minicomputer by which the library can be manipulated.

Foltz et al. [62] also developed a rapid method for the detection of drugs in body fluids from suspected overdose cases. Similar to that of Finkle et al. [58], their method utilizes a computerized GC-MS system. Initial identification is based on the chemical ionization mass spectrum of the drug or the drug's metabolite. Confirmation can be provided by comparison of the GC retention time with that of a known standard, or by recording its electron-impact mass spectrum. Using methane as the reactant gas, CI mass spectra were obtained for 375 drugs, drug metabolites, and other compounds encountered in body fluid extracts.

Using prescribed extraction procedures and a single general-purpose gas chromatographic column operated with temperature programming, the GC conditions found satisfactory for such drug identification studies were as follows:

Gas chromatograph: Varian Aerograph model 1740

Column: 6-ft by 2-mm-i.d. glass column packed with 3% OV-17 coated on 100-120 mesh Gas Chrom Q

Column temperature: 150 to 280°C at 10°C/min

Carrier gas: nitrogen, 30 ml/min flow rate

Injector temperature: 280°C

Detector temperature: 290°C

A duplicate column was used in combination with the mass spectrometer and operated under the same conditions, except that either methane or helium was used as the carrier gas at flow rates of approximately 18 ml/min.

The computerized GC-MS system utilized in their project consisted of a Varian 1740 gas chromatograph coupled to a Finnigan 1015 quadrupole mass spectrometer which in turn was interfaced to a System Industries 250 data system containing a Digital Equipment PDP-8/E computer.

The report of Foltz et al. contained both CI-MS and EI-MS mass spectral information for several diuretic agents as listed below:

Methane CI-MS Data

Compound	M.W.	MH^+ (RI)	Prominent fragment ions > m/e 50
Mannitol	182	183 (47)	129 (100), 69 (65), 111 (61), 99 (55)
Acetazolamide	220	223 (100)	181 (27)
Triamterene	253	254 (100)	
Chlorothiazide	294	296 (100)	279 (5), 295 (4), 281 (2)

EI-MS Data

Compound	Prominent fragment ions > m/e 30
Triamterene	253 (100), 252 (90), 43 (21), 254 (17), 104 (15)
Chlorothiazide	295 (100), 268 (70), 297 (44), 97 (43), 57 (35)
Ethacrynic acid	247 (100), 189 (62), 249 (61), 243 (47), 191 (42)
Methylclothiazide	310 (100), 64 (58), 36 (54), 28 (44), 312 (43)
Spironolactone	341 (100), 55 (56), 91 (40), 340 (30), 374 (15)

In compiled retention index data for 480 drugs using SE-30 as the liquid stationary phase, Moffat [59] included several diuretics whose retention indices were given as amisometradine, 2025; ethoxzolamide, 2550.

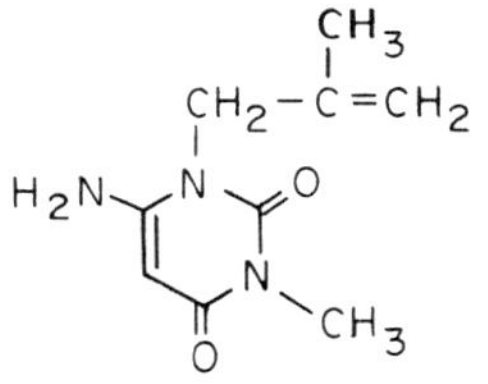

Amisometradine

A. Acetazolamide [58, 62, 167, 341, 342]

In 1977, Wallace et al. [341] developed an electron-capture GC assay for acetazolamide in blood, plasma, and saliva following oral administration to normal subjects. The purpose of their study was threefold: (1) to develop a rapid, sensitive method for quantitating acetazolamide in biological fluids; (2) to determine the feasibility of monitoring acetazolamide dosage in glaucoma patients by measurements of saliva concentrations; and (3) to establish the relationship between plasma, saliva, and erythrocyte (red blood cell) concentrations of acetazolamide after oral administration of a single 250-mg dose to humans.

Sample preparation was rather straightforward:

Aliquots of blood, plasma (50 to 100 µl), and saliva (1 to 2 ml), adjusted to approximately pH 5 by the addition of 0.5 ml of 0.1 M acetate buffer, were extracted with 10 ml of organic solvent (six volumes of ether, four volumes of dichloromethane, and two volumes of

2-propanol). The tubes were centrifuged for 15 min at 1500 rpm. The lower aqueous phase was frozen in a dry ice-acetone bath, and the upper organic layer was decanted quantitatively. Alternatively, if the concentration of acetazolamide in plasma or saliva exceeded the linear range of the standard curve (100 ng of acetazolamide/50 μl of methylating reagent), an aliquot of the organic layer was removed. The organic extract was evaporated to dryness under a slow stream of nitrogen.

The internal standard, fluoranthene (2.5 μg in an ether solution), was added to the dried organic extract of plasma and saliva samples. The solvent was evaporated to dryness under nitrogen. After addition of 50 μl of methylating reagent (0.1 M trimethylphenylammonium hydroxide or 0.2% tetramethylammonium hydroxide in methanol), 2-μl aliquots were chromatographed.

GC separations were performed with a Varian Aerograph model 1200 gas chromatograph equipped with a ^{63}Ni electron capture detector and 1.8-m by 0.3-cm-o.d. glass columns packed with 3% OV-17 on 100-120 mesh Gas Chrom Q. Using a carrier-gas (95:5 argon:methane mixture) flow rate of 30 ml/min and injector, column, and detector temperatures of 280, 215, and 340°C, respectively, the retention times of fluoranthene and methylated acetazolamide were 2.0 and 2.5 min, respectively.

Whereas the minimum detectable amount of acetazolamide was reported to be 10 ng/sample, the recovery of actazolamide from blood, plasma, and saliva via the single extraction into the organic solvent mixture was 96 to 104%; based on calibration curves prepared daily by plotting the peak height ratio of acetazolamide to internal standard versus acetazolamide concentration. On the other hand, the concentration of drug in the red blood cell fraction was calculated using the hemacrit:

$$C_B = C_{RBC}(H) + C_p(1 - H) \tag{1.25}$$

$$C_{RBC} = \frac{C_B - C_p(1 - H)}{H} \tag{1.26}$$

where C_B is the concentration in the blood, C_p is the concentration in the plasma, C_{RBC} is the concentration in the red blood cells, and H is the hematocrit.

Based on their GC data, they concluded that:

Peak plasma levels of 10 to 18 μg/ml were reached 1 to 3 hr after the dose (a single 250-mg dose administered to 5 volunteers). At least 1 hr later, erythrocyte levels reached peak concentrations of

13 to 29 µg/ml. Over 31 hr, plasma levels declined more rapidly than erythrocyte levels. Saliva concentrations averaged 1% of those in plasma and decreased at a rate equal to that of plasma. Saliva levels were proportional to, but not equal to, plasma water concentration. Saliva-to-plasma ratios were consistent for any given individual and, therefore, offer a means of monitoring drug dosage without resorting to frequent blood sampling.

For a specific patient receiving a 250-mg dose of acetazolamide, Figure 1.54 shows semilogarithmic plots of plasma, blood, and red blood cell (A) and plasma, plasma water, and saliva (B) levels of acetazolamide versus time; the data for the other four volunteers are listed in Table 1.43.

Also, in 1977, Wallace and Riegelman [342] studied in vitro the binding of acetazolamide to human erythrocytes. In this investigation, blood and plasma samples were analyzed by electron-capture gas chromatography [341] with the erythrocyte concentration calculated from the difference using the hematocrit. Wallace and Riegelman noted that:

Since erythrocyte uptake of acetazolamide is concentration dependent, it is assumed to be partially composed of a saturable process. The total erythrocyte concentration can be expressed as:

$$RBC_{tot} = RBC_b + RBC_f \quad (1.27)$$

At equilibrium, the diffusible free drug concentration, RBC_f, within the erythrocytes is assumed to be equal to the concentration of the free drug in the plasma, C_f, therefore:

$$RBC_b = RBC_{tot} - C_f \quad (1.28)$$

The total uptake curve is a sum of two processes: a linear, presumably diffusion-controlled process such that RBC_f is equal to C_f and a nonlinear, saturable binding process such that the relationship of RBC_b to C_f changes with the free concentration. The curve for RBC_b is obtained by subtracting the values for RBC_f from the experimental curve, RBC_{tot}.

The bound concentration, RBC_b, as calculated from Eq. [1.28], can also be expressed in terms of the law of mass action for the reversible macromolecule-ligand interaction:

$$RBC_b = \frac{nMk_a C_f}{1 + k_a C_f} \quad (1.29)$$

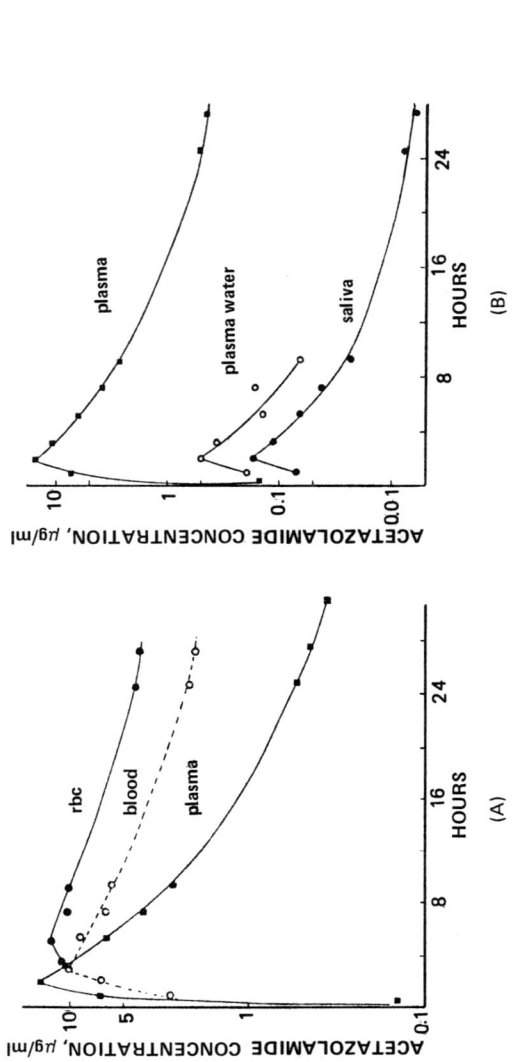

Figure 1.54. A. Semilogarithmic plot of plasma, blood, and red blood cell levels of acetazolamide in subject I after a 250-mg dose. B. Semilogarithmic plot of plasma, plasma water, and saliva levels of acetazolamide in subject I. Adapted from Wallace et al. [341].

TABLE 1.43

Blood, Plasma, and Red Blood Cell Levels (μg/ml) of Acetazolamide in Four Normal Subjects Following Oral Administration of a 250-mg Tablet[a]

	Hours										
	0.25	0.5	1	2	3	5	7	9	24	27	31
Subject II											
Blood	0	0	0	4.79	8.42	10.54	10.65	9.61	2.91	2.68	
Plasma	0	0	0	8.74	10.61	8.92	8.04	6.26	1.06	0.76	0.63
Red blood cell	0	0	0	0.16	5.85	12.44	13.71	13.54	5.09	4.93	
Subject III											
Blood	1.40	9.16	14.53	19.37		12.92	11.26	8.26	2.47	2.05	
Plasma	1.20	7.91	13.77	12.95	9.12	8.97	5.97	5.24	0.84	0.78	0.35
Red blood cell	1.69	11.04	15.66	29.00		14.70	19.20	12.79	4.92	3.95	
Subject IV											
Plasma	0	7.90	12.95	18.12	10.43	7.01	6.61	4.60	0.74	0.64	0.45
Subject V											
Blood	0	0.29	5.34	11.71	11.12	7.89	7.12	6.41	1.87	1.73	1.61
Plasma	0	0.60	6.66	13.31	7.95	4.41	4.41	3.58	0.80	0.67	0.45
Red blood cell	0	0	3.51	9.49	15.47	12.71	10.86	10.12	3.40	3.19	3.21

[a] Adapted from Wallace et al. [341].

Since the macromolecule concentration is unknown, only the product of the number of binding sites, n, and the macromolecule concentration, M, can be calculated. However, the product nM is a useful parameter, because it represents the maximum binding capacity of the protein.

Linear transformation of Eq. [1.29] yields:

$$\frac{RBC_b}{C_f} = nMk_a - k_a RBC_b \qquad (1.30)$$

Thus, for a plot of RBC_b/C_f versus RBC_b, the absolute value of the slope is the association constant, k_a, and the intercept on the abscissa, the maximum binding capacity, nM. The dissociation constant, k_d, is the reciprocal of the association constant.

Based on four experiments performed with different units of whole blood, the values (average) obtained for the maximum binding capacity (nM, µg/ml) and dissociation constant (k_d, µg/ml) for acetazolamide were 28 ± 3.6 and 0.35 ± 0.11, respectively.

B. Chlorthalidone [28, 343]

In 1974, Ervik and Gustavii [343] converted the polar molecule chlorthalidone to its tetramethyl derivative by a process called extractive alkylation. This process takes place when the substrate in anionic form is extracted as an ion pair with a quarternary ammonium ion into an organic solvent such as dichloromethane in the presence of methyl iodide.

Ervik and Gustavii divided the methylation process into two reactions such that:

$$A^- + Q^+ = QA_{org} \qquad (1.31)$$

$$QA_{org} + CH_3I_{org} = CH_3\text{-}A_{org} + QI_{org} \qquad (1.32)$$

From the partition ratio of the ion pair,

$$D_{QA} = E_{QA}[Q^+] \qquad (1.33)$$

it is rather obvious that Eq. (1.31) is enhanced by a high partition ratio.

In their study, the symbols used were as follows:

HA, A^- = chlorthalidone in protonized and unprotonized forms, respectively

Q^+ = quarternary ammonium ion

$[\ ]$, $[\ ]_{org}$ = actual concentration in the aqueous and organic phase, respectively

$$E_{QA} = \frac{[QA]_{org}}{[Q^+][A^-]} = \text{extraction constant of the ion pair QA}$$

$$D_{QA} = \frac{[QA]_{org}}{[A^-]} = E_{QA}[Q^+] = \text{partition ratio of } A^- \text{ as ion pair}$$

$$P = \frac{100}{1 + [V_{aq}/D_{QA}V_{org}]} = \text{percentage degree of extraction}$$

V_{aq}, V_{org} = volume of aqueous and organic phase, respectively

The method described for the preparation of the sample for GC analysis was as follows:

The deep-frozen sample (plasma, serum, or urine) is allowed to thaw at room temperature. After shaking, 2 ml (maximum) of the sample is weighed into a 15-ml centrifuge tube and 0.2-0.3 g of sodium hydrogen carbonate and 5.00 ml of methyl isobutyl ketone are added. The tube is shaken for 10 min. After centrifugation, 4.00 ml of the organic layer is transferred to a 15-ml centrifuge tube, 2.50 ml of 0.1 M sodium hydroxide is added, and the tube is shaken for 10 min. After centrifugation, 2.00 ml of the aqueous layer is transferred to a 15-ml centrifuge tube with a screw cap (with Teflon-faced rubber liner).

Next 50 µl of 0.1 M tetrahexylammonium hydrogen sulfate solution (neutralized with an equivalent amount of sodium hydroxide) in water and 5.00 ml of 0.5 M methyl iodide in dichloromethane are added. The tube is shaken at 50°C for 20 min. After centrifugation for 5 min at 2500 rpm, 4.00 ml of the organic layer is transferred to a 15-ml centrifuge tube with a conical bottom and evaporated to dryness at room temperature with a gentle stream of nitrogen.

To the residue, a suitable amount of hexane containing the tetraethyl derivative of chlorthalidone (the internal standard) is added. The tube is capped and placed in an ultrasonic bath for 5 min.

After centrifugation for 5 min at 2500 rpm, 1 to 2 μl of the solution are injected into the gas chromatograph using "on-column" technique.*

For the determination of chlorthalidone in plasma in nanogram quantities, the analyses were performed with a Varian 1740 gas chromatograph equipped with a 8.5 mC ^{63}Ni electron capture detector (operated at a dc electrode voltage of 90 V) and a 170-cm by 2-mm-i.d. glass column packed with 3% JXR on 100-120 mesh Gas Chrom Q and operated as follows: injector temperature, 240°C; column temperature, 240°C; detector temperature, 250°C; nitrogen carrier-gas flow rate, 40 ml/min. Capable of detecting chlorthalidone down to 2 ng/ml of plasma with a relative standard deviation below 6%, the retention times obtained for the methyl and ethyl derivatives of chlorthalidone using the above GC conditions were approximately 3.14 and 4.60 min, respectively.

C. Hydrochlorothiazide [28,344-347]

In 1975, Vanden Heuvel et al. [344] successfully applied electron-capture detection to the analysis of hydrochlorothiazide in human blood and plasma with a sensitivity (0.05 μg/ml) suitable for use with persons on therapeutic dosage levels. The main steps of a detailed procedure devised for isolation of the drug and the internal standard, the bromo analog of hydrochlorothiazide (6-bromo-3,4-dihydro-2H-1,2,4-benzothiadiazine-7-sulfonamide 1,1-dioxide) in a form suitable for GC analysis consisted of the following: (1) addition of the internal standard, (2) removal of extraneous substances with benzene extraction, (3) extraction with ethyl acetate, (4) back-titration into ammonium hydroxide, (5) adjustment to pH 3.7 and extraction with ethyl acetate, (6) evaporation of the extract to dryness, (7) dissolution of the residue in trimethylanilinium hydroxide in methanol, and (8) analysis by gas chromatography.

In this study, Vanden Heuvel et al. used a Hewlett-Packard model 7610A gas chromatograph equipped with an automatic sampler, an electron-capture detector (8 mCi ^{63}Ni, 50-μsec pulse width, 310°C), and a 1.2-m by 2.5-mm-i.d. U-shaped glass column packed with a 1% mixture of OV-1 and polycyclohexanedimethanol adipate (6:1). Operated with an argon-methane (95:5) carrier-gas flow rate of 60 ml/min and injector and column

---

*From Ervik and Gustavii [343], reproduced with permission from Analytical Chemistry.

temperatures of 280 and 235°C, respectively, the retention times of the tetramethylated derivatives of hydrochlorothiazide and the internal standard were about 14.60 and 19.25 min, respectively.

In Table 1.44 are listed the range of plasma levels (n = 3) after dosages of 50 and 100 mg of hydrochlorothiazide as well as drug blood levels (n = 1) for a patient receiving a 50-mg dose.

Lindstrom et al. [345] reported in 1975 a GC procedure for the determination of hydrochlorothiazide in plasma, blood corpuscles, and urine using an extractive alkylation technique which has been described previously for the diuretics chlorthalidone [343] and furosemide [349]. The analytical data were obtained with a Varian 1400 gas chromatograph equipped with a ^{63}Ni electron-capture detector (300°C) for plasma and blood

TABLE 1.44

Hydrochlorothiazide Levels in Plasma and Blood[a]

Number of subjects	Dose (mg)	Hours (postdose)	Range of plasma levels (μg/ml)	Blood level (μg/ml)
1	50	1.5		0.36
		2.0		0.51
		3.0		0.62
		4.0		0.64
		6.0		0.44
		24.0		0.10
3	50	1.5	0.05-0.23	
		2.0	0.11-0.35	
		3.0	0.28-0.29	
		4.0	0.18-0.24	
3	100	1.5	0.15-0.71	
		2.0	0.34-0.51	
		3.0	0.33-0.43	
		4.0	0.22-0.35	

[a]Adapted from Vanden Heuvel et al. [344].

corpuscle specimens, whereas a Packard-Becker 409 gas chromatograph equipped with a flame ionization detector (270°C) was employed for urine samples. With both instruments, similar operating conditions and columns were used: 1.5-m by 2-mm-i.d. silanized glass column packed with 1% Sephadex SE-30 on 80-100 mesh Gas Chrom Q; injector temperature, 230°C; column temperature, 225°C; nitrogen carrier-gas flow rate, 30 to 40 ml/min.

In their procedure, chlorthalidone is added as an internal standard to plasma or urine samples before the extractions are performed; derivatization of the drug and internal standard is accomplished by the use of tetrahexylammonium hydrogen sulfate in the presence of methyl iodide in dichloromethane. In the case of samples prepared from blood corpuscles, the internal standard is added after one extraction. Using the above instruments and operating conditions, the retention times of the methylated derivatives of chlorthalidone and hydrochlorothiazide were approximately 4.2 and 5.2 min, respectively.

The recovery of hydrochlorothiazide and chlorthalidone extracted from an aqueous phase into 4-methyl-2-pentanone (checked with ^{14}C-labeled hydrochlorothiazide) at pH 6 was about 91% after one extraction for each compound with the minimum amount of hydrochlorothiazide that could be quantitatively determined being just slightly below 10 ng/ml for plasma (2 to 3 ng/ml if 3 ml of plasma were extracted).

Using a GC procedure similar to that proposed by Lindstrom et al. [349], Beermann et al. [346] were concerned with the absorption, metabolism, and excretion of hydrochlorothiazide. An abstract of their findings contained the following:

^{14}C-Hydrochlorothiazide was administered orally (n = 4) and i.v. (n = 2) to healthy subjects. The gastrointestinal absorption ranged between 60 and 80%, most of it took place in the duodenum and the upper jejunum. The radioactivity was eliminated mainly in the urine, while no significant biliary excretion was observed. Chromatographic analysis of the urinary radioactivity demonstrated that > 95% of the absorbed or injected ^{14}C-hydrochlorothiazide was excreted unchanged. The radioactivity in plasma during the first 10 hr after oral administration declined with a fast phase but the levels of label thereafter suggested a slower phase. The existence of such a phase was verified in one subject given 75 mg of hydrochlorothiazide orally. His plasma levels of hydrochlorothiazide (determined by GC) declined according to a two-compartment model, the half-lives of the α- and β-phases being 1.7 and 13.1 hr, respectively. Hydrochlorothiazide accumulated in the blood cells and the ratio between the radioactivity in cells and that in plasma averaged 3.5. The fate of a single dose of ^{14}C-hydrochlorothiazide in two hypertensive patients treated with the

drug chronically was similar to that in the healthy subjects. A third
patient, who had slightly elevated serum creatinine, eliminated
hydrochlorothiazide more slowly than the others. Like the healthy
subjects, the patients eliminated hydrochlorothiazide to >95% in
unchanged form.

D. Bumetanide [347,348]

In 1973, Feit et al. [347] developed a GC procedure for the determination
and urinary recovery of butetamide (3-n-butylamino-4-phenoxy-5-sulfa-
mylbenzoic acid), a potent "high-ceiling" diuretic, based on flash-heater
methylation. In this method, a mixture of tetramethylammonium hydroxide
and trimethylanilinium hydroxide was advantageously used as the methylation reagent. The procedure used to prepare urinary samples for GC
analysis was as follows:

Urine, 5 to 10 ml, was adjusted to pH 2 by addition of 1 N hydrochloric acid. Then 20 μl of internal reference solution (25 μg of
4-benzyl-3-n-butylamino-5-sulfamylbenzoic acid/ml in ether) and
15 ml of ether were added, and the mixture was shaken in a separator for 2 min. The organic layer was washed with three 5-ml portions of water and then filtered into a tapered centrifuge tube (10 ml)
through a small cotton plug, previously washed with ether, and
covered with a thin layer of anhydrous sodium sulfate. Then 50 μl
of methylation reagent (two parts of an approximately 1 M aqueous
solution of trimethylanilinium hydroxide mixed with one volume of a
10% methanolic solution of tetramethylammonium hydroxide solution)
was added, and the tube was shaken for 2 min. After centrifugation,
1 to 2 μl of the aqueous layer was injected into the gas chromatograph.

Feit et al. used for their GC determinations a Perkin-Elmer model 900
gas chromatograph equipped with a flame ionization detector and a 2-m by
3.3-mm-o.d. stainless steel column packed with 1.5% OV-17 coated on
100-120 mesh Diatomite CQ. Using the specified operating conditions
(injector temperature, 370°C; column temperature, 270°C; detector temperature, 300°C; nitrogen carrier-gas flow rate, 30 ml/min), the retention
times of methylated bumetamide and internal standard (sequence of reactions during flash-heater methylation of bumetanide given below) were
about 12.0 and 16.4 min, respectively.

In the methylation reaction sequence given below, compounds II, III, and
IV were identified as methyl 3-n-butylamino-5-dimethylsulfamyl-4-
phenoxybenzoic acid, methyl 3-(N-n-butylanilino)-5-dimethylsulfamyl-
4-hydroxybenzoic acid, and methyl 3-(N-n-butylanilino)-5-dimethylsulfamyl-
4-methoxbenzoic acid, respectively. As shown, formation of IV involves

Smiles rearrangement and methylation of the intermediate phenolic hydroxyl of III.

Capable of detecting concentrations as low as 0.1 µg/ml of human urine with recoveries of bumetanide added to urine samples (between 0.1 and 0.5 µg/ml) ranging from 90 to 105%, the mean urinary excretion in healthy volunteers during the periods of collection following oral administration of 0.5 and 1.0 mg bumetanide is shown in Table 1.45 as well as the urinary excretion of electrolytes using standard procedures. Over the total period of response, a parallelism is shown between bumetanide excretion and saluretic action.

In 1974, using the GC procedure developed by Feit et al. [347], Davies et al. [348] studied the diuretic activity of bumetanide in 16 normal subjects and 40 hospitalized patients with fluid retention. Based on analytical data, they noted that "the drug produced a rapid diuretic response with a pattern of salt and water excretion resembling that of furosemide. At the time of maximal natriuresis, which amounted to 13 to 23% of the filtered load of sodium, urinary calcium and magnesium also increased. Urinary urate was unchanged in the first 2 hr after bumetanide, following which there was a phase of urate retention. Free water clearance during maximal hydration was not significantly altered. Comparative studies in edematous patients showed that 1 mg of bumetanide was equivalent to 60 mg of furosemide. Oral doses of 15 mg of bumetanide evoked effective diuresis without adverse effects in three edematous patients with advanced renal disease. Prolonged therapy over 7 to 14 weeks with daily doses of 0.25 to 4 mg of bumetanide plus potassium supplements controlled edema in 12 patients; asymptomatic hyperuricemia occurred in most, and decreased carbohydrate tolerance in one. There was no evidence of significant metabolism of bumetanide in vivo. The drug was distributed in a

TABLE 1.45

Mean Urinary Excretion in Healthy Volunteers During the Periods of Collection Following Oral Administration of 0.5 and 1 mg of Bumetanide[a]

Excretion[b]	0-6 hr			6-24 hr			0-24 hr		
	Control[c]	0.5 mg	1 mg	Control[c]	0.5 mg	1 mg	Control[c]	0.5 mg	1 mg
Bumetanide (μg)		166.7	404.3		10.0	23.2		176.7	427.5
		±9.9	±39.5		±4.2	±6.0		±8.9	±35.1
Sodium (meq)	53.7	131.1	188.5	99.7	62.5	41.7	153.3	193.5	230.2
	±12.6	±23.7	±22.7	±11.0	±11.0	±5.7	±21.6	±34.2	±23.0
Potassium (meq)	28.2	45.7	51.0	40.0	41.0	34.0	68.2	86.7	85.0
	±2.0	±3.4	±5.1	±5.7	±7.2	±7.4	±6.3	±8.1	±11.3
Chloride (meq)	65.0	159.0	219.7	80.2	49.2	24.7	145.2	208.2	244.3
	±11.8	±20.4	±18.8	±11.4	±10.7	±3.4	±22.4	±28.9	±20.0
Volume (ml)	442.8	1469.2	2042.5	834.2	805.0	546.7	1277.0	2274.2	2589.2
	±49.5	±90.6	±156.2	±93.4	±134.7	±69.9	±113.1	±135.9	±177.9

[a] From Feit et al. [347], courtesy of the Journal of Pharmaceutical Sciences.
[b] Values represent the mean ±SD for six volunteers.
[c] Mean values calculated from the day before administration.

"central" compartment of approximately 5 liters. The overall elimination rate constant was high and indicated that despite rapid renal drug clearance, a substantial part of injected drug left the central compartment by one or more extrarenal routes.

E. Furosemide [349,350]

In 1974, Lindstrom and Molander [349] developed a GC method for the determination of furosemide in plasma using an extractive alkylation technique and an electron-capture detector. Analogous to the procedure described for chlorthalidone [343], the preparation of the sample for GC analysis consisted of diluting a 1-ml plasma sample with 2 ml of water, and then acidifying with 0.15 ml of 4 M HCl. Following the extraction of the mixture with two 5-ml aliquots of diethyl ether and centrifugation, the ether phases are combined and transferred to a screw-capped tube. To the residue resulting from the evaporation of the solvent with a stream of nitrogen, 2 ml of 0.2 M NaOH solution, 50 μl of 0.1 M tetrahexylammonium hydrogen sulfate solution, and 5.0 ml of 0.5 M methyl iodide in dichloromethane were added. This mixture was then shaken for 20 min at 50°C and, after centrifugation, 4.0 ml of the organic phase were transferred to another tube and evaporated to dryness at room temperature under a flow of nitrogen. To the residue was added 0.2 ml of the internal standard solution (concentration of triethyl derivative of furosemide in n-hexane not specified); this resulting solution was then placed in an ultrasonic bath for 5 min and, after centrifugation, 5 μl were withdrawn and injected into the gas chromatograph.

Quantitative analyses were obtained using a Packard-Becker model 409 gas chromatograph equipped with a ^{63}Ni electron-capture detector and 1.8-m by 2-mm-i.d. glass columns packed with 3% JXR coated on 100-120 mesh Gas Chrom Q. Using injector, column, and detector temperatures of 260, 245, and 275°C, respectively (carrier gas and its flow rate not specified), the retention times of trimethylfurosemide and the internal standard (triethylfurosemide) were about 4.19 and 5.81 min, respectively. Under the GC operating conditions used, the method was capable of determining furosemide down to 0.1 μg/ml of plasma. On the other hand, the extraction of furosemide from plasma, according to the procedure described above, yielded 98% of the substance in the organic phase after one extraction. Furthermore, in the range investigated (0.3 to 5.4 μg/ml), the calibration curve (prepared by plotting the ratio of peak areas of the peaks of trimethylfurosemide and the internal standard versus furosemide concentration) was linear.

Using the GC procedure of Lindstrom and Molander [349] with modification (1% SE-30, 1-m column operated at 220°C; injector temperature,

230°C; detector temperature, 300°C) and high-performance liquid chromatography, Beermann et al. [350] investigated the elimination of furosemide in healthy subjects and in those with renal failure.

In their study, "furosemide was administered intravenously to 5 healthy volunteers and 15 patients with various degrees of renal failure. Two patients were given the drug orally. The plasma half-life of furosemide averaged 0.79 hr in the healthy subjects. Although most patients with kidney disease had a prolonged half-life ($t_{1/2}$), up to 24.58 hr, some with advanced renal failure had an almost normal $t_{1/2}$. The plasma clearance of furosemide, which in the normal subjects averaged 194 ml/min, decreased proportionally with decreasing creatinine clearance, as did the renal clearance, which in the healthy subjects averaged 95 ml/min. There was no correlation between kidney function and the apparent volume of distribution or of nonrenal clearance. One patient was given ^{35}S-labeled furosemide intravenously. Although the furosemide plasma $t_{1/2}$ was essentially normal, the elimination rate of metabolites was decreased. Unlike that of healthy subjects, the main route of excretion of label was in the feces."

With regard to pharmacokinetic calculations, the elimination rate constant (k) of the terminal portion of the plasma concentration/time curve for furosemide was determined by least-squares regression analysis; the area under the furosemide plasma concentration/time curve (AUC_∞) being estimated by the trapezoidal rule and extrapolated to infinity.

The apparent volume of distribution (V_d) was obtained by

$$V_d = \frac{dose}{AUC_\infty} \times k \qquad (1.34)$$

The plasma clearance (Cl_p) was calculated as

$$Cl_p = \frac{dose}{AUC} \qquad (1.35)$$

On the other hand, Beermann et al. estimated the renal clearance of furosemide by dividing the urinary recovery by the area under the plasma concentration versus time curve during the corresponding time.

F. Tienilic Acid [351]

In 1976, Desager et al. [351] described a GC procedure for the determination of tienilic acid {[2,3-dichloro-4-(2-thienyl)phenoxy]-acetic acid}, a diuretic with uricosuric properties, in human urine and plasma. Related to ethacrynic acid, in which the ketone function is linked to the 2-position of a thiophene ring, the compound is chromatographed as its methyl ester (diazomethane used as methylating reagent). For its determination in plasma and urine, 2-chloro-10-(3'-dimethylaminopropyl)-phenothiazine-S-oxide and cholesterol were used as internal standards, respectively.

For the determination of tienilic acid (TA) in plasma, the extraction procedure used was as follows:

> To a 20-ml stoppered tube were added successively 0.5 ml of plasma, 0.5 ml of distilled water, 0.5 ml of 3 N HCl, and 10 ml of diethyl ether. After manual extraction for 30 sec and separation of the two layers, 8 ml of the upper layer were transferred to a second tube. To this extract, 1 ml of ethereal diazomethane were added and the mixture was allowed to stand for 15 min. Evaporation on a Rotavapor without warming afforded the residue for the GC analysis. Before injection, solubilization was effected with 1 ml of methanol containing 4.6 or 10 μg of internal standard (the S-oxide compound) and 4 μl were injected into the gas chromatograph.

On the other hand, TA was extracted from urine as follows:

> In a 60-ml stoppered flask, 1 ml of methanolic cholesterol solution (75 μg/ml) was evaporated to dryness. To the residue, a 2-ml urine sample, 2 ml of 3 N HCl, and 10 ml of diethyl ether were added. After manual extraction for 1 min and separation of the two phases, 8 ml of the upper phase were transferred to a second tube. This extract was evaporated to dryness and the residue was mixed with 2 ml of methanol-diethyl ether (1:9, v/v) and methylated with 2 ml of ethereal diazomethane. After 15 min, a final evaporation afforded the residue for the GC analysis. After addition of 2 ml of light petroleum (B.P. 40-60°C), 8 μl were injected into the gas chromatograph.

In their investigation, two different GC instruments were used to determine TA in plasma and urine. For the analysis of the plasma extract, the determination of TA was performed with a Varian model 2100 gas chromatograph equipped with an electron-capture detector (^{3}H-Sc) and a 5-ft by 2-mm-i.d. U-shaped glass column packed with 3% OV-225 coated on acid-washed, DMCS-treated Chromosorb W-HP (mesh size not specified). To obtain retention times of 3.0 and 2.0 min for the internal standard (S-oxide compound) and the methyl ester of TA, respectively, the following GC conditions were maintained: injector temperature, 280°C; column temperature, 262°C; detector temperature, 285°C; ^{3}H-Sc foil temperature, 267°C; nitrogen carrier-gas flow rate, 45 ml/min. Using peak height ratio measurements, the recovery of TA from plasma was 95 ± 3%, whereas the sensitivity was approximately 50 ng/ml.

With regard to the analysis of TA in urine, Desager et al. used a Pye 104 gas chromatograph equipped with a flame ionization detector and a 5-ft by 4-mm-i.d. coiled glass column packed with 3% OV-225 on AW-DMCC-treated Chromosorb W-HP. With the specified instrument settings (injector temperature, 295°C; column temperature, 280°C; detector temperature, 310°C; nitrogen carrier-gas flow rate, 60 ml/min), the retention times for cholesterol (internal standard) and the methyl derivative of TA were 2.35 and 3.20 min, respectively; these GC conditions permitting TA to be detected in urine down to a level of 1 μg/ml.

When applied to the analysis of TA administered to a volunteer, the first results showed that the drug is rapidly cleared from the plasma (half-life = 1.5 hr) and is highly transformed (18% recovery from 24-hr urine).

G. Spironolactone [62,352,353]

Since the metabolism of spironolactone is rather extensive (see Fig. 1.55), investigators [352,353] have concentrated on the analysis of one of its primary metabolites (aldadiene or canrenone) in human plasma [352] or urine [352,353].

In 1971, Chamberlain [352] developed a specific and sensitive GC method for the determination of aldadiene in human plasma and urine after therapeutic doses of spironolactone. Sample preparation for GC analysis from both biological media consisted of the following:

1. Urine sample: To each analysis tube was added 200 μl of the internal standard solution (androst-4-ene-3,6,17-trione, 1 μg/ml in ethanol), 5 ml of urine, and 5 ml of dichloromethane with shaking after each addition. After the layers were allowed to separate, the upper aqueous phase was removed and the organic extract (lower phase) washed again with 1 ml of water, dried by filtration through Whatman no. 1 filter paper, and evaporated to dryness. The residue was dissolved in 1 ml of methanol and a 10- to 15-μl aliquot was withdrawn and used for GC analysis.

2. Plasma sample: The procedure was the same as above except that 1 ml of plasma was used and 0.25% NaOH added also to the tube containing the internal standard.

The extracts with the internal standard were analyzed with a Pye 104 gas chromatograph equipped with a ^{63}Ni electron-capture detector and a 1.5-m by 4-mm-i.d. silanized glass column packed with 2% OV-1 coated on 80-100 mesh CQ solid support. Using a column temperature and nitrogen carrier-gas flow rate of 250°C and 120 ml/min, respectively (no other

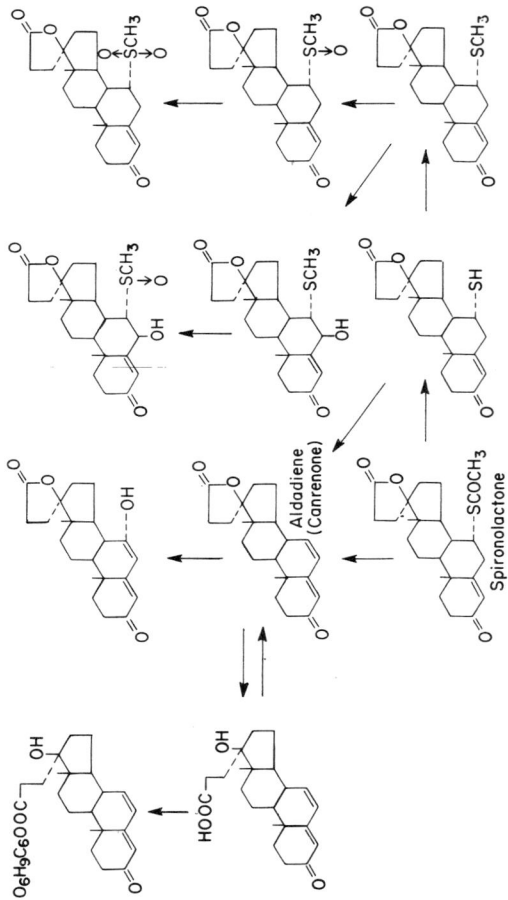

Figure 1.55. Metabolism of spironolactone.

GC conditions specified), the retention times of androst-4-ene-3,6,17-trione and aldadiene were approximately 4.0 and 12.0 min, respectively. Using the extraction procedures discussed above, the mean recovery of aldadiene added to urine and plasma was 96% (range, 89 to 101%) with a standard deviation of ±4%.

Based on plasma and urine specimens collected from male volunteers who ingested 100 mg of spironolactone (blood samples drawn at 0, 0.5, 1, 2, 4, 6, and 24 hr; urine samples collected at 0, 2, 4, 6, and 24 hr), Chamberlain noted that plasma levels of aldadiene reached a peak of 10 to 15 µg/100 ml about 3 hr after spironolactone administration with urinary excretion of the metabolite reflecting the plasma levels; about 4 mg being excreted in the 24 hr after the 100-mg dose.

Feher et al. [353] in 1976 proposed a simple GC method with flame detection for the determination of aldadiene in human urine. The extraction procedure was rather simple:

To a 10-ml aliquot of 24-hr urine, 10.0 µg of Δ^1-testololactone (TL, D-homo-17α-oxaandrosta-1,4-diene-3,17-dione) was added as internal standard, and the urine was extracted with 10 ml of diethyl ether. The extract was washed with 1 ml of 10% NaOH solution and two 1-ml volumes of water, dried over anhydrous Na_2SO_4, and evaporated to dryness. The residue was transferred with small volumes of ether into a capillary tube, the solution evaporated to dryness, and the residue redissolved in exactly 10 µl of dioxane.

Quantitative measurements of 0.2- to 1.0 µl aliquots of the above solution were performed with a Pye-Unicam series 104 gas chromatograph equipped with a flame ionization detector and a 1.5-m by 4-mm-i.d. glass column packed with 1% SE-30 on 80-100 mesh Diatomit CQ. With the specified GC operating conditions (injector temperature, not specified; column temperature, 230°C; detector temperature, 260°C; nitrogen carrier-gas flow rate, 60 ml/min), the retention time of aldadiene relative to the internal standard was 1.94, whereas the recoveries of aldadiene and internal standard from urine were 70.8 ± 1.8% and 71.4 ± 1.4%, respectively, in 12 determinations following addition of 0.1- to 1.0 µg/ml amounts to urine specimens. Having a lower limit of detection of about 20 ng, the average recovery of aldadiene excreted in 24-hr urines during three consecutive days following administration of 200 mg of spironolactone as a single dose to four subjects was 3.52 ± 0.31%.

VI. ANTISCLEROSIS (ANTIHYPERLIPIDEMIA) DRUGS

The three major drugs in this category investigated by gas chromatographic techniques are illustrated in Figure 1.56.

A. Clofibrate [28,58,59,62,354-367,369]

As early as 1970, Silvestri [354] developed a GC method for the determination of clofibrate (ethyl p-chlorophenoxyisobutyrate) in biological fluids that relied on the extraction of the drug from acidified plasma into a mixture of diethyl ether-light petroleum. After washing, drying over sodium sulfate, and evaporation of the mixed solvent, the residue was subjected to GC analysis on a 5% butanediol succinate column. With regard to clofibrate itself, it was noted that the residue was esterified after adsorption on Amberlite IRA-400 resin by treatment with dry HCl in methanol. Although chromatograms of the chemicals were given, those of biological extracts were not illustrated in the report.

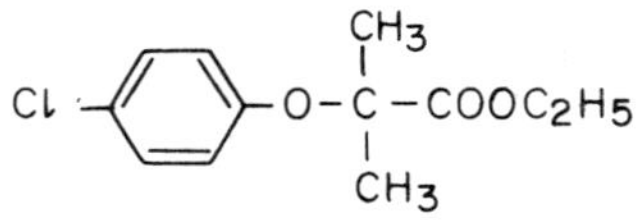

Clofibrate

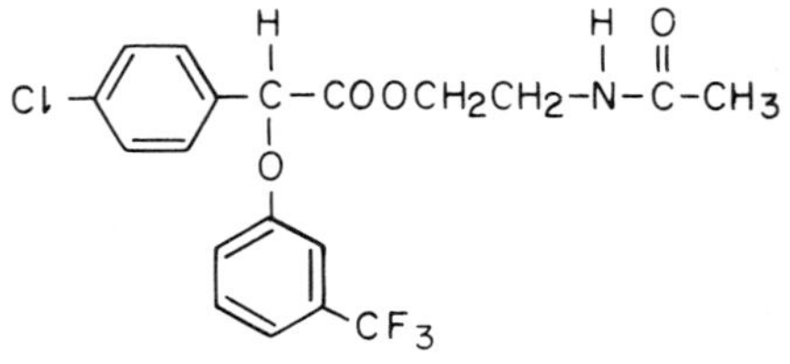

Halofenate

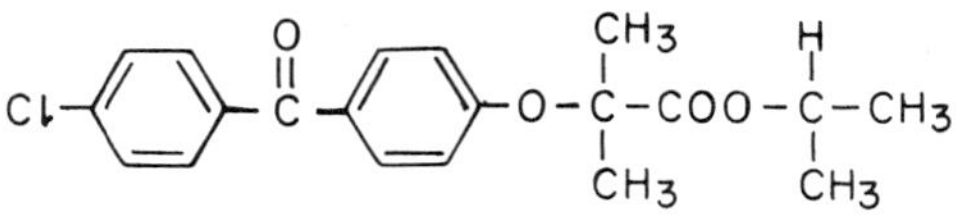

Procetofene

Figure 1.56. Structures of several antisclerosis drugs.

ANTISCLEROSIS (ANTIHYPERLIPIDEMIA) DRUGS 219

Qualitatively, Finkle and co-workers [28,58], Foltz et al. [62], and Moffat [59] examined clofibrate by gas chromatography as well as integrated GC-MS.

Whereas Finkle et al. [28] noted that clofibrate yielded a RRT of 0.50 using column system I, Moffat [59] included clofibrate among the 480 drugs examined with SE-30 columns, reporting for it a retention index of 1560. On the other hand, using the GC-MS system previously discussed in this chapter, Finkle et al. [58] listed clofibrate via the alphabetical index as shown below:

```
CLOFIBRATE
MOL. WT.  242      BASE PEAK 128
    41  59  75  87  99 111 128 141    0 169    0    0    0    0 242
   244   0   0   0   0   0   0   0    0   0    0    0    0    0   0
```

In addition to the EI-MS spectral data listed for clofibrate, Foltz et al. [62] recorded methane CI-MS data for this compound as indicated below:

Clofibrate EI-MS Data

Prominent fragment ions > m/e 30
128 (100), 130 (32), 169 (21), 87 (55), 169 (27)

Methane CI-MS Data

M.W.	MH^+ (RI)	Prominent fragment ions > m/e 50
242	243 (100)	115 (78), 87 (55), 169 (27)

Horning et al. [355] studied the effect of chronic administration of ethyl p-chlorophenoxyisobutyrate (CPIB) on the excretion of bile lipids in four dogs with surgically implanted Thomas cannulae for periods of 2 to 7 months and also measured the concentration of cholesterol, triglycerides, and p-chlorophenoxyisobutyric acid (CPIBA) in serum and of bile acids, cholesterol, and phospholipids (phosphatidyl cholines) in bile.

In serum, CPIBA concentrations were determined by GC as the trimethylsilyl (TMSi) derivative whose structure was confirmed by integrated GC-MS.

Sample preparation prior to GC analysis consisted of the following:

One milliliter of serum was diluted to 20 ml with glass-distilled water, and after adjusting the pH to 4.0-4.5 with acetic acid, the

$$Cl-\underset{}{\bigcirc}-O-\underset{CH_3}{\overset{CH_3}{\underset{|}{\overset{|}{C}}}}-COOH$$

p−Chlorophenoxybutyric Acid
(CPIBA)

sample was transferred to a 10-cm by 1-cm DEAE-Sephadex column. Neutral and basic fractions, including proteins, were washed from the column with water, and the acids were eluted with a solution of 150 ml of 1.5 M pyridine-acetic acid. After lyophilization the residue was transferred with methanol to a graduated centrifuge tube; the volume of methanol was reduced to approximately 0.2 ml with a nitrogen stream. The solution was transferred quantitatively to a 1-ml vial; 10 μl of pyridine was added, and the solution was evaporated (nitrogen stream). The pyridine salt of CPIBA was redissolved in 50 μl of pyridine, and 100 μl of bis-(trimethylsilyl)trifluoroacetamide was added. The contents of the vial were mixed (Vortex mixer) and allowed to stand overnight.

For quantitative work, an internal standard (methyl myristate) was added to the sample.

Horning et al. performed the chromatographic separations using Barber-Colman model 5000 gas chromatographs equipped with two different column systems: system A for the analysis of bile acids; 6-ft by 3.4-mm-i.d. U-shaped columns packed with 1% SE-30 or 1% OV-17 on 100-120 mesh Gas Chrom P; injector temperature 260°C; column temperature programmed from 200°C at 1°C/min; detector temperature 300°C; carrier gas and its flow rate not specified; system B for the analysis of the TMSi derivative of CPIBA; 12-ft by 3.4-mm-i.d. W-shaped glass column packed with 5% SE-30 on 80-100 mesh Gas Chrom P; injector temperature 260°C; column temperature programmed from 100°C at 2°C/min; detector temperature 300°C; carrier gas and its flow rate not given.

Confirmational and mass spectral studies were carried out with a LKB 9000 integrated GC-MS instrument equipped with a 9-ft by 3.4-mm-i.d. coiled glass column packed with 1% OV-17 or 1% SE-30 on 100-120 mesh Gas Chrom P. The other conditions specified were accelerating voltage, 70 eV; current, 60 μA; ion source temperature, 250°C.

For the separation and derivatization of the bile acids, 50 ml of a chloroform:methanol solution (2:1) were added to a separatory funnel containing a 1-ml sample of bile and 10 ml of distilled water, the mixture was then shaken vigorously for 10 min, and finally placed in a cold room (4°C) overnight to complete the separation of the two phases. Following the separation of the upper water-methanol layer containing the bile salts and its concentration at 40°C via a rotary evaporator by the removal of most of the alcohol, the water was removed by lyophilization.

To prepare the sample for GC analysis, Horning et al. used the following procedure:

> The residue was dissolved in glass-distilled water and hydrolyzed enzymatically with cholylglycine hydrolase. To an aliquot (0.10 ml) of the lophilized methanol phase there was added 0.1 ml of sodium acetate solution (0.1 M, pH 5.6), 0.2 ml of EDTA solution (1.86% of the disodium salt), 0.10 ml of 0.2 M Cleland's reagent, and 0.1 ml of enzyme. The reaction mixture was incubated at 37°C for 30 min and then acidified with 0.5 ml of glacial acetic acid. The bile acids were extracted four times with 4-ml portions of benzene-acetone (2:1). The combined benzene-acetone extracts were taken to dryness under reduced pressure (rotary evaporator); the residue was dissolved in 0.5 ml of methanol. The overall recovery of cholic acid-^{14}C from taurocholic acid (carbonyl-^{14}C) added to bile was $90 \pm 4\%$.
>
> The bile acids were converted to methyl ester-trimethylsilyl (ME-TMSi) derivatives for analysis by gas chromatography. An ethereal solution of diazomethane was added to the methanolic solution (0.5 ml) of bile acids until the yellow color persisted. After standing at room temperature for 30 min, the excess ether, methanol, and diazomethane were removed with a nitrogen stream. The residue of bile acid methyl esters was dissolved in 0.1 ml of pyridine and 0.1 ml of bis(trimethylsilyl)trifluoroacetamide or N-trimethylsilylimidazole and 0.05 ml of trimethylchlorosilane was added. The mixture was allowed to stand overnight at room temperature to ensure complete silylation of all hydroxyl groups. An aliquot of the solution was analyzed directly by gas chromatography.

Using the GC conditions described above, a typical GC analysis of the acid fraction isolated from plasma of Dog 530 is shown in Figure 1.57, whereas the chromatogram of urinary acids isolated from the urine of a dog treated with CPIB is illustrated in Figure 1.58.

Based on their findings, Horning et al. concluded that chronic administration of CPIB resulted in a marked increase in the concentration of cholesterol, bile acids, and phosphatidyl cholines in the bile of all dogs, and a decrease in serum cholesterol and triglyceride concentration in serum in three of the four dogs. Serum concentrations of CPIBA were monitored to ensure the presence of the drug in the dogs; however, no correlation between serum levels of CPIBA and the concentration of biliary lipids was noted.

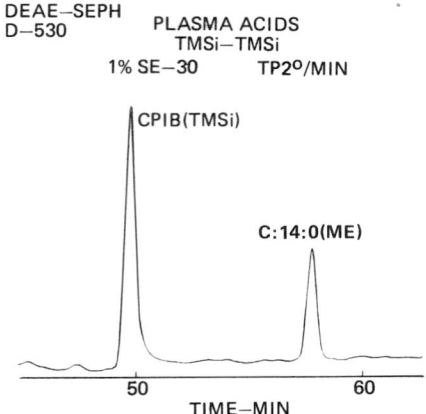

Figure 1.57. Gas chromatographic analysis of the acid fraction isolated from plasma of Dog 530. The major metabolite of CPIB, p-chlorophenoxyisobutyric acid, was separated as the trimethylsilyl ester derivative; the internal standard was methyl myristate (C:14:0, ME). The separation was carried out with a 12-ft 5% SE-30 column with temperature programming at 2°C/min from 100°C. From Horning et al. [355], courtesy of Lipids.

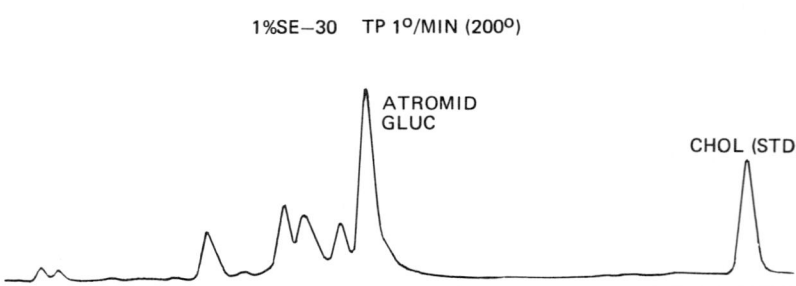

Figure 1.58. Gas chromatographic (GC) analysis of urinary acids isolated from the urine of a dog treated with ethyl p-chlorophenoxyisobutyrate (CPIB). The acids were separated as the methyl ester-trimethylsilyl ether derivatives. Separation was carried out on a 12-ft 1% SE-30 column by temperature programming at 1°C/min from 200°C. The ester glucuronide of CPIB acid (ATROMID GLUC) was separated by GC as the intact glucuronide. The structure was confirmed by GC-MS techniques. From Horning et al. [355], courtesy of Lipids.

In 1974, Sedaghat et al. [357] described a specific and sensitive method for the detection of clofibrate (CPIB) in biological fluids (plasma, urine, bile, and feces) as the free acid (CPIBA).

The procedure recommended for extraction and derivatization of CPIBA were as follows:

One milliliter of plasma, urine, or bile or 1 g of feces was mixed with 10 ml of methanol in a 125-ml glass-stoppered bottle, and 200 µl of the internal recovery standard (methyl ester of p-chlorophenoxypropionic acid, 260 µg/200 µl methanol) was added. This mixture was refluxed for 1 hour with 1 ml of 10 N NaOH in order to hydrolyze any conjugated CPIB that might be present.

After cooling, the mixture was acidified with 1 ml of concentrated HCl. Twenty milliliters of chloroform and 30 ml of chloroform:methanol (2:1) were then added successively, and the mixture was shaken for 1 min; 10 ml of water was added and the shaking was continued for 1 min. After centrifugation (5 min at 1000g), the lower phase containing CPIBA and CPP (p-chlorophenoxypropionic acid) was transferred to a 500-ml round-bottomed flask. Twenty milliliters of chloroform was added to the upper phase, and the procedure was repeated twice in order to assure a quantitative transfer. The combined lower phases were evaporated to dryness with a rotary evaporator.

Five milliliters of 5% HCl-methanol was added to the dried residue and the mixture was left overnight; the methyl esters were concentrated by rotary evaporation. Because of the volatility of the methyl esters of CPIBA and CPP, the evaporation must be carried out at room temperature; care must be taken to stop the evaporation as soon as the residue appears dry.

After dissolving the above residue in chloroform:methanol (2:1), the esters were quantitatively transferred to TLC plates where a clean separation of the methyl esters of CPIBA and CPP from the other fatty acids was possible. The portion of the plate corresponding to the CPIBA-CPP esters was recovered and the solutes were eluted into a 100-ml round-bottomed flask. Following the addition of 200 µl of internal standard (methyl ester of arachidic acid, 140 µg/200 µl of methanol), the mixture was cautiously evaporated to dryness and redissolved in 1 ml of methanol.

For GC analysis, a 5-µl aliquot was withdrawn and injected into a F&M model 400 gas chromatograph equipped with a hydrogen flame ionization detector and a 6-ft by 4-mm-i.d. glass column packed with 10% EGSS-X on Gas Chrom Q. Using the specified GC conditions (injector temperature, 220°C; nitrogen carrier-gas flow rate, 24 ml/min), the retention times of the methyl esters of CPIBA, CPP, and arachidic acid were about 8.83, 12.50, and 16.50 min, respectively.

Capable of detecting clofibrate at levels less than 10 µg/ml of plasma, urine, or bile or per gram of feces, recovery of the drug is greater than 90% from urine and plasma and greater than 80% from feces and bile.

In 1975, Karmen and Haut [359] also developed an assay for CPIBA in serum based on gas chromatography of its methyl ester. Two internal standards (chlorophenoxyacetic acid and p-chlorophenoxypropionic acid), similar in chemical structure to CPIBA, are added; the compounds are extracted, converted to methyl esters with diazomethane as methylating reagent, and analyzed by GC using an alkali flame ionization detector selectively sensitive to halogen.

Extraction of the drug from serum and its subsequent derivatization is accomplished as follows:

> One hundred micrograms of CPP and 500 µg of CPA in 0.1 ml of acetone are added to 1.0 ml of serum in a 15-ml test tube. The serum is then acidified with 1 ml of 1 N H_2SO_4, and extracted three times with 5 ml of diethyl ether. The extracts are combined in another 15-ml test tube over 0.1 g of anhydrous Na_2SO_4 to remove water and the combined extract is decanted into a second tube. Two milliliters of alcohol-free diazomethane are added, and the solution is allowed to stand for 5 min at room temperature. Then 0.2 ml of isooctane are added and the solution is carefully concentrated to 0.2 ml by evaporation with a stream of nitrogen. One- to three-microliter aliquots of the concentrate are then injected into the GC column.

GC separations were carried out with a Packard model 802 gas chromatograph equipped with a dual-flame, alkali flame ionization detector (FID-AFID), and 183-cm by 4-mm glass columns packed with 10% ethylene glycol adipate polyester (EGA) on 80-100 mesh Chromosorb W or 3% SE-30 on 80-100 mesh Supelcoport. Although no GC operating parameters were listed, chromatograms were shown which indicated the retention times of the methyl esters of CPIBA, CPP, and CPA to be about 12.90, 13.35, and 16.60 min, respectively, on the 10% EGA column, whereas their respective retention times with the SE-30 column were 0.47, 0.42, and 0.45 min. With recovery of CPIBA close to 90%, Karmen and Haut noted that the serum CPIBA levels in three persons at intervals after administration of a 2-g oral dose could be conveniently assayed; the CPIBA results of one subject based on the use of each standard with the AFID detector are listed in Table 1.46.

Gugler, Shoeman, Huffman, Cohlmia, and Azarnoff [360] studied the pharmacokinetics of three drugs (clofibrate, antipyrine, and diphenylhydantoin) in patients with hypoalbuminemia secondary to the nephrotic syndrome, but with relatively normal renal function, since the binding of

TABLE 1.46

Serum CPIBA Concentrations Following Oral Administration[a,b]

Hours after 2-g dose of clofibrate	AFID	
	CPP standard	CPA standard
Patient I: 75 kg		
1	19.2 ± 0.8	16.2 ± 2.2
2	39.8 ± 6.4	39.4 ± 5.2
3	46.8 ± 3.2	48.2 ± 11.9
4	54.8 ± 1.5	49.4 ± 0.8
6	63.8 ± 5.8	62.4 ± 0.4
12	99.2 ± 19.2	79.4 ± 6.7
24	68.7 ± 11.3	69.0 ± 15.0

[a] Adapted from Karmen and Haut [359].
[b] CPIBA concentration in micrograms per milliliter of serum.

drugs to plasma proteins can significantly alter the intensity of pharmacological and toxicological effects of drugs. Since clofibrate, during absorption and in plasma, is rapidly hydrolyzed to CPIBA, CPIBA and CPIBA-glucuronide were determined using a Barber-Colman model 5000 gas chromatograph equipped with a flame ionization detector and 6-ft columns packed with 3% SE-30 coated on 80-100 mesh Gas Chrom Q.

For GC analysis of CPIBA, Gugler et al. isolated the drug from plasma or urine in the following manner:

To 1 ml of plasma or urine, 1 ml of 0.5 N HCl was added and the CPIBA extracted into 8 ml of chloroform. After shaking and centrifuging the sample, the aqueous layer was aspirated and 7 ml of the organic layer was transferred to another tube and evaporated to dryness. The residue was dissolved in 1 ml of freshly prepared 0.5% K_2CO_3 in methanol (w/v) and 0.1 ml of dimethyl sulfate added. Methylation was achieved by heating the mixture for 10 min in a water bath at 70°C. After addition of 1 ml of 0.2 M acetate buffer, pH 5.6, the CPIBA was extracted into 8 ml of chloroform containing clofibrate as an internal standard (1 µg/ml). After shaking, centrifugation, and aspiration of the aqueous phase, 7 ml of the organic phase was transferred into conical tubes and evaporated under a gentle stream of air to a volume of 0.1 to 0.2 ml.

Using 1- to 3-µl aliquots of the final solution, the methyl ester of CPIBA and clofibrate yielded retention times of 2.0 and 2.5 min, respectively, when the GC operating conditions were maintained as follows: injector temperature, 240°C; column temperature, 185°C; detector temperature, 270°C; carrier gas and its flow rate not specified. Concentrations as low as 3 µg/ml were easily detectable, with recovery of CPIBA reported to be 94 ± 2%. On the other hand, CPIBA-glucuronide was measured as CPIBA after enzymatic hydrolysis of urine samples diluted 1:10 with 0.1 M acetate buffer, pH 5.0. To 4 ml of diluted urine, 0.1 ml of β-glucuronidase-sulfatase solution from Helix pomatia was added and incubated at 37°C for 12 hr.

With regard to the pharmacokinetic parameters determined after chronic administration of clofibrate, Gugler et al. noted that:

Plasma protein binding was reduced from 96.4 to 88.8% in nephrotic patients, a change qualitatively similar to that observed with diphenylhydantoin. The half-life ($t_{1/2}$) of CPIBA was considerably shortened in nephrotic patients to as low as 5.2 hr in one patient in whom protein binding was reduced to 83%. No data were obtained for plasma clearance and the apparent volume of distribution since single-intravenous dose studies could not be performed due to a lack of an intravenous dosage form of clofibrate.

The steady-state plasma concentration of CPIBA was lower in nephrotic patients; however, the concentration of unbound drug was similar in both groups (5.1 ± 0.6 versus 4.7 ± 0.5 µg/ml). In normal volunteers receiving 1 g of clofibrate twice daily, an inverse correlation was found between body weight and steady-state plasma concentration.

No significant difference was found between nephrotic patients and and the controls in the excretion in urine of either CPIBA, CPIBA-glucuronide, or CPIBA/CPIBA-glucuronide ratio in the steady state.

Bruderlein, Robinson, Kraml, and Dvornik [361] developed a GC procedure for the determination of CPIBA in serum and urine of laboratory animals and man.

For the analysis of CPIBA in serum, sample preparation was carried out as follows:

To 10.0 ml of chloroform in a glass-stoppered (40-ml) centrifuge tube are added 0.1 ml of 3-MPA (3-methoxyphenylacetic acid, internal standard prepared by dissolving 5 mg of 3-MPA in 10 ml of methanol), 1.0 ml of serum, and 4.0 ml of 0.5 N HCl. The tube is shaken for 10 min and centrifuged for 10 min at 1000 rpm. The aqueous layer is aspirated and discarded, and 8.0 ml of the chloroform transferred to a clean tube. After the addition of 5.0 ml of 0.1 N NH_4OH, the tube is shaken for 20 min and centrifuged. A 4.0-ml aliquot of the aqueous phase is transferred to a third tube containing an equal volume of methanol and evaporated to dryness under reduced pressure. The residue is transferred in a small volume of acetone to a 0.5-ml Reactivial and dried in a stream of nitrogen. Methylation is achieved in 30 min at room temperature by the addition of 0.1 ml of the methanolic HCl (a 3% w/v solution of HCl prepared by bubbling dry HCl gas into 50 ml of methanol at 0°C). Excess reagent is removed in a stream of nitrogen; it is of critical importance that evaporation is stopped as soon as the residue appears to be dry. The residue is dissolved in 50 μl of acetone and aliquots, usually 2 μl, are used for injection into the gas chromatog chromatograph.

GC separation and quantitation of the methylated extract is carried out with a Varian Aerograph model 2100 gas chromatograph equipped with a flame ionization detector and 6-ft by 2-mm-i.d. U-shaped glass columns packed with 3.5% SE-30 on 100-120 mesh Gas Chrom Q; the instrumental conditions for analysis were injector temperature, 250°C; column temperature, 138°C; detector temperature, 250°C; nitrogen carrier-gas flow rate, 10.0 ml/min. With these operating parameters, the retention times for the methyl esters of 3-MPA and CPIBA were 5.5 and 8.5 min, respectively.

In the GC procedure, Brunderlein et al. noted that the recovery of CPIBA based on its extraction from serum (obtained by adding 3-MPA after extraction) was 90.0 ± 1.3% (n = 15) and was independent of the CPIBA concentration in the 5- to 100-μg/ml range. In practice, the minimal detectable amount of CPIBA in serum is approximately 1 μg/ml. Furthermore, GC scans of the extracts of several normal urine samples contained no interfering peaks with retention times similar to those of CPIBA or 3-MPA. Hence, the method is also applicable to urine samples.

Compared to the UV spectrophotometric method of Barrett and Thorp [372], both methods are specific when used to determine CPIBA levels in normal sera from laboratory animals or humans (Fig. 1.59) treated with clofibrate. Serum from patients treated with other drugs or abnormal sera from patients affected with a variety of diseases will often contain high and fluctuating levels of nonspecific absorbing substances, and this will usually preclude the use of the UV procedure. This is vividly illustrated by the data given in Table 1.47, where both methods were used to analyze CPIBA in sera from uremic patients.

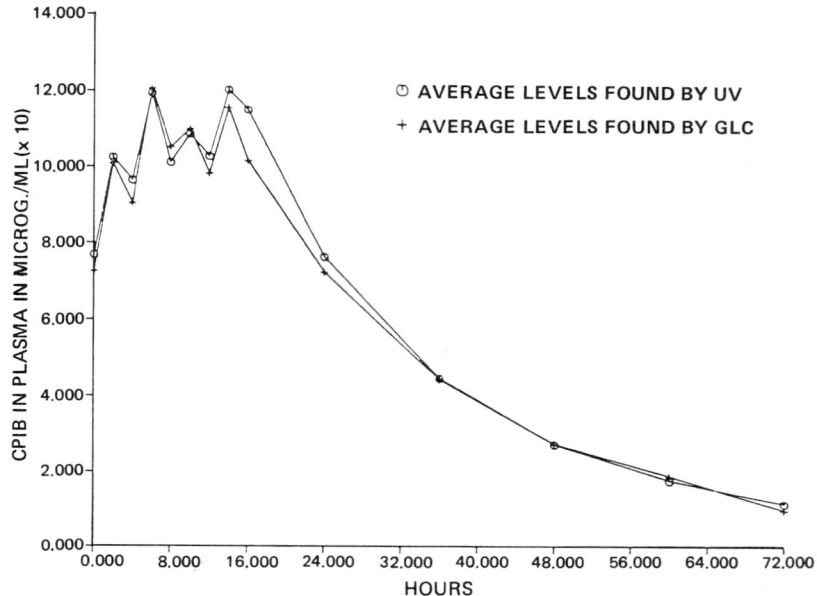

Figure 1.59. Analysis of sera from human volunteers given 0.5 g of Atromid-S (every 4 hr, q.i.d.). Each point represents the average value for 5 volunteers. From Bruderlein et al. [361], courtesy of Clinical Biochemistry.

In 1975, two other GC studies were reported relative to the determination of CPIBA in blood plasma [362,363]. In the method proposed by Tuong and Tuong [362], CPIBA is extracted from acidified plasma into benzene, the extract is evaporated to dryness, and the residue is methylated with an alcohol-free solution of diazomethane and submitted to chromatography for analysis. They recommended the use of the following extraction-methylation procedure for sample preparation prior to its analysis:

A volume of 1.0 or less of plasma was diluted with distilled water to a final volume of 2.0 ml. The mixture was acidified with 1.0 ml of 0.4 M perchloric acid and extracted with 5.0 ml of benzene by gentle shaking for 15 min in an Omni-Shaker at 20 cycles/min. After centrifugation for 15 min at 1000 g, 4.0 ml of the organic phase were transferred into a tapered 7-ml sample vial and evaporated to dryness under a stream of nitrogen in a water bath at 40°C.

TABLE 1.47

Application of the UV and GLC Methods to the Analyses of
CPIB in Sera from Uremic Patients [a,b]

	CPIB (μg/ml serum)					
	Patient 1			Patient 2		
Time (hr)	UV	GLC	Δ	UV	GLC	Δ
0				26	n.d.	26
1	101	n.d.	101	66	2	64
2	48	14	34	121	64	57
3	128	15	113	113	48	65
4				96	29	67
5				73	26	47
6				76	22	54
7	182	54	128	61	8	53
8				67	7	60
9				61	n.d.	61
10				51	2	49
11	157	45	112	49	n.d.	49
21	152	57	95			
31.5	147	70	77			
47	131	81	50			
58	127	63	64			

[a] From Brunderlein et al. [361], courtesy of Clinical Biochemistry.
[b] Each patient received 1.0 g of Atromid-S, orally.

An alcohol-free ethereal solution of diazomethane was prepared according to de Boer [373], but scaled down tenfold. This methylating agent was added dropwise to the above dry residue until a persistent yellow color was obtained. The mixture was kept for 10 min in an ice bath. The solvent and the excess of diazomethane were then carefully removed under vacuum, while the sample vial was cooled to -10°C in an ice-salt mixture. The residue was immediately dissolved in an appropriate volume of octadecane (external standard prepared by dissolving either 100 or 250 mg/liter of n-hexane) and 1 to 4 μl of the solution were injected into the chromatograph by means of a 10-μl microsyringe.

The chromatographic conditions used with a Hewlett-Packard model 5751G gas chromatograph equipped with a flame ionization detector, a laboratory data system, consisting of an HP 2100A computer, 16-bit word 12K of core memory, and an HP 2752A teleprinter, and 6-ft by 2-mm-i.d. coiled glass columns packed with 3% OV-17 on 100-120 mesh Chromosorb W-HP were injector temperature, 180°C; column temperature, held isothermally for 6 min at 150°C, then programmed to 195°C at 10°C/min and held at the final temperature for 5 min; helium carrier-gas flow rate, 25 ml/min. Under these operating conditions, the retention times of the methyl ester of CPIBA and the external standard (octadecane) were about 3 and 5 min, respectively, with the sensitivity of the FID detector toward pure CPIBA methyl ester being 1 ng, but with plasma extracts the limit of detection increasing considerably to 50 ng injected, that is, 250 ng/ml in plasma.

With an apparent recovery of CPIBA from plasma of nearly 70%, two animal studies were conducted in which (1) the CPIBA level in male rats after oral administration of Atherolip (aluminum salt of CPIBA) with or without addition of vitamin B_6 and (2) the CPIBA level in male and female rats after prolonged oral administration of Atherolip with or without addition of vitamin B_6 were determined chromatographically. Summarizing their data, they noted that in the first investigation the addition of vitamin B_6 did not have a clear influence on the absorption of Atherolip. At 5 hr, the overall mean plasma level was about 139 μg/ml for a dose of 360 mg/kg of Atherolip and reached 183 μg/ml for the 450-mg/kg dose.

After prolonged administration (a study in which both male and female animals were treated for 7 weeks, 5 days/week, the first 2 weeks with 450 mg/kg/day of Atherolip with or without 10 mg/kg/day of vitamin B_6, the last 5 weeks with 1350 mg/kg/day of Atherolip with or without 10 mg/kg/day of vitamin B_6, before receiving the last dose), again no influence of vitamin B_6 occurred, but female rats showed a significantly lower CPIBA acid plasma concentration (481 μg/ml) than male rats (724 μg/ml), 2 hr after the last dose of 450 mg/kg of Atherolip.

Berlin [363] also quantitatively analyzed CPIBA in plasma by GC in order to evaluate therapeutic plasma concentrations and pharmacokinetics of CPIBA. In this investigation, a Varian 1200 gas chromatograph equipped with a flame ionization detector and 6-ft by 3-mm-i.d. silanized glass columns packed with 3% OV-17 on 80-100 mesh Gas Chrom Q was used in conjunction with the following conditions: injector temperature, 232°C; column temperature, 131°C; detector temperature, 240°C; nitrogen carrier-gas flow rate, 40 ml/min. The procedure used to isolate the CPIBA from plasma was as follows:

> To blood plasma (200 µl) is added 50 µl of 2 M H_3PO_4 and 0.5 ml of internal standard solution [2-(4-chloro-3-methylphenoxy)-2-methylpropionic acid, 9 µg/ml of toluene]. After shaking (10 min), the organic phase is transferred to a 3-ml tapered glass tube and the plasma is reextracted with 0.5 ml of toluene. To the combined organic phases is added 0.5 ml of 0.5 M Na_2HPO_4 and the mixture is shaken for 10 min. The organic phase is removed and the aqueous phase is made acidic with 50 µl of 5 M H_3PO_4. One hundred microliters of methylene chloride is added and the mixture is extracted on a whirl-mixer for 30 sec. After removal of the aqueous phase, diazomethane in ether (50 µl) is added and the solution is evaporated under nitrogen to about one-fifth of its volume. One microliter is analyzed by gas chromatography.

Using the GC conditions given above, the retention times for the methyl esters of CPIBA and the internal standard were 4.3 and 6.7 min, respectively.

Reportedly capable of determining CPIBA plasma levels down to 1 µg/ml, Berlin noted that the values of the partition coefficients for CPIBA indicate that a single extraction is not sufficient to achieve a quantitative extraction as acid into toluene. However, a second extraction will increase the recovery to the 98% level.

Connor, Johnson, and Solomon [365] described a GC method for CPIBA in which the drug and internal standards [p-chlorophenoxyacetic acid (150 µg/ml of methanol) and 3-(p-chlorophenoxy)propionic acid (150 µg/ml of methanol)] are separated from serum or saliva by a double extraction procedure and converted to the corresponding butyl esters by reaction with iodobutane in a mixture of methanol and N,N-dimethylacetamide containing tetramethylammonium hydroxide.

The GC instrument used by Connor et al. was a Hewlett-Packard model 5711A unit equipped with dual flame ionization detectors and 120-cm by 2-mm-i.d. glass columns packed with 3% OV-17 on 100-120 mesh Gas Chrom Q; the other operating parameters maintained for quantitation were injector temperature, 250°C; column temperature, programmed from 130 to 240°C at a rate of 16°C/min; detector temperature, 300°C; nitrogen carrier-gas flow rate, 50 ml/min. The retention times of the butyl derivatives of CPIBA, CPAA, and CPPA were approximately 2.88, 3.26, and 3.87 min, respectively.

Using their procedure for CPIBA analysis, Connor et al. found that the absolute recoveries of CPIBA, CPAA, and CPPA from serum were 89.1%, 95.9%, and 99.8%, respectively, and from saliva were 91.5%, 90.9%, and

95.3%, respectively. Within-run coefficient of variation of this assay at a serum CPIBA concentration of 79.2 mg/liter was 2.3% and at a salivary CPIBA concentration of 2.5 mg/liter was 2.1%. Precision during 4 months of the serum and salivary assays at these concentrations was 4.1% and 6.2%, respectively. The mean serum concentration of CPIBA (12 hr after dose) in patients receiving the drug at an average dose of 28.0 mg/kg/day was 109 mg/liter. Serum and salivary concentrations of CPIBA were used to calculate the unbound fraction of drug in human serum. Such measurements can be used to monitor therapy in patients with renal disease, where drug toxicity may arise from high concentrations of unbound CPIBA. The formula used to estimate the unbound fraction in serum is

$$\text{percent unbound drug} = \frac{\text{(saliva)}}{\text{(serum)}} \times \frac{1 + 10^{7.4 - pK_a}}{1 + 10^{pH \text{ saliva} - pK_a}} \times 100 \quad (1.36)$$

Using Eq. (1.36), they noted that in an individual with normal renal function, the bound fraction of CPIBA was about 96.4%. In an individual with severe renal insufficiency (creatinine clearance less than 5 ml/min) the bound fraction was 88.8%.

In 1976, Gugler and Jensen [366] also developed a GC method for the determination of CPIBA (active metabolite of clofibrate) in plasma and urine; a procedure which involved an extraction of CPIBA into toluene and back-extraction of the CPIBA and 2-naphthoic acid (internal standard) into the methylating reagent (trimethylanilinium hydroxide). Concentration of 1 μg/ml in plasma and urine could easily be measured with a Hewlett-Packard model 5750 gas chromatograph equipped with a flame ionization detector and silanized 6-ft by 4-mm-i.d. glass columns packed with 3% SE-30 on 80-100 mesh Gas Chrom Q. Retention times of 1.5 and 2.5 min for the methyl esters of CPIBA and 2-naphthoic acid, respectively, were obtained using the following GC conditions: injector temperature, 290°C; column temperature, 150°C; detector temperature, 270°C; nitrogen carrier-gas flow rate, 25 ml/min.

With regard to the proposed procedure, Gugler and Jensen reported that:

1. The coefficient of variation was determined by assaying six samples at each of the concentrations 10, 20, 50, 100, and 200 μg/ml in both plasma and urine. The CV was 3.3% for plasma and 2.7% for urine; that is, reproducibility was good.

2. The one extraction into toluene proved to be sufficient to obtain good recovery; the recovery was 71 ± 2% (n = 10) from plasma and 91 ± 2% (n = 10) from urine.

3. The specificity of the method was assessed by assaying plasma and urine samples from patients taking other drugs. Butylbiguanide, digoxin, ethacrynic acid, furosemide, glibenclamide, α-methyldopa, oxifedrine, reserpine, and spironolactone were tested and did not interfere with the assay when administered in normal therapeutic doses.

Using the GC method of Bruderlein et al. [361], Goldberg, Sherrard, Haas, and Brunzell [367] designed an investigation to determine (1) the rate of plasma clofibrate disappearance in patients with long-term renal failure and patients with the nephrotic syndrome, and (2) whether an appropriate reduction in clofibrate dosage would reduce or eliminate the previously reported toxicity [374-376] while retaining the hypolipidemic effect of the drug in the treatment of hypertriglyceridemia in patients receiving maintenance hemodialysis.

Summarizing their results, Goldberg et al. found that:

A daily dose of 1.5 to 2.0 g of clofibrate lowers serum triglyceride levels in patients with normal renal function but causes muscle toxicity and elevated creatine phosphokinase levels in patients with long-term renal failure. Plasma clofibrate disappearance is prolonged as much as seven times normal in severely uremic patients (plasma clofibrate half-life in the nonuremic control, uremic, and nephrotic groups being 16.5 ± 4.7, 109.6 ± 35.9, and 8.7 ± 3.5 hr, respectively). A marked reduction in the standard 14 g/week clofibrate dose to a total dose of 1.0 to 1.5 g/week effectively lowered serum triglyceride levels (-28%, $p < 0.02$) in hypertriglyceridemic hemodialysis patients without toxicity. The serum clofibrate level at this dose was comparable to that in hypertriglyceridemic nonuremic patients receiving 14 g/week of clofibrate (about 77 ± 19 μg/ml). The dose of clofibrate administered to hemodialysis patients can be adjusted to avoid toxicity and provide the desired therapeutic effect by monitoring serum creatine phosphokinase and triglyceride levels.

B. Halofenate [368-370]

In 1971, Hucker et al. [368] studied the metabolism of halofenate in the rat, dog, rhesus monkey, and man. As noted by the investigators, lower concentrations of the primary metabolite, (p-chlorophenyl) (m-trifluoromethylphenoxy)acetic acid (CPTFA) were determined by gas chromatography as follows:

(p-Chlorophenyl)(m-trifluoromethyl-phenoxy)acetic Acid

An analog of CPTFA [2,4-dichlorophenyl)(3-trifluoromethylphenoxy) acetic acid] was used as an internal standard. A sample of 0.2 to 3.0 ml of plasma was added to a glass-stoppered centrifuge tube containing 10 ml of heptane (containing 2% isoamyl alcohol), internal standard (1 ml of a 30 μg/ml solution in 0.05 M phosphate buffer, pH 7.4) and 2 N HCl (half the sample volume). The tube was shaken for 10 min and centrifuged, and 9 to 10 ml of the heptane were transferred to another tube containing 1.5 ml of 0.1 N NaOH. After shaking for 5 min, the heptane was removed by aspiration. Methylene choride (1 ml) and 2 N HCl (0.2 ml) were added to the aqueous layer; the tube contents were agitated on a Vortex mixer for 1 min. After centrifugation, the methylene chloride was transferred to a glass-stoppered centrifuge tube with a pointed tip. Diazomethane in ether (20 μl of a 0.5 M solution, generated from N-nitroso-N-methylurea) was added. The tube was kept at room temperature for 5 min and the volume of solvent then reduced to 10 to 15 μl by placing the tube in warm water. A 1-μl aliquot was injected into the chromatograph.

(2,4-Dichlorophenyl)(3-trifluoromethylphenoxy)acetic Acid

Quantitative data were obtained with a F&M model 810 or 5750 gas chromatograph equipped with a flame ionization detector and 6-ft by 1/4-in.-i.d. coiled glass columns packed with 1% QF-1 on 80-100 mesh Gas Chrom Q. Retention times of 3.5 and 4.3 min for the methyl esters of

CPTFA and the internal standard, respectively, were obtained by maintaining the following GC conditions: injector temperature, 190°C; column temperature, 170°C; detector temperature, 250°C; helium carrier-gas flow rate, 50 ml/min.

Using halofenate-carboxyl-^{14}C and radioactive counting, Hucker et al. summarized their findings in the following manner:

> Administration of ^{14}C-labeled halofenate to rats resulted in distribution of radioactivity to various tissues but highest concentrations of label were found in plasma. A large fraction of the dose was excreted in rat bile followed by extensive reabsorption of the biliary radioactivity. Biliary excretion in the dog was less extensive. The dose was excreted equally in rat urine and feces but predominantly in dog feces. A major metabolite in urine of both species was hydroxylated in the trifluoromethylphenoxy ring. Chronic administration of halofenate to dogs resulted in a slow increase in plasma levels. Administration of halofenate-^{14}C to the rhesus monkey and man gave similar excretion patterns, 46 to 56% of the dose being excreted in urine and 25 to 27% in feces in 5 to 6 days. Halofenate was evidently rapidly converted on absorption to the corresponding acid (CPTFA) since only the latter was found in plasma of all species after administration of halofenate. The plasma half-life ($t_{1/2}$) was approximately 16 hr in the monkey and 24 hr in man, with a slower phase (post-24-hr) with a $t_{1/2}$ of nearly 48 hr. About 70% of the urinary radioactivity in both species was represented by CPTFA with the remainder present as CPTFA-glucuronide.

Dujovne et al. [369] compared the hypolipidemic as well as other laboratory and clinical effects of halofenate, clofibrate, and placebo in 29 patients with type IV hyperlipoproteinemia in a double-blind, controlled, therapeutic trial of one year duration. Whereas clofibrate levels in plasma was monitored by the method of Gugler et al. [360], halofenate was determined using a gas chromatograph equipped with an electron-capture detector and an all-glass 6-ft by 1/4-in. column packed with 2.5% SE-30 on 80-100 mesh Gas Chrom Q; the other GC conditions were injector temperature, 215°C; column temperature, 200°C; detector temperature, 225°C; carrier-gas flow rate not specified. The procedure used for the preparation of the sample for subsequent GC analysis consisted of adding 1 ml of 0.5 N HCl to 1 ml of plasma and then extracting the mixture with 8 ml of chloroform containing 75 µg of trichlorophenoxypropionic acid as internal standard. Seven milliliters of the chloroform layer was evaporated and the residue dissolved in 1 ml of a freshly prepared mixture of 0.5% K_2CO_3 in 90% methanol. Then 0.1 ml of dimethyl sulfate was added and the solution heated at 70°C for 10 min. Following the evaporation of the solution to approximately 0.1 ml under a stream of air, 1 ml of 0.2 N acetate buffer, pH 5.6, and 4 ml of heptane were added. After shaking and separation of the phases, 1 µl of the heptane phase was injected onto the GC column.

Their analytical data suggested that "clofibrate and halofenate lowered serum triglycerides to a similar extent. The hypotriglyceridemic effect of halofenate was significant only when data from noncompliant patients were discarded. Only clofibrate lowered baseline levels of plasma cholesterol (a reduction of approximately 19%). Very low-density lipoproteins were decreased and low-density lipoproteins were increased by clofibrate but not by halofenate. Halofenate had a marked hypouricemic effect that was greater than that of clofibrate. The hypouricemic effect of halofenate and clofibrate were paralleled with a concomitant decrease in serum bilirubin. Abnormal increases in serum creatine phosphokinase were observed with both drugs primarily in patients who had abnormal initial levels.

Huffman et al. [370] also used the GC method of Dujovne et al. [369] to study the effect of halofenate on β-adrenergic blockade by propranolol in four subjects during chronic drug administration in a randomized, double-blind study. They noted that propranolol concentration (measured by fluorometry) was significantly lower during treatment with halofenate than with placebo. The reduction in propranolol levels correlated with a decrease in β-adrenergic blockade.

C. Procetofene

Elsom, Hawkins, and Chasseaud [371] identified in 1976 a major metabolite of the new hypolipidemic agent procetofene, isopropyl 2-[4'-(p-chlorobenzoyl)phenoxy]-2-methylpropionate, in humans by integrated

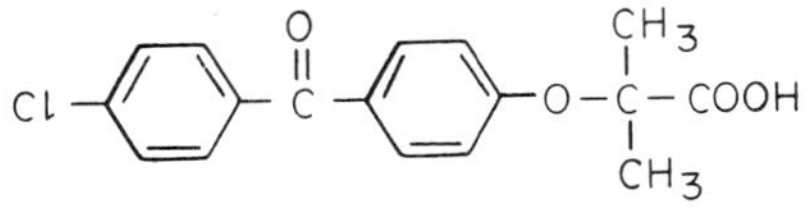

Structure A

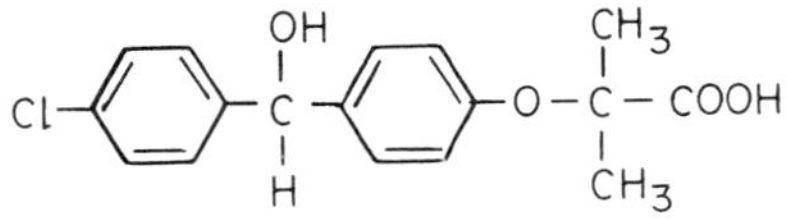

Structure B

ANTISCLEROSIS (ANTIHYPERLIPIDEMIA) DRUGS

GC-MS in which a Pye 104 gas chromatograph was interfaced to a VG Micromass 16F mass spectrometer via a single-stage jet separator. Equipped with a 200-cm by 0.4-cm-i.d. glass column packed with 1% Carbowax 20M on 80-100 mesh Gas Chrom Q, the other GC-MS conditions used were helium carrier-gas flow rate, 40 ml/min; column temperature, 220°C; jet separator temperature, 200°C; ion source temperature, 220°C; electron beam energy, 70 eV; trap current, 100 μA; ion voltage supply for multiple ion monitoring of up to eight ions in the mass range 0 to 300% of the lowest mass being programmable.

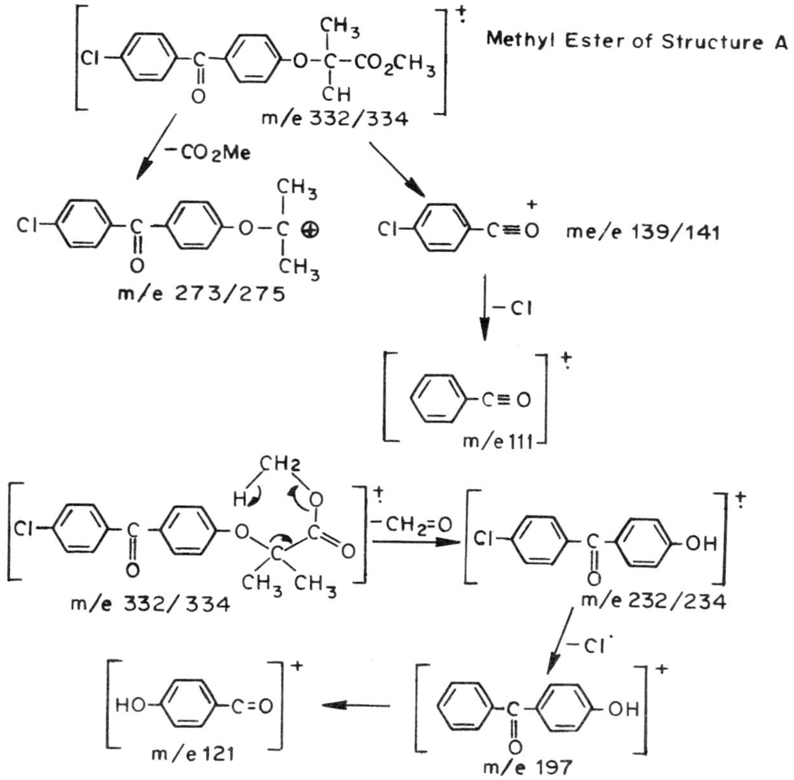

In both human plasma and urine samples, the major metabolites sought were the corresponding carboxylic acid (structure A) and the benzhydrol (structure B) shown above. Methylation of both metabolites by treatment with diazomethane in methanol yielded methyl esters whose mass spectra showed significant differences from the parent drug procetofene with its molecular ion at m/e 360 and a corresponding isotope peak (due to ^{37}Cl) at m/e 362. The mass spectrum of structure A had a molecular ion at m/e 332 and fragment ions at m/e 273 and 232, all associated with isotope peaks as indicated from its postulated fragmentation pattern illustrated above.

On the other hand, the methyl ester of the benzhydrol metabolite yielded a molecular ions at m/e 334 and 336.

By monitoring three ions, namely m/e 336, 334, and 332 (the ions m/e 334 and 332 representing the molecular ion of methylated structure A and m/e 334 and 332 those of the methylated benzhydrol compound), Elsom et al. noted that there was no compound corresponding to structure B with a retention time of 8 min, whereas a peak appeared at a retention time of 15 min which corresponded to the carboxylic metabolite (this being detected unequivocally in either urine or plasma).

REFERENCES

1. Goth, A., Medical Pharmacology: Principles and Concepts, 7th ed., C. V. Mosby, St. Louis, 1974.
2. Chow, M. S. S. and Ronfeld, R. A., J. Clin. Pharmacol., 15, 405 (1975).
3. Smith, T. W. and Haber, E., N. Engl. J. Med., 289, 1063 (1973).
4. Gjerdum, K., Acta Med. Scand., 191, 25 (1972).
5. Lukas, D. S., Ann. N. Y. Acad. Sci., 179, 338 (1971).
6. Storstein, L., Clin. Pharmacol. Ther., 16, 14 (1974).
7. Rasmussen, K., Jervell, J., Storstein, L., and Gjerdum, K., Clin. Pharmacol. Ther., 13, 6 (1972).
8. Lukas, D. S. and Martino, A. G., J. Clin. Invest., 48, 1041 (1969).
9. Greenblatt, D. J., Duhme, D. W., Koch-Weser, J., and Smith, T. W., N. Engl. J. Med., 289, 651 (1973).
10. Wagner, J. G., Christensen, M., Sakmar, E., Blair, D., Yates, J. D., Willis, P. W., Sedman, A. J., and Stoll, R. G., J. Amer. Med. Ass., 224, 199 (1973).
11. Doherty, J. E. and Perkins, W., Amer. J. Cardiol., 15, 170 (1965).
12. Reuning, R. H., Sams, R. A., and Notari, R. E., J. Clin. Pharmacol., 13, 127 (1973).
13. Jelliffe, R. W., Ann. Int. Med., 69, 703 (1968).
14. Van Heuvel, W. J. A. and Horning, E. C., J. Org. Chem., 26, 634 (1961).
15. Friedman, M., Bine, R., Jr., Byers, S. O., and Bland, C., Circulation, 2, 749 (1950).

REFERENCES

16. Jelliffe, R. W. and Blankenhorn, D. H., J. Chromatog., 12, 268 (1963).
17. Wilson, W. E., Johnson, S. A., Perkins, W. H., and Ripley, J. E., Anal. Chem., 39, 40 (1967).
18. Richey, J. M., Richey, H. G., Jr., and Schraer, R., Anal. Biochem., 9, 272 (1964).
19. Lau, H. L., J. Gas Chromatog., 4, 136 (1966).
20. Maume, B., Wilson, W. E., and Horning, E. C., Anal. Lett., 1, 401 (1968).
21. Tan, L., J. Chromatog., 45, 68 (1969).
22. Sawlewicz, L., Linde, H. H. A., and Meyer, K., Helv. Chim. Acta, 51, 1353 (1968).
23. Sakurai, K., Yoshii, E., Hashimoto, H., and Kubo, K., Chem. Pharm. Bull., 16, 1140 (1968).
24. Wilson, W. E. and Ripley, J. E., Anal. Chem., 41, 810 (1969).
25. Jelliffe, R. W., Circulation, 28, 743 (1963).
26. Watson, E and Kalman, S. M., J. Chromatog., 56, 209 (1971).
27. Watson, E., Tramell, P., and Kalman, S. M., J. Chromatog., 69, 157 (1972).
28. Finkle, B. S., Cherry, E. J., and Taylor, D. M., J. Chromatog. Sci., 9, 393 (1971).
29. Kibbe, A. H. and Araujo, O. E., J. Pharm. Sci., 62, 1703 (1973).
30. Anbar, M and St. John, G. A., Anal. Chem., 48, 198 (1976).
31. Brown, P., Bruschweiler, F., Pettit, G. R., and Reichstein, T., Org. Mass Spectrom., 5, 573 (1971).
32. Knight, J. C., J. Chromatog., 133, 222 (1977).
33. Rozanski, A., Analyst (London), 97, 968 (1972).
34. Moss, A. J. and Patton, R. D., Antiarrhythmic Agents, Charles C. Thomas, Springfield, Ill., 1973.
35. Glazko, A. J., in B. B. Brodie and W. M. Heller (Eds.), Bioavailability of Drugs, S. Karger, Basel, 1972, pp. 163-177.
36. Odar-Cederlof, A. and Borga, O., Eur. J. Clin. Pharmacol., 7, 31 (1974).
37. Arnold, K. and Gerber, N., Clin. Pharmacol. Ther., 11, 121 (1970).
38. Bigger, J. T., Schmidt, D. H., and Kutt, H., Circulation, 38, 363 (1968).
39. Scott, D. B., in D. B. Scott and D. B. Julian (Eds.), Lidocaine in the Treatment of Ventricular Arrhythmias, Livingstone, Edinburgh and London, 1971.
40. Rowland, M., Thomson, P., Guichard, A., Melmon, K., and Pate, D., Ann. N. Y. Acad. Sci., 179, 383 (1971).
41. Sung, C. Y. and Truant, A. P., J. Pharmacol. Exp. Ther., 112, 432 (1954).

42. Eriksson, E., Acta Chir. Scand., Suppl., 358, 1 (1966).
43. Giannelly, R. J., N. Engl. J. Med., 277, 1215 (1967).
44. Koch-Weser, J. and Klein, S. W., J. Amer. Med. Ass., 215, 1454 (1971).
45. Koch-Weser, J., Ann. N. Y. Acad. Sci., 179, 370 (1971).
46. Evans, G. H. and Shand, D. G., Clin. Pharmacol. Ther., 14, 487 (1973).
47. Evans, G. H., Nies, A. S., and Shand, D. G., J. Pharmacol. Exp. Ther., 186, 114 (1973).
48. Coltart, D. J., Gibson, D. G., and Shand, D. G., Brit. Med. J., 1, 490 (1971).
49. Houston, A. B. and Perry, W. F., Can. Med. Ass. J., 63, 556 (1950).
50. Bellet, S., Roman, L. R., and Boza, O., Amer. J. Cardiol., 27, 368 (1971).
51. Ronfeld, R. A. and Chow, M. S. S., unpublished work.
52. Kessler, K. M., Lowenthal, D. T., Warner, H., Gibson, T., Briggs, W., and Reidenberg, M., N. Engl. J. Med., 290, 706 (1974).
53. Reidenberg, M. M. and Affrime, M., Ann. N. Y. Acad. Sci., 226, 115 (1973).
54. Conn, H. L. and Luchi, R. J., Amer. J. Med., 37, 685 (1964).
55. Brochmann-Hanssen, E. and Fontan, C. R., J. Chromatog., 119, 296 (1965).
56. Palmer, K. H., Martin, B., Baggett, B., and Wall, M. E., Biochem. Pharmacol., 18, 1845 (1969).
57. Finkle, B. S., Taylor, D. M., and Bonelli, E. J., J. Chromatog. Sci., 10, 312 (1972).
58. Finkle, B. S., Foltz, R. L., and Taylor, D. M., J. Chromatog. Sci., 12, 304 (1974).
59. Moffat, A. C., J. Chromatog., 113, 69 (1975).
60. Laurie, W. A. and Field, F. H., J. Amer. Chem. Soc., 94, 2913 (1972).
61. Field, F. H., J. Amer. Chem. Soc., 91, 6334 (1969).
62. Foltz, R. L., Clarke, P. A., Knowlton, D. A., and Hoyland, J. R., Rapid Identification of Drugs from Mass Spectra, Batelle, Columbus Laboratories, Columbus, Ohio, Jan 1974.
63. Smith, E., Barkan, S., Ross, B., Maienthal, M., and Levine, J., J. Pharm. Sci., 62, 1151 (1973).
64. Midha, K. K. and Charette, C., J. Pharm. Sci., 63, 1244 (1974).
65. Valentine, J. L., Driscoll, P., Hamburg, E. L., and Thompson, E. D., J. Pharm. Sci., 65, 96 (1976).
66. Huffman, D. H. and Hignite, C. E., Clin. Chem., 22, 810 (1976).
67. Brodie, B. B. and Udenfriend, S., J. Pharmacol. Exp. Ther., 78, 154 (1943).

REFERENCES

68. Hartel, G. and Korhonen, A., J. Chromatog., 37, 70 (1968).
69. Kern, H., Schilling, P., and Muller, S. H., Gas Chromatographic Analysis of Pharmaceuticals and Drugs, Varian, Walnut Creek, Calif., 1968.
70. Atkinson, A. J., Jr., Parker, M., and Strong, J., Clin. Chem., 18, 643 (1972).
71. Meola, J., P-E Lab. Med. Newsl., 5(1), 9 (1973).
72. Karlsson, E., Eur. J. Clin. Pharmacol., 6, 245 (1973).
73. Sterling, J., Cox, S., and Haney, W. G., J. Pharm. Sci., 63, 1744 (1974).
74. Karlsson, E., Molin, L., Norlander, B., and Sjoqvist, F., Brit. J. Clin. Pharmacol., 1, 467 (1974).
75. Drayer, D. E., Reidenberg, M. M., and Sevy, R. W., Proc. Soc. Exp. Biol. Med., 146, 358 (1974).
76. Simons, K. J. and Levy, R. H., J. Pharm. Sci., 64, 1968 (1975).
77. Frislid, K., Bredesen, J. E., and Lunde, P. K. M., Clin. Chem., 21, 1180 (1975).
78. Poet, R. B. and Radin, H., in K. Florey (Ed.), Analytical Profiles of Drug Substances, Vol. 4, Academic Press, New York, 1975.
79. Graffner, C., Johnsson, G., and Sjogren, J., Clin. Pharmacol. Ther., 17, 414 (1975).
80. Graffner, C., J. Pharmacokin. Biopharmaceut., 3, 69 (1975).
81. Simons, K. J., Levy, R. H., Cutler, R. E., Christopher, G. T., and Lindner, A., Res. Commun. Chem. Pathol. Pharmacol., 11, 173 (1975).
82. Gibson, T. P., Matusik, J., Matusik, E., Nelson, H. A., Wilkinson, J., and Briggs, W. A., Clin. Pharmacol. Ther., 17, 395 (1975).
83. Elson, J., Strong, J. M., Lee, W. K., and Atkinson, A. J., Jr., Clin. Pharmacol. Ther., 17, 134 (1975).
84. Strong, J. M., Dutcher, J. S., Lee, W. K., and Atkinson, A. J., Jr., J. Pharmacokin. Biopharmaceut., 3, 223 (1975).
85. Strong, J. M., Dutcher, J. S., Lee, W. K., and Atkinson, A. J., Jr., Clin. Pharmacol. Ther., 18, 613 (1975).
86. Galeazzi, R. L., Sheiner, L. B., Lockwood, T., and Benet, L. Z., Clin. Pharmacol. Ther., 19, 55 (1976).
87. Galeazzi, R. L., Benet, L. Z., and Sheiner, L. B., Clin. Pharmacol. Ther., 20, 278 (1976).
88. Atkinson, A. J., Jr., Krumlovsky, F. A., Huang, C. M., and del Greco, F., Clin. Pharmacol. Ther., 20, 585 (1976).
89. Drayer, D. E., Strong, J. M., and Reidenberg, M. M., in Advances in Mass Spectrometry in Biochemistry and Medicine, Vol. 1, Spectrum Publ., New York, 1976.
90. Keenaghan, J. B., Anesthesiology, 29, 110 (1968).

91. Mather, L. E. and Tucker, G. T., J. Pharm. Sci., 63, 306 (1974).
92. Baer, D. T. and Barkus, J. C., Jr., Res. Commun. Chem. Pathol. Pharmacol., 17, 333 (1977).
93. Elson, J., Strong, J. M., and Atkinson, A. J., Jr., Clin. Pharmacol. Ther., 15, 204 (1974).
94. Mark, L. C., Kaydan, H. J., Steele, J. M., Cooper, J. R., Berlin, I., Rovenstine, E. A., and Brodie, B. B., J. Pharmacol. Exp. Ther., 102, 5 (1951).
95. Reidenberg, M. M., Drayer, D. E., Levy, M., and Warner, H., Clin. Pharmacol. Ther., 17, 722 (1975).
96. Sitar, D. S., Graham, D. N., Rango, R. E., Dufresne, L., and Ogilvie, R. I., Pharmacologist, 16, 175 (1974).
97. Manion, C. V., Lalka, D., Baer, D. T., and Meyer, M. B., J. Pharm. Sci., 66, 981 (1977).
98. Scott, E. M. and Wright, R. C., J. Lab. Clin. Med., 70, 355 (1967).
99. Benet, L. Z., J. Pharm. Sci., 61, 536 (1972).
100. Teorell, T., Arch. Int. Pharmacodyn., 57, 205 (1937).
101. Berman, M. and Weiss, M. F., SAAM Manual (PHS Publication No. 1703), U.S. Government Printing Office, Washington, D.C., 1967.
102. Kazyak, L. and Knoblock, E. C., Anal. Chem., 35, 1448 (1963).
103. Cometti, A., Bagnasco, G., and Maggi, N., J. Pharm. Sci., 60, 1074 (1971).
104. Vessman, J. and Schill, G., Svensk. Farm. Tidskr., 66, 601 (1962).
105. Koehler, H. M., and Hefferen, J. J., J. Pharm. Sci., 53, 745 (1964).
106. Vessman, J., Acta Pharm. Suecica, 1, 183 (1964).
107. Byars, B., Aerograph Res. Notes, Fall Issue, 1964, p. 1.
108. Svinhufvud, G., Ortengren, B., and Jacobsson, S. E., Scand. J. Clin. Invest., 17, 162 (1965).
109. Beckett, A. H., Boyes, R. N., and Parker, J. B. R., Anesthesia, 20, 294 (1965).
110. Katz, J., Anesthesiology, 27, 835 (1966).
111. Pratt, E. L., Warrington, H. P., and Grego, J., Anesthesiology, 28, 432 (1967).
112. Reynolds, F. and Beckett, A. H., J. Pharm. Pharmacol., 20, 704 (1968).
113. Tompsett, S. L., Clin. Chem., 15, 591 (1969).
114. DiFazio, C. A. and Brown, R. E., Anesthesiology, 34, 86 (1971).
115. Breck, G. D. and Trager, W. F., Science, 173, 544 (1971).
116. Rowland, M., Thomson, P. D., Guichard, A., and Melmon, K. L., Ann. N. Y. Acad. Sci., 179, 383 (1971).

REFERENCES

117. Strong, J. M. and Atkinson, A. J., Jr., Anal. Chem., 44, 2287 (1972).
118. Keenaghan, J. B. and Boyes, R. N., J. Pharmacol. Exp. Ther., 180, 454 (1972).
119. Blumer, J., Strong, J. M., and Atkinson, A. J., Jr., J. Pharmacol. Exp. Ther., 186, 31 (1973).
120. Strong, J. M., Parker, M., and Atkinson, A. J., Jr., Clin. Pharmacol. Ther., 14, 67 (1973).
121. Benowitz, N. and Rowland, M., Anesthesiology, 39, 639 (1973).
122. Levy, R. H. and Rowland, M., J. Pharmacokin. Biopharmaceut., 2, 313 (1974).
123. Patel, I. H. and Levy, R. H., J. Pharmacokin. Biopharmaceut., 2, 337 (1974).
124. Greenwood, N. D. and Nursten, H. E., J. Chromatog., 92, 323 (1974).
125. Adjepon-Yamoah, K. K. and Prescott, L. F., J. Pharm. Pharmacol., 26, 889 (1974).
126. Strong, J. M. and Atkinson, A. J., Jr., Finnigan Spectra, 4 (4) (December 1974).
127. Cameron, J. D., Clin. Chim. Acta, 56, 307 (1974).
128. Strong, J. M., Mayfield, D. E., Atkinson, A. J., Jr., Burris, B. C., Raymon, F., and Webster, L. T., Jr., Clin. Pharmacol. Ther., 17, 184 (1975).
129. Ballard, B. E., J. Pharm. Sci., 64, 781 (1975).
130. Halkin, H., Meffin, P., Melmon, K. L., and Rowland, M., Clin. Pharmacol. Ther., 17, 669 (1975).
131. Collinsworth, K. A., Strong, J. M., Atkinson, A. J., Jr., Winkle, R. A., Periroth, F., and Harrison, D. C., Clin. Pharmacol. Ther., 18, 59 (1975).
132. Irgens, T. R., Henderson, W. M., and Shelver, W. H., J. Pharm. Sci., 65, 608 (1976).
133. Nelson, S. D., Nelson, M. B., and Trager, W. F., paper presented at 172nd National American Chemical Society Meeting, San Francisco, Calif., Aug. 30-Sept. 3, 1976.
134. Hucker, H. B. and Stauffer, S. C., J. Pharm. Sci., 65, 926 (1976).
135. Nau, H. and Biemann, K., Anal. Chem., 46, 426 (1974).
136. Patel, J. A., Amer. J. Hosp. Pharm., 27, 411 (1970).
137. Sandberg, D. H., Resnick, G. L., and Bacallao, C. Z., Anal. Chem., 40, 736 (1968).
138. Chang, T. and Glazko, A. J., Clin. Res., 16, 339 (1968).
139. Machata, G. and Battista, H., Mikrochim. Acta, 11, 866 (1968).
140. Sabih, K. and Sabih, K., Anal. Chem., 41, 1452 (1969).

141. Erdey, L., Kaplar, L., Takacs, J., and Dessouky, Y. M., J. Chromatog., 45, 63 (1969).
142. Grimmer, G. and Gillen, H. W., Clin. Chem., 15, 582 (1969).
143. Street, H. V., J. Chromatog., 41, 358 (1969).
144. Pippenger, C. E., Scott, J. E., and Gillen, H. W., Clin. Chem., 15, 255 (1969).
145. MacGee, J., Anal. Chem., 42, 421 (1970).
146. Barrett, J., Clin. Chem. Appl. Study No. 33, Perkin-Elmer Corp., Norwalk, Conn., October 1970.
147. Evenson, M. A., Jones, P., and Darcey, B., Clin. Chem., 16, 107 (1970).
148. Van Meter, J. C., Buckmaster, H. S., and Shelley, L. L., Clin. Chem., 16, 135 (1970).
149. Baylis, E. M., Fry, D. E., and Marks, V., Clin. Chim. Acta, 30, 93 (1970).
150. Kupferberg, H. J., Clin. Chim. Acta, 29, 283 (1970).
151. Sabih, K. and Sabih, K., J. Pharm. Sci., 60, 1216 (1971).
152. Hammer, R. H., Wilder, B. J., Streiff, R. R., and Mayersdorf, A., J. Pharm. Sci., 60, 327 (1971).
153. Sampson, D., Harasymiv, I., and Hensley, W. J., Clin. Chem., 17, 382 (1971).
154. Van Meter, J. C., Clin. Chem., 17, 460 (1971).
155. Proelss, H. F. and Lohmann, H. J., Clin. Chem., 17, 222 (1971).
156. Mule, S. J., J. Chromatog., 55, 255 (1971).
157. Chin, D., Fastlich, E., and Davidow, B., J. Chromatog., 71, 545 (1972).
158. Cooper, R. G., Greaves, M. S., and Owen, G., Clin. Chem., 18, 1343 (1972).
159. Skinner, R. F., Gallaher, E. G., Knight, J. B., and Bonelli, E. J., J. Forensic Sci., 17, 189 (1972).
160. Sine, H. E., McKenna, M. J., Law, M. R., and Murray, M. H., J. Chromatog. Sci., 10, 297 (1972).
161. Riedmann, M., Naturwissenschaften, 59, 306 (1972).
162. Toseland, P. A., Grove, J., and Berry, D. J., Clin. Chim. Acta, 38, 321 (1972).
163. Adams, R. F., Perkin-Elmer Clin. Chem. Newsl., 4(1), 15 (1972).
164. Larsen, N. E., Naestoft, J., and Hvidberg, E., Clin. Chim. Acta, 40, 171 (1972).
165. Gardner-Thorpe, C., Parsonage, M. J., Smethurst, P. F., and Toothill, C., Clin. Chim. Acta, 36, 223 (1972).
166. Kupferberg, H. J., J. Pharm. Sci., 61, 284 (1972).
167. Gardner-Thorpe, C., Parsonage, M. J., and Toothill, C., Clin. Chim. Acta, 35, 39 (1972).

REFERENCES

168. Kananen, G., Osiewicz, R., and Sunshine, I., J. Chromatog. Sci., 10, 283 (1972).
169. Papadopoulos, A. S., Baylis, E. M., Fry, D. E., and Marks, V., Clin. Chim. Acta, 48, 135 (1973).
170. Goudie, J. H. and Burnett, D., Clin. Chim. Acta, 43, 423 (1973).
171. Patterson, D. A., in H. Purnell (Ed.), New Developments in Gas Chromatography, Vol. 11, Wiley, New York, 1973.
172. Chang, T. and Glazko, A. J., J. Lab. Clin. Med., 75, 145 (1970).
173. Cremers, H. M. H. G. and Verheesen, P. E., Clin. Chim. Acta, 48, 413 (1973).
174. Griffiths, W. C., Oleksyk, S. K., and Diamond, I., Clin. Biochem., 6, 124 (1973).
175. Friel, P. and Green, J. R., Clin. Chim. Acta, 43, 69 (1973).
176. Horning, M. G., Nowlin, J., Lertratanangkoon, K., Stillwell, R. N., Stillwell, W. G., and Hill, R. M., Clin. Chem., 19, 845 (1973).
177. Skinner, R. F., Gallaher, E. G., and Predmore, D. B., Anal. Chem., 45, 574 (1973).
178. Solow, E. B., Metaxas, J. M., and Summers, T. R., J. Chromatog. Sci., 12, 256 (1974).
179. Cimbura, G. and Kofoed, J., J. Chromatog. Sci., 12, 261 (1974).
180. Horning, M. G., Gregory, P., Nowlin, J., Stafford, M., Lertratanangkoon, K., Butler, C., Stillwell, W. G., and Hill, R. M., Clin. Chem., 20, 282 (1974).
181. Horning, M. G., Lertratanangkoon, K., Nowlin, J., Stillwell, W. G., Stillwell, R. N., Zion, T. E., Kellaway, P., and Hill, R. M., J. Chromatog. Sci., 12, 630 (1974).
182. Brachet-Liermann, A., Trezeguet, C., Versille, C., and Dubois, M., Applications Note GC 5-74, Hewlett-Packard, Palo Alto, Calif., 1974.
183. Driessen, O. and Emonds, A., Proc. Kon. Ned. Akad. Wetensch., 77, No. 2 (1974).
184. Friel, P. and Troupin, A. S., Clin. Chem., 21, 751 (1975).
185. Pecci, J. and Giovanniello, T. J., J. Chromatog., 109, 163 (1975).
186. Blaschke, T. F., Neflin, P. J., Melmon, K. L., and Rowland, M., Clin. Pharmacol. Ther., 17, 685 (1975).
187. Garrettson, L. K. and Jusko, W. J., Clin. Pharmacol. Ther., 17, 481 (1975).
188. Toseland, P. A., Albani, M., and Gauchell, F. D., Clin. Chem., 21, 98 (1975).
189. Meijer, J. W. A., Epilepsia, 12, 341 (1971).
190. Grimmer, G., Jacob, J., and Schafer, H., Arzneim.-Forsch., 19, 1287 (1969).
191. Solow, E. B. and Green, J. B., Neurology, 22, 540 (1972).

192. Friel, P., Green, J. R., and Kupferberg, H. J., Epilepsia, 13, 273 (1972).
193. Berlin, A., Agurell, S., Borga, O., Lund, L., and Sjoqvist, F., Scand. J. Clin. Lab. Invest., 29, 281 (1972).
194. Perchalski, R. J., Scott, K. N., Wilder, B. J., and Hammer, R. H., J. Pharm. Sci., 62, 1735 (1973).
195. Estas, A. and Dumont, P. A., J. Chromatog., 82, 307 (1973).
196. Davis, H. L., Falk, K. J., and Bailey, D. G., J. Chromatog., 107, 61 (1975).
197. Ritz, D. P. and Warren, C. G., Clin. Toxicol., 8, 311 (1975).
198. Horning, M. G., Butler, C., Nowlin, J., Stillwell, W. G., Stillwell, R. N., and Hill, R. M., in R. S. Melville and V. F. Dobson (Eds), Selected Approaches to Gas Chromatography-Mass Spectrometry in Laboratory Medicine, DHEW Publ. No. (NIH) 75-762, Washington, D.C., 1975.
199. Walle, T., J. Chromatog., 114, 345 (1975).
200. Least, C. J., Jr., Johnson, G. F., and Solomon, H. M., Clin. Chem., 21, 1658 (1975).
201. Booker, H. E. and Darcey, B. A., Clin. Chem., 21, 1766 (1975).
202. Hoppel, C., Garle, M., and Elander, M., J. Chromatog., 116, 53 (1976).
203. Midha, K. K., McGilveray, I. J., and Wilson, D. L., J. Pharm. Sci., 65, 1240 (1976).
204. Orme, M., Borga, O., Cook, C. E., and Sjoqvist, F., Clin. Chem., 22, 246 (1976).
205. Spiehler, V., Sun, L., Miyada, D. S., Sarandis, S. G., Walwick, E. R., Klein, M. W., Jordan, D. B., and Jessen, B., Clin. Chem., 22, 749 (1976).
206. Abraham, C. V. and Joslin, H. D., Clin. Chem., 22, 769 (1976).
207. Soldin, S. J. and Hill, J. G., Clin. Chem., 22, 856 (1976).
208. Vandemark, F. L. and Adams, R. F., Clin. Chem., 22, 1062 (1976).
209. Schwartz, P. A., Rhodes, C. T., and Cooper, J. W., Jr., J. Pharm. Sci., 66, 994 (1977).
210. Serfontein, W. J. and De Villiers, L. S., J. Chromatog., 130, 342 (1977).
211. Hill, R. E. and Latham, A. N., J. Chromatog., 131, 341 (1977).
212. Sheehan, M. and Haythorn, P., J. Chromatog., 132, 237 (1977).
213. Abraham, C. V. and Gresham, D., J. Chromatog., 136, 332 (1977).
214. Sengupta, A. and Peat, M. A., J. Chromatog., 137, 206 (1977).
215. Gordos, J., Schaublin, J., and Spring, P., J. Chromatog., 143, 171 (1977).

REFERENCES

216. Hoppel, C., Garle, M., Rane, A., and Sjoqvist, F., Clin. Pharmacol. Ther., 21, 294 (1977).
217. Horning, M. G., Stratton, C., Nowlin, J., Wilson, A., Horning, E. C., and Hill, R. M., in L. O. Boreus (Ed.), Fetal Pharmacology, Raven Press, New York, 1973, pp. 355-373.
218. Rane, A., Garle, M., Borga, O., and Sjoqvist, F., Clin. Pharmacol. Ther., 15, 39 (1974).
219. Krauer, B., Draffan, G. H., Williams, F. M., Clare, R. A., Dollery, C. T., and Hawkins, D. F., Clin. Pharmacol. Ther., 14, 442 (1973).
220. Sjoqvist, F., Bergfors, P. G., Borga, O., Lind, M., and Ygge, H., J. Pediatr., 80, 496 (1972).
221. Jalling, B., Boreus, L. O., Kallberg, N., and Agurell, S., Eur. J. Clin. Pharmacol., 6, 234 (1973).
222. Levy, G., J. Pharm. Sci., 54, 959 (1965).
223. Mirkin, B. L., J. Pediatr., 78, 329 (1971).
224. Hill, R. M., Clin. Pharmacol. Ther., 14, 654 (1973).
225. Hammar, C. G., Holmstedt, B., and Ryhage, R., Anal. Biochem., 25, 532 (1968).
226. Brooks, C. J. W., and Middleditch, B. S., Clin. Chim. Acta, 34, 145 (1971).
227. Horning, M. G., Stillwell, W. G., Nowlin, J., Lertratanangkoon, K., Carroll, D., Dzidic, I., Stillwell, R. N., and Horning, E. C., J. Chromatog., 91, 413 (1974).
228. Horning, M. G., Nowlin, J., Hickert, P., Stillwell, W. G., and Hill, R. M., in C. Galli, G. Jacine, and A. Pecile (Eds.), Dietary Lipids and Postnatal Development, Raven Press, New York, 1973, pp. 257-269.
229. Horning, M. G., Stillwell, W. G., Nowlin, J., Lertratanangkoon, K., Stillwell, R. N., and Hill, R. M., in Modern Problems in Pediatrics, Karger, Basel (in press).
230. Horning, E. C., Horning, M. G., Carroll, D. I., Dzidic, I., and Stillwell, R. N., Anal. Chem., 45, 936 (1973).
231. Stillwell, W. G., Hung, A., Stafford, M., and Horning, M. G., Anal. Lett., 6, 407 (1973).
232. Carroll, D. I., Dzidic, I., Stillwell, R. N., Horning, M. G., and Horning, E. C., Anal. Chem., 46, 706 (1974).
233. Pippenger, C. E. and Gillen, H. W., Clin. Chem., 15, 582 (1969).
234. Larsen, N. E. and Naestoft, J., J. Chromatog., 92, 157 (1974).
235. Milne, G. W. A., Fales, H. M., and Axenrod, T., Anal. Chem., 42, 1432 (1970).
236. Law, N. C., Aandahl, V., Fales, H. M., and Milne, G. W. A., Clin. Chim. Acta, 32, 221 (1971).

237. Dill, W. A., Chucot, L., Chang, T., and Glazko, A. J., Clin. Chem., 17, 1200 (1971).
238. Saitoh, Y., Nishihara, K., Nakagawa, F., and Suzuki, T., J. Pharm. Sci., 62, 206 (1973).
239. Albert, K. S., Sakimar, E., Hallmark, M., Weidler, D., and Wagner, J. G., Clin. Pharmacol. Ther., 16, 727 (1974).
240. MacGee, J., Clin. Chem., 17, 587 (1971).
241. Greeley, R. H., Clin. Chem., 20, 192 (1974).
242. Tigelaar, R. E., Rapport, R. L., Inman, J. K., and Kupferberg, H. J., Clin. Chim. Acta, 43, 231 (1973).
243. Cook, C. E., Kepler, J. A., and Christensen, H. D., Res. Commun. Chem. Pathol. Pharmacol., 5, 767 (1973).
244. Goldbaum, L. R., Anal. Chem., 24, 1604 (1952).
245. Bogan, J. and Smith, H., J. Forensic Sci. Soc., 7, 37 (1967).
246. Wallace, E., Anal. Chem., 40, 978 (1968).
247. Sherwin, A. L., Eisen, A. A., and Sokolowski, C. D., Arch. Neurol. (Chicago), 29, 73 (1973).
248. Wilensky, A. J. and Lowden, J. A., Neurology, 23, 318 (1973).
249. Tindell, G. L., Walle, T., and Gaffney, T. E., Life Sci., 11, 1029 (1972).
250. Walle, T., Ishizaki, T., Saelens, D., Privitera, P. J., Gartiez, D., and Gaffney, T. E., paper presented at Fifth International Congress on Pharmacology, San Francisco, Calif., 1972.
251. Walle, T. and Gaffney, T. E., J. Pharmacol. Exp. Ther., 182, 83 (1972).
252. Walle, T., Ishizaki, T., and Gaffney, T. E., J. Pharmacol. Exp. Ther., 183, 508 (1972).
253. DiSalle, E., Baker, K. M., Bareggi, S. R., Watkins, W. D., Chidsey, C. A., Frigerio, A., and Morselli, P. L., J. Chromatog., 84, 347 (1973).
254. Saelens, D. A., Walle, T., Privitera, P. J., Knapp, D. R., and Gaffney, T. E., in E. Costa and B. Holmstedt (Eds.), Advances in Biochemical Psychopharmacology, Vol. 7, Raven Press, New York, 1973.
255. Saelens, D. A., Walle, T., Privitera, P. J., Knapp, D. R., and Gaffney, T. E., J. Pharmacol. Exp. Ther., 188, 86 (1974).
256. Walle, T., Morrison, J. I., and Tindell, G. L., Res. Commun. Chem. Pathol. Pharmacol., 9, 1 (1974).
257. Walle, T., J. Pharm. Sci., 63, 1885 (1974).
258. Walle, T., Morrison, J., Walle, K., and Conradi, E., J. Chromatog., 114, 351 (1975).
259. Ervik, M., Acta Pharmacol. Toxicol., 36, Suppl. 5, 136 (1975).
260. Desager, J. P. and Harvengt, C., J. Pharm. Pharmacol., 27, 52 (1975).

REFERENCES

261. Wagner, J. G., Weidler, D. J., and Lin, Y. J., Res. Commun. Chem. Pathol. Pharmacol., 13, 9 (1976).
262. Abramson, F. P., in R. S. Melville and V. F. Dobson (Eds.), Selected Approaches to Gas Chromatography-Mass Spectrometry in Laboratory Medicine, DHEW Publ. No. (NIH) 75-762, Washington, D.C., 1975.
263. Koslow, S. H., Catabeni, F., and Costa, E., Science, 176, 177 (1972).
264. Narasimhachari, N. and Vouros, P., Anal. Biochem., 45, 154 (1972).
265. Gartiez, D. A. and Walle, T., J. Pharm. Sci., 61, 1728 (1972).
266. Saelens, D. A., Walle, T., and Privitera, P. J., J. Chromatog., 123, 185 (1976).
267. Parker, K. D., Fontan, C. R., and Kirk, P. L., Anal. Chem., 34, 1345 (1962).
268. Anthony, G. M., Brooks, C. J. W., Maclean, I., and Sangster, I., J. Chromatog. Sci., 7, 623 (1969).
269. Anthony, G. M., Brooks, C. J. W., and Middleditch, B. S., J. Pharm. Pharmacol., 22, 205 (1970).
270. Lebish, P., Finkle, B. S., and Brackett, J. W., Jr., Clin. Chem., 16, 195 (1970).
271. Lhuguenot, J. C. and Maume, B. F., J. Chromatog. Sci., 12, 411 (1974).
272. Donike, M., Chromatographia, 7, 651 (1974).
273. Curtius, H. C., Wolfensberger, M., Steinmann, B., Redweik, U., and Siegfreid, J., J. Chromatog., 99, 529 (1974).
274. Watson, J. R. and Lawrence, R. C., J. Pharm. Sci., 66, 560 (1977).
275. Ranney, R. E., Dean, R. R., Karim, A., and Radzialowski, F. M., Arch. Int. Pharmacodyn. Ther., 191, 162 (1971).
276. Hutsell, T. C. and Stachelski, S. J., J. Chromatog., 106, 151 (1975).
277. Duchateau, A. M. J. A., Merkus, F. W. H. M., and Schobben, F., J. Chromatog., 109, 432 (1975).
278. Hinderling, P. H. and Garrett, E. R., J. Pharmacokin. Biopharmaceut., 4, 199 (1976).
279. Hinderling, P. H. and Garrett, E. R., J. Pharmacokin. Biopharmaceut., 4, 231 (1976).
280. Zacchei, A. G. and Weidner, L., J. Pharm. Sci., 64, 814 (1975).
281. Rutherford, B. S. and Bishara, R. H., J. Pharm. Sci., 65, 1322 (1976).
282. Acta Cardiol., Suppl., 18, 131, 177, 195, 233 (1974).
283. Van Durme, J. P., Bogaert, M. G., and Rosseel, M. T., Brit. J. Clin. Pharmacol., 1, 461 (1974).

284. Van Durme, J. P., Bogaert, M. G., and Rosseel, M. T., Eur. J. Clin. Pharmacol., 7, 343 (1974).
285. Kelly, J. G., Nimmo, J., Rae, R., Shanks, R. G., and Prescott, L. F., J. Pharm. Pharmacol., 25, 550 (1973).
286. Kiddie, M. A., Royds, R. B., and Shaw, T. R. D., Brit. J. Pharmacol., 47, 674P (1973).
287. Kiddie, M. A. and Kaye, C. M., Brit. J. Clin. Pharmacol., 1, 86 (1974).
288. Willox, S. and Singh, B. N., J. Chromatog., 128, 196 (1976).
289. Beckett, A. H. and Chidomere, E. C., J. Pharm. Pharmacol., 29, 281 (1977).
290. Camera, E. and Pravisani, D., Anal. Chem., 36, 2109 (1964).
291. Fossel, E. T., J. Gas Chromatog., 3, 179 (1965).
292. Williams, A. F., Murray, W. J., and Gibb, B. H., Nature, 210, 816 (1966).
293. Sherber, P. A., Marcus, M., and Kleinberg, S. I., Enzymol. Biol. Clin., 10, 365 (1969).
294. Trowell, J. M., Anal. Chem., 42, 1440 (1970).
295. Sherber, P. A., Marcus, M., and Kleinberg, S., Biochem. Pharmacol., 19, 607 (1970).
296. Gobbeler, K. H., Pharm. Z., 27, 961 (1971).
297. Davidson, I. W. F., Dicarlo, F. J., and Szabo, E. I., J. Chromatog., 57, 345 (1971).
298. Rosseel, M. T. and Bogaert, M. G., J. Chromatog., 64, 364 (1972).
299. Rosseel, M. T. and Bogaert, M. G., J. Pharm. Sci., 62, 754 (1973).
300. Malbica, J. O., Monson, K., Neilson, K., and Sprissler, R., J. Pharm. Sci., 66, 385 (1977).
301. Chin, D. A., Prue, D. G., Michelucci, J., Kho, B. T., and Warner, C. R., J. Pharm. Sci., 66, 1143 (1977).
302. Sisenwine, S. F. and Ruelius, H. W., J. Pharmacol. Exp. Ther., 176, 296 (1971).
303. Fanelli, R. and Frigerio, A., J. Chromatog., 93, 441 (1974).
304. Regnier, G., Canevari, R. J., Laubie, M. J., and Le Douarec, J. C., J. Med. Chem., 11, 1151 (1968).
305. Laubie, M., Schmitt, H., and Le Douarec, J. C., Eur. J. Pharmacol., 6, 75 (1969).
306. Corrodi, H., Fuxe, K., and Ungerstedt, U., J. Pharm. Pharmacol., 23, 989 (1971).
307. Corrodi, H., Farnebo, L. O., Fuxe, K., Hamberger, B., and Ungerstedt, U., Eur. J. Pharmacol., 20, 195 (1972).
308. Garattini, S., Fanelli, R., Jori, A., Consolo, S., Ladinsky, H., and Samanin, R., in Proceedings of International Symposium "Trivastal", Monastir, 1972.

REFERENCES

309. Higuchi, S., Sasaki, H., and Sado, T., J. Chromatog., 110, 301 (1975).
310. Mardente, S. and De Marchi, F., J. Pharm. Sci., 64, 1866 (1975).
311. Hucker, H. B. and Stauffer, S. C., J. Pharm. Sci., 65, 1253 (1976).
312. Miyazaki, H., Ishibashi, M., Izawa, T., Takayama, H., and Idzu, G., Chem. Pharm. Bull., 23, 837 (1975).
313. Miyazaki, H., Ishibashi, M., Takayama, H., Abuki, H., Idzu, G., Morishita, N., and Ando, M., paper presented at 4th Symposium on Drug Metabolism and Action, Sendai, Japan, September 1972.
314. Crombez, E., Van Den Bossche, W., and De Moerloose, P., J. Chromatog., 117, 161 (1976).
315. Brown, S. A. and Shyluk, J. P., Anal. Chem., 34, 1058 (1962).
316. Brown, S. A., National Research Council, Saskatoon, Canada, unpublished work, 1962.
317. Karlsen, J., von Hagen, P., and Svendsen, A. B., Medd. Norsk Farm. Selskap, 29, 153 (1967).
318. Furuya, T. and Kojima, H., J. Chromatog., 29, 382 (1967).
319. Steck, W. and Bailey, B. K., Can. J. Chem., 47, 2425 (1969).
320. Steck, W. and Bailey, B. K., Can. J. Chem., 47, 3577 (1969).
321. Pellizzari, E. D., Chuang, C. M., Kuc, J., and Williams, E. B., J. Chromatog., 40, 285 (1969).
322. Deckert, F. W., J. Chromatog., 64, 355 (1972).
323. Deckert, F. W., J. Chromatog., 69, 201 (1972).
324. Hoque, M. and Dutta, J., J. Indian Chem. Soc., 49, 871 (1972).
325. Kaiser, D. G. and Martin, R. S., J. Pharm. Sci., 63, 1579 (1974).
326. Midha, K. K., McGilveray, I. J., and Cooper, J. K., J. Pharm. Sci., 63, 1725 (1974).
327. Schuppel, R. V., Konig, R., Steinhilber, E., and Deckert, F. W., Naunyn.-Schmiedebergs Arch. Pharmakol., 282, Suppl. R87 (1974).
328. Bianchetti, G., Latini, R., and Morselli, P. L., J. Chromatog., 124, 331 (1976).
329. Yacobi, A., Udall, J. A., and Levy, G., Clin. Pharmacol. Ther., 19, 552 (1976).
330. Midha, K. K., Hubbard, J. W., Cooper, J. K., and McGilveray, I. J., J. Pharm. Sci., 65, 387 (1976).
331. Heni, N. and Glogner, P., Naunyn.-Schmiedebergs Arch. Pharmakol., 293, 183 (1976).
332. Schmitt, K. F. and Jahnchen, E., J. Chromatog., 130, 418 (1977).
333. Midha, K. K. and Cooper, J. K., J. Pharm. Sci., 66, 799 (1977).
334. Svendsen, A. B. and Ottestad, E., Pharm. Acta Helv., 32, 457 (1957).
335. Welling, P. G., Lee, K. P., Khanna, U., and Wagner, J. G., J. Pharm. Sci., 59, 1621 (1970).

336. Trager, W. F., Lewis, R. J., and Garland, W. A., J. Med. Chem., 13, 1196 (1970).
337. Pohl, L. R., Haddock, R. E., Garland, W. A., and Trager, W. F., J. Med. Chem., 18, 513 (1975).
338. Haddock, R. E., Trager, W. F., and Pohl, L. R., J. Med. Chem., 18, 519 (1975).
339. Li, H. and Cervoni, P., J. Pharm. Sci., 65, 1352 (1976).
340. Milne, G. W. A., Fales, H. M., and Axenrod, T., Anal. Chem., 43, 1815 (1971).
341. Wallace, S. M. and Riegelman, S., J. Pharm. Sci., 66, 729 (1977).
342. Wallace, S. M., Shah, V. P., and Riegelman, S., J. Pharm. Sci., 66, 527 (1977).
343. Ervik, M. and Gustavii, K., Anal. Chem., 46, 39 (1974).
344. Vanden Heuvel, W. J. A., Gruber, V. F., Walker, R. W., and Wolf, F. J., J. Pharm. Sci., 64, 1309 (1975).
345. Lindstrom, B., Molander, M., and Groschinsky, M., J. Chromatog., 114, 459 (1975).
346. Beermann, B., Groschinsky-Grind, M., and Rosen, A., Clin. Pharmacol. Ther., 19, 531 (1976).
347. Feit, P. W., Roholt, K., and Sorensen, H., J. Pharm. Sci., 62, 375 (1973).
348. Davies, D. L., Lant, A. F., Millard, N. R., Smith, A. J., Ward, J. W., and Wilson, G. M., Clin. Pharmacol. Ther., 15, 141 (1974).
349. Lindstrom, B. and Molander, M., J. Chromatog., 101, 219 (1974).
350. Beermann, B., Dalen, E., and Lindstrom, B., Clin. Pathol. Ther., 22, 70 (1977).
351. Desager, J. P., Vanderbist, M. Hwang, B., and Levandoski, P., J. Chromatog., 123, 379 (1976).
352. Chamberlain, J., J. Chromatog., 55, 249 (1971).
353. Feher, T., Bodrogi, L., and Varadi, A., J. Chromatog., 123, 460 (1976).
354. Silvestri, S., Farmaco, Ed. Prat., 25, 197 (1970).
355. Horning, M. G., Hebert, R. M., Roth, R. J., Davis, D. L., Horning, E. C., Fischer, E. P., and Jordan, G. L., Jr., Lipids, 7, 114 (1971).
356. Horning, M. G., Hebert, R. M., Roth, R. J., Davis, D. L., Horning, E. C., Fischer, E. P., and Jordan, G. L., Jr., paper presented at "Recent Advances in Drugs Affecting Lipid Metabolism," AOAC Mtg., Houston, Tex., May 1971.
357. Sedaghat, A., Nakamura, H., and Ahrens, E. H., Jr., J. Lipid Res., 15, 352 (1974).
358. Knuchel, V. F. and Ochs, H., Arzneim.-Forsch., 24, 576 (1974).

REFERENCES

359. Karmen, A. and Haut, H., Biochem. Med., 12, 154 (1975).
360. Gugler, R., Shoeman, D. W., Huffman, D. H., Cohlmia, J. B., and Azarnoff, D. L., J. Clin. Invest., 55, 1182 (1975).
361. Bruderlein, H., Robinson, W. T., Kraml, M., and Dvornik, D., Clin. Biochem., 8, 261 (1975).
362. Tuong, T. C. and Tuong, A., J. Chromatog., 106, 97 (1975).
363. Berlin, A., J. Pharm. Pharmacol., 27, 54 (1975).
364. Houin, G., Thebault, J. J., and d'Athis, P., Eur. J. Clin. Pharmacol., 8, 433 (1975).
365. Connor, J. N., Johnson, G. F., and Solomon, H. M., Clin. Chem., 22, 884 (1976).
366. Gugler, R. and Jensen, C., J. Chromatog., 117, 175 (1976).
367. Goldberg, A. P., Sherrard, D. J., Haas, L. B., and Brunzell, J. D., Clin. Pharmacol. Ther., 21, 317 (1977).
368. Hucker, H. B., Grady, L. T., Michniewicz, B. M., Stauffer, S. C., White, S. E., Maha, G. E., and McMahon, F. G., J. Pharmacol. Exp. Ther., 179, 359 (1971).
369. Dujovne, C. A., Azarnoff, D. L., Huffman, D. H., Pentikainen, P., Hurwitz, A., and Shoeman, D. W., Clin. Pharmacol. Ther., 19, 352 (1976).
370. Huffman, D. H., Azarnoff, D. L., Shoeman, D. W., and Dujovne, C. A., Clin. Pharmacol. Ther., 19, 807 (1976).
371. Elsom, L. F., Hawkins, D. R., and Chasseaud, L. F., J. Chromatog., 123, 463 (1976).
372. Barrett, A. M. and Thorp, J. M., Brit. J. Pharmacol., 32, 381 (1968).
373. de Boer, T. J., Rec. Trav. Chim. Pays-Bas, 73, 229 (1954).
374. Bridgman, J. F., Rosen, S. M., and Thorp, J. M., Lancet, 2, 506 (1972).
375. Dosa, S., Mallick, N. P., and Slotki, I. N., Lancet, 1, 250 (1974).
376. Pierides, A. M., Alvarez-Ude, K., Kerr, D. N. S., and Skillen, A. W., Lancet, 2, 1279 (1975).

Chapter 2

ANTIHYPERTENSIVE, HYPOGLYCEMIC, AND THYROID-RELATED DRUGS

I. ANTIHYPERTENSIVE DRUGS

Many antihypertensive drugs have been examined by GC or GC-MS, including all those shown in Figure 2.1, as well as some others such as mebutamate [1-7] (see Chapter 2, Volume 2), pargyline [2,3,8-15] (see Chapter 2, Volume 3, and Chapter 1, Volume 4, phentolamine [16] (see Chapter 1, Volume 4), propranolol (see Chapter 2, Volume 4, and Chapter 1 of this volume) and the diuretics discussed in Chapter 1 of this volume (chlorothiazide, chlorthalidone, furosemide, etc.).

Several more qualitative studies have also included antihpyertensive drugs among a wide variety of compounds examined. Moffat [13] reported retention indices of 1530 and 1410 for hydralazine and pheniprazine [(1-methyl-2-phenylethyl)hydrazine], respectively, whereas Finkle et al. [2] tabulated relative retention data using specific column systems (see Chapter 1 of Volume 2 for column, GC operating, extraction, and coding details) for alseroxylon (a fat-soluble alkaloidal fraction extracted from Rauwolfia serpentina) and hydralazine: hydralazine, RRT = 0.44, column system I; alseroxylon, RRT = 1.43, column system VII. On the other hand, the GC-MS report of Foltz et al. [4] contained methane CI-MS and EI-MS data for pheniprazine and deserpidine, respectively; as tabulated below:

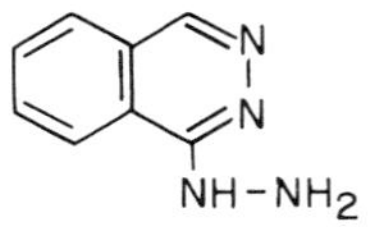

Hydralazine

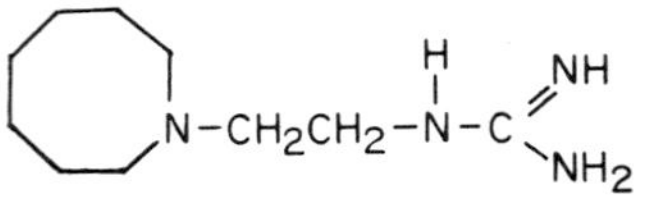

Guanethidine

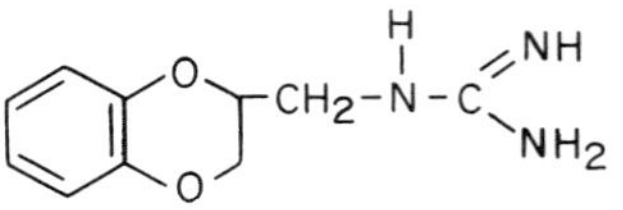

Guanoxan

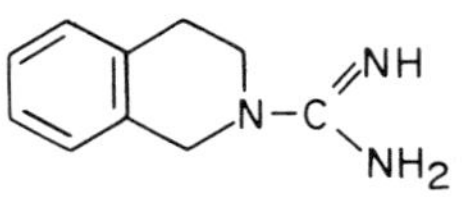

Debrisoquin

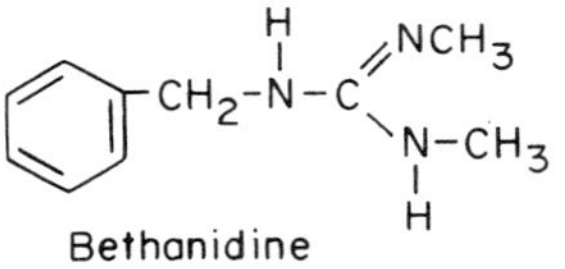

Bethanidine

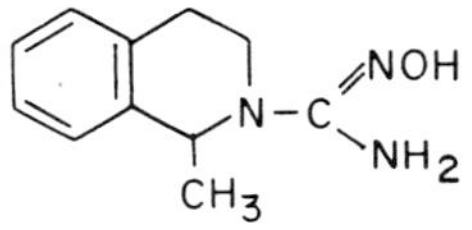

3,4-Dihydro-1-methyl-2(1H)-isoquinoline carboxamidoxime

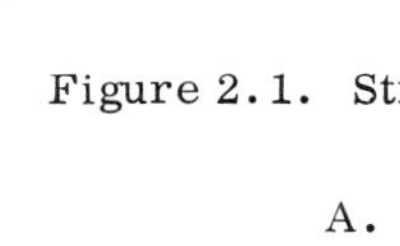

Clonidine

[2-(2,6-Dichloroanilino)-2-imidazoline]

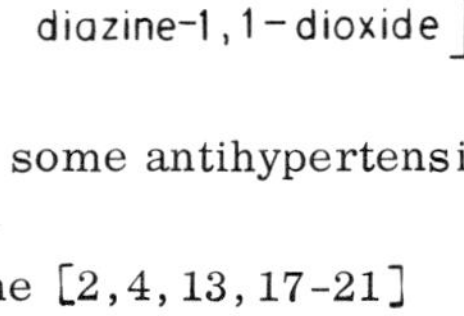

Diazoxide

[7-Chloro-3-methyl-2H-1,2,4-benzothiadiazine-1,1-dioxide]

Figure 2.1. Structures of some antihypertensive drugs

A. Hydralazine [2,4,13,17-21]

In 1975, Jack et al. [17] described a GC method for the determination of hydralazine in plasma in which, on treatment with nitrous acid, hydralazine is converted into tetrazolo(1,5-a)phthalazine, a stable compound that can be extracted from biological material with organic solvent and determined quantitatively by gas chromatography. The 4-methyl analog of hydralazine serves as internal standard for derivatization, extraction, and gas chromatography.

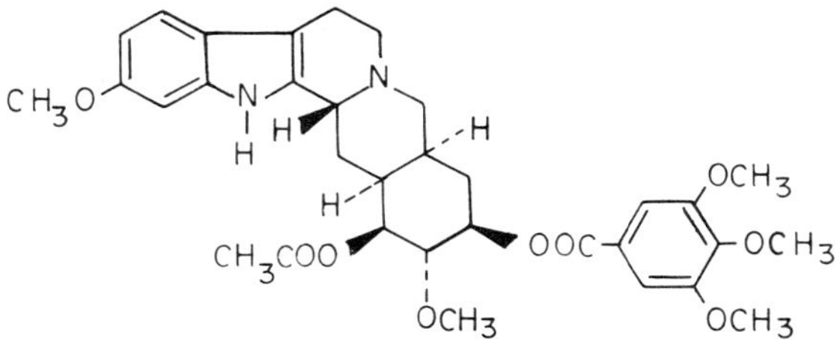

Reserpine

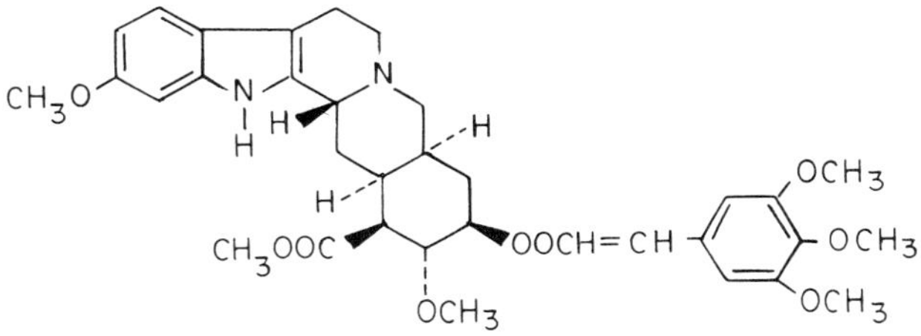

Rescinnamine

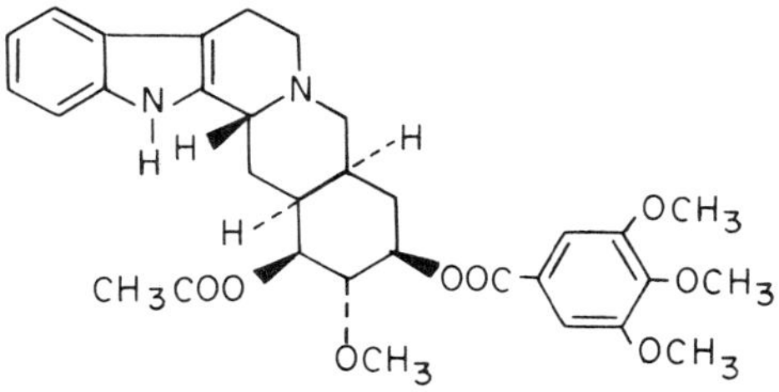

Deserpidine

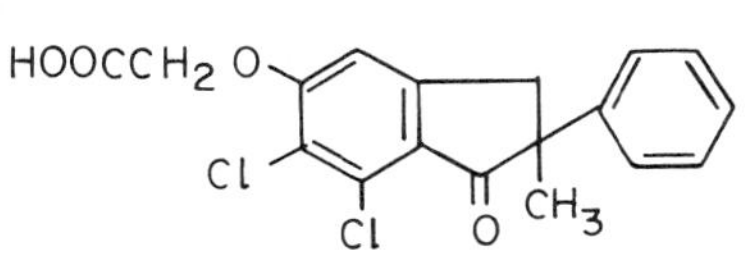

(6,7-Dichloro-2-methyl-1-oxo-2-phenyl-5-indanyloxy)-acetic acid

Figure 2.1 (continued)

Methane CI-MS Data

Compound	M.W.	MH$^+$ (RI)	Prominent fragment ions > m/e 50
Pheniprazine	150	151 (82)	59 (100), 91 (84), 119 (78), 134 (22)
Hydralazine	160	161 (100)	160 (37)

EI-MS Data

Compound	M.W.	Prominent fragment ions > m/e 30
Deserpidine	578	365 (100), 195 (57), 221 (57), 28 (44), 366 (41)

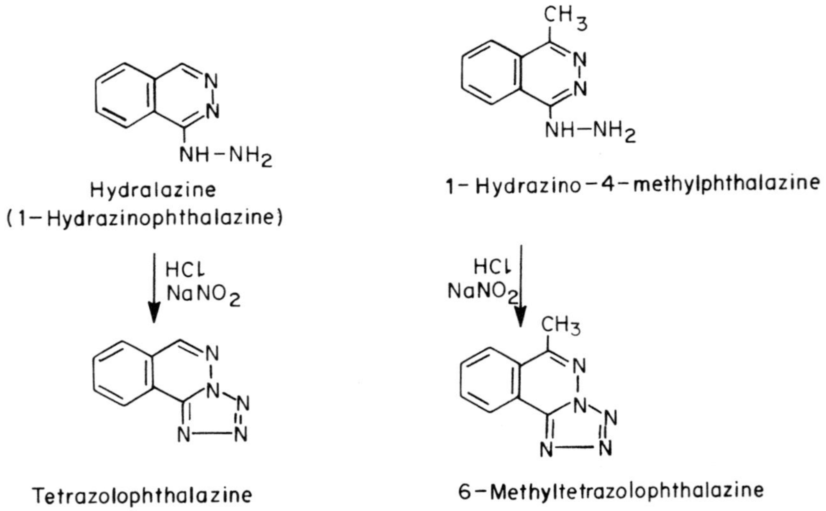

Hydralazine
(1-Hydrazinophthalazine)

1-Hydrazino-4-methylphthalazine

HCl
NaNO$_2$

HCl
NaNO$_2$

Tetrazolophthalazine

6-Methyltetrazolophthalazine

The procedure recommended for sample preparation for subsequent analysis by GC is as follows:

The internal standard, 1-hydrazino-4-methylphthalazine, (50 ng in 0.1 ml of 0.1 N HCl) is added to 1 ml (or less) of plasma, then 1 ml of 2 N HCl and 0.1 ml of 50% aqueous sodium nitrite are added. The solution is mixed and left to react for 15 min at room temperature, then the pH is adjusted to 10 ($\pm$1) by adding 2 ml of 1 N NaOH and 4 ml of buffer of pH 10 (0.03 M borax and 0.04 M NaOH). The derivatives are then extracted with 3 ml of benzene by shaking for 5 min; after centrifugation, the organic phase is removed and evaporated under a stream of dry nitrogen at 45°C. Immediately after all the benzene has evaporated, the vials are removed from the water bath and refrigerated until GC analysis can be carried out. (Excessive long evaporation results in loss of the derivatives.) The dry residue is redissolved in 300 to 900 μl of toluene (depending on concentration), and approximately 5 μl of this solution are injected into the gas chromatograph.

Jack et al. performed all chromatographic studies using a Pye Unicam model 74 (series 104) gas chromatograph equipped with an electron-capture detector (pulsed, 150 μsec) and a 5-ft by 2-mm-i.d. borosilicate glass column packed with 3% OV-225 on 80-100 mesh Chromosorb W-HP. To obtain retention times of 6.4 and 9.1 min for tetrazolophthalazine and 6-methyltetrazolophthalazine, respectively, the GC conditions were maintained as follows: injector temperature, 220°C; column temperature, 220°C; detector temperature, 300°C; nitrogen carrier-gas flow rate, 30 ml/min.

With a sensitivity of 10 ng/ml of plasma, which was sufficient to monitor plasma levels in man after administration of single oral doses of 50 mg of hydralazine, plasma levels of unchanged drug in samples collected from a healthy human male volunteer at intervals of 0.0, 0.5, 1.0, 2.0, 3.0, 4.0, 6.0, 8.0, 10.0, and 24.0 hr after ingestion of the dose were 0.0, 266.0, 226.0, 155.0, 115.0, 67.0, 44.0, 32.0, 21.0, and 8.0 ng/ml, respectively.

Using the procedure proposed by Jack et al. [17], Melander et al. [18] examined in five healthy males the influence of food on the bioavailability of hydralazine in noncoated and coated tablets. The plasma concentrations of unchanged drug were plotted against time, and the peak concentration (C_{max}), time of peak concentration (t_{max}), elimination half-life ($t_{1/2}$), and area under the plasma concentration curves (AUC) were assessed. Estimates of these kinetic parameters of hydralazine were made from GC results, as indicated in Table 2.1.

Melander et al. summarized their findings by noting that each subject received an oral 50-mg dose on four different occasions; two 25-mg noncoated tablets with and without food and one 50-mg coated tablet with

TABLE 2.1

Estimates of Kinetic Parameters of Hydralazine in Five Healthy Male Subjects Given an Oral Dose Under Four Different Conditions[a,b]

Condition	C_{max} (ng/ml)				t_{max} (min)				Kinetic
	A	B	C	D	A	B	C	D	
Subject no.									
1	220	360	170	700	30	28	45	27	
2	160	256	131	214	31	61	50	121	
3	158	385	280	414	61	29	59	29	
4	290	383	192	380	63	46	45	88	
5	110	280	165	220	49	46	44	90	

[a]Adapted from Melander et al. [18].
[b]Condition A: 2 X 25 mg, fasting; condition B: 2 X 25 mg, nonfasting; condition C: 1 X 50 mg, fasting; condition D: 1 X 50 mg, nonfasting.
Note: conditions A and B used noncoated tablets; conditions C and D used coated tablets.

and without food. The meal was a standardized breakfast of 440 cal (150 ml of low-fat milk, 100 ml of orange juice, 1 egg, 2 pieces of crisp bread, 5 mg of margarine, 20 g of cheese). Venous blood samples were obtained during a 6-hr period, and the plasma concentrations of unmetabolized hydralazine were assessed by a selective and sensitive GC method. The results indicated that food enhances the bioavailability of hydralazine two- to threefold both when noncoated and coated tablets were used.

In 1976, Haegele and co-workers [19] investigated by in vivo and in vitro studies the metabolism of hydralazine (HP) using integrated GC-MS, a deuterium-labeled internal standard (d_3-MTP, d_3-3-methyl-s-triazolo [3,4-a]phthalazine) for quantification, ^{14}C-labeled internal standards to demonstrate recoveries from the biological samples, and synthesized standards to identify the metabolic products illustrated in Figure 2.2; namely, 3-methyl-s-triazolo(3,4-a)phthalazine (MTP), s-triazolo(3,4-a) phthalazine (TP), 1-hydrazinophthalazine acetone hydrazone (HPAH), 1-hydrazinophthalazine pyruvic acid hydrazone (HPPAH), and phthalazine (P).

Parameters							
$t_{1/2}$ (hr)				AUC (ng-ml/min)			
A	B	C	D	A	B	C	D
1.58	2.47	1.92	1.65	26,890	53,220	22,067	54,471
1.55	1.55	1.48	1.87	18,221	35,972	16,402	49,405
1.25	2.45	2.37	2.45	14,935	39,066	44,552	50,661
2.93	2.98	3.00	2.47	24,607	64,869	27,542	71,656
1.25	1.62	1.25	1.83	12,830	45,357	21,119	42,774

In the two investigations reported (the in vitro HP metabolism as studied by rat liver homogenate and the in vivo HP metabolites in rat urine), the underivatized HP was converted to tetrazolophthalazine (TZOP) with a 50% $NaNO_2$ solution immediately prior to extraction. In the case of the in vitro sample, the extractions were first made at the acidic pH and then again at a pH of 10 to 11. The extraction procedure involved transferring the aqueous sample to a conical centrifuge tube with 25 ml of chloroform-isopropanol (3:1), shaking the contents on a Vortex mixer for 1 min, centrifuging, removing the lower organic phase, and filtering into a round-bottom flask. After reextracting the aqueous phase two more times with 10 ml of the mixed solvent mixture, the organic phases were combined and then evaporated to dryness under vacuum at 35°C. The aqueous phase was then adjusted to pH 10-11 and extracted again as described. As noted by Haegele et al., further processing of the samples for GC-MS analysis was carried out via the procedure for the in vivo experiments described below.

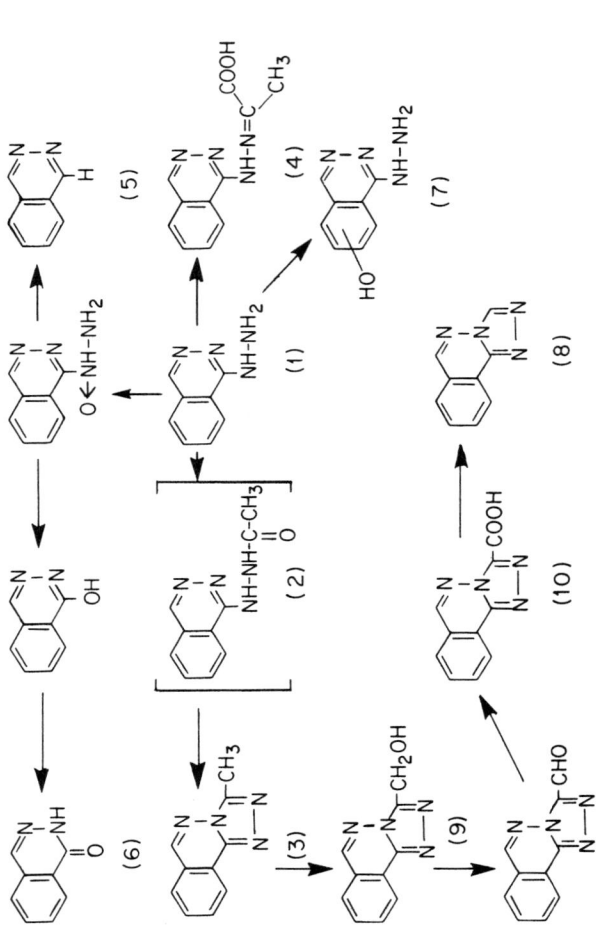

Figure 2.2. Metabolic pathways of hydralazine for some products reported in the literature. 1, Hydralazine (HP); 2, 1-hydrazinophthalazine acetone hydrazone (HPAH); 3, methyltriazolophthalazine (MTP); 4, 1-hydrazinophthalazine pyruvic acid hydrazone (HPPAH); 5, phthalazine (P); 6, phthalazinone (PO); 7, hydroxylated phenyl ring hydralazine; 8, triazolophthalazine (TP); 9, 3-hydroxymethyltriazolophthalazine (HMTP); 10, 3-carboxytriazolophthalazine (CTP). Adapted from Haegele et al. [19].

Processing of the urine samples consisted of the following:

Urine was collected for 4 to 5 hr. Upon termination of the procedure, the urine was either analyzed directly or frozen immediately for subsequent analysis within 24 hr. Before acidification of the urine (2 to 3 ml), 1 mg of EDTA was added. This was followed by 1 ml of 2 N HCl and 0.2 ml of a 50% $NaNO_2$ solution. The reaction mixture was allowed to stand for 15 min. Extraction was carried out with three 10-ml portions of chloroform-isopropanol (3:1). The urine was then adjusted to pH 10 with 4 N NaOH solution and reextracted with three portions of chloroform-isopropanol. The extracts were combined and dried over Na_2SO_4.

Aliquots of this solution were transferred to Reacti-Vials and evaporated to dryness. The sample was redissolved with 50 μl of acetonitrile. Then 50 μl of Regisil-TMCS (trimethylchlorosilane) were added and the sample heated at 100°C for 15 min. After addition of the deuterium-labeled internal standard (d_3-MTP), aliquots were injected onto the GC column for analysis by GC-MS.

GC-MS studies were performed on a Hewlett-Packard GC-MS-COMP system equipped with a 3-ft by 4-mm-i.d. coiled glass column packed with 3% OV-17 on 80-100 mesh Chromosorb W. The other GC-MS conditions used were helium carrier-gas flow rate, 40 ml/min; column temperature, programmed from 170 to 240°C at a rate of 4°C/min; ion source temperature, 210°C; ionizing energy, 25 eV. Using these operating parameters, the retention times for phthalazine (P), phthalazinone (PO), 1-hydrazinophthalazine acetone hydrazone (HPAH), triazolophthalazine (TP), tetrazolophthalazine (TZOP), 3-methyl-s-triazolo(3,4-a)phthalazine (MTP), the internal standard (d_3-MTP), and the TMSi derivative of 1-hydrazinophthalazine pyruvic acid hydrazone (HPPAH) were 1.7, 2.3, 4.9, 8.0, 8.9, 9.6, 9.6, and 17.0 min, respectively. The m/e ions used for single-ion monitoring (SID) for the determination of the various metabolites as well as the base peak of each in their respective mass spectrum are listed in Table 2.2. In addition to this GC-MS data, it was reported that the TMSi derivative of 3-hydroxymethyltriazolophthalazine (HMTP) had a retention time of approximately 14.8 min with m/e ions in its mass spectrum occurring at 272 (M^+), 257 ($M-CH_3^+$), 183 ($M-TMSi-0^+$), and 115. The peak at 18.8 min yielded a similar mass spectrum with m/e 272 as the base peak; this compound was postulated to be an hydroxylated phenyl ring MTP compound. The carboxyl derivative of MTP (identified in Fig. 2.2 as component 10 or CTP) was also tentatively identified by the occurrence of m/e 286 (M^+), 271 ($M-CH_3^+$), and 197 ($M-TMSi-0^+$).

Using ^{14}C-labeled standards, the recovery of HP, MTP, TP, TZOP, and HPPAH was 79.4 (after incubation with glusulase, 88.7), 98, 99, 95, and 76%, respectively.

TABLE 2.2

Ions for SIM and Base Peaks of Standards (GC-MS Analysis)[a]

Compound	Ions for SIM (m/e)	Base peak (25 eV)
Phthalazine (P)	103, 130	130
Phthalazinone (PO)	117, 146	146
1-Hydrazinophthalazine acetone hydrazone (HPAH)	115, 185, 200	185
Triazolophthalazine (TP)	115, 170	170
Tetrazolophthalazine (TZOP)	115	115
3-Methyl-s-triazolo-(3,4-a) phthalazine (MTP)	115, 184	184
d_3-MTP (IS)	115, 187	187
TMSi ester of 1-hydrazinophthalazine pyruvic acid hydrazone (HPPAH)	115, 184, 212	212

[a] Adapted from Haegele et al. [19].

Typical results for the analysis of urinary extract and liver homogenate samples are given in Table 2.3.

Using the procedure developed by Jack et al. [17], Talseth [21] studied the kinetics of hydrazine elimination. In his investigation, "hydralazine was given orally in single doses of 10, 25, and 50 mg to two slow-acetylating subjects, while two rapid-acetylating subjects also received 100- and 150-mg doses on different occasions. Administration of the 50-mg dose to the subjects who were slow acetylators and the 150-mg dose to those who were rapid acetylators caused a disproportionately large increase in the amount of unchanged drug appearing in the systemic circulation as judged from the increases in the ratios of areas under concentration-time curves (AUC) to dose. A modification of the GC hydralazine assay allowed the simultaneous determination of hydralazine and its acetylated metabolite, 3-methyl-s-triazolo(3,4-a)-phthalazine, in serum. It was found that the disproportionately large increases in the AUC/dose ratio of hydralazine upon intake of 50 or 150 mg doses by the slow- and the rapid-acetylating subjects, respectively, were paralleled by a decrease in the ratio AUC^{MTP}/AUC^{HP} during a 6-hr observation period. It is

TABLE 2.3

GC-MS Results for Typical Urinary Extracts and Liver Homogenate Samples[a]

Compound	Percent found		
	Liver homogenate		Urinary extract
	A[b]	B[c]	
Phthalazine	0.2	1.6	6.9
Phthalazinone	7.0	4.5	3.4
Hydralazine	0.4	0.2	2.0
3-Methyltriazolophthalazine	69.5	70.8	31.8
3-Hydroxymethyltriazolophthalazine	12.2	9.5	4.3
3-Carboxytriazolophthalazine	0.1	0.6	0.2
Triazolophthalazine	6.8	5.1	20.5
Hydroxylated phenyl ring 3-methyltriazolophthalazine	3.1	8.0	29.5
1-Hydrazinophthalazine acetone hydrazone	0.8	0.6	0.8
1-Hydrazinophthalazine pyruvic acid hydrazone	0.1	0.1	0.6
	100.2	100.0	100.0

[a]Adapted from Haegele et al. [19].
[b]A: no cofactors added.
[c]B: with cofactors added (glucose-6-phosphate, NADPH, NADH).

concluded that the acetylation of hydralazine is a capacity-limited process." In Table 2.4 are listed the hydralazine doses and some of the corresponding pharmacokinetic parameters derived from healthy subjects.

In 1977, Smith et al. [20] also described a GC method for the determination of hydralazine in various tablet formulations based on the quantitative reaction of hydralazine with 2,4-pentanedione to yield 1-(3,5-dimethylpyrazole)phthalazine. Sample preparation for GC analysis was carried out in the following manner:

TABLE 2.4

Hydralazine Doses and Corresponding Pharmacokinetic Data Derived from Healthy Subjects[a]

Parameter	Subject 1 (slow acetylator)			Subject 2 (slow acetylator)		
	10 mg	25 mg	50 mg	10 mg	25 mg	50 mg
A. Hydralazine						
Peak conc. (ng/ml)	58	200	356	58	167	457
$t_{1/2}$ (hr)	1.82	1.54	2.82	2.06	1.62	1.78
B. 3-Methyl-s-triazolo-(3,4-a)phthalazine						
Peak conc. (ng/ml)		30	39		20	43
$t_{1/2}$ (hr)		0.88	2.04		3.77	1.39
$\left[AUC^{MTP}/AUC^{HP} \right]$		0.11	0.08		0.09	0.07
$\left\{ \dfrac{\text{Peak conc.}^{MTP}}{\text{Peak conc.}^{HP}} \right\}$		0.15	0.11		0.12	0.10

[a]Adapted from Talseth [21].

Hydralazine + 2,4-Pentanedione → 1-(3,5-Dimethylpyrazole)-phthalazine

The average weight of 10 tablets was obtained and the tablets were ground to a fine powder. A powdered amount equivalent to the tablet potency was weighed out and transferred quantitatively to a 35-ml screw-cap centrifuge tube. An appropriate amount of water was added to the tube, resulting in a hydralazine concentration of 2 mg/ml. The solution was sonified for 5 min and shaken for 30 min, then allowed to stand at room temperature for 10 min. A 10-ml aliquot of the suspension was removed and added to a 35-ml centrifuge containing 1.0-ml of 2,4-pentanedione. The resulting mixture was shaken for 30 min and left to react at room temperature for an additional 30 min. Ten milliliters of internal standard solution (0.6 mg of phenanthrene/ml of ethyl acetate) was then added and the tube was placed on a mechanical shaker for 10 min to extract the resulting hydralazine derivative. Approximately 1 μl of the ethyl acetate layer was injected into the GC unit without further treatment.

Smith et al. performed GC analyses with a Tracor MT-220 and a Varian 2100 gas chromatograph equipped with flame ionization detectors and 6-ft by 4-mm-i.d. U-shaped glass columns packed with 10% SE-30 on 80-100 mesh Gas Chrom Q. Using the specified GC conditions (injector temperature, 210°C; column temperature, 200°C; detector temperature, 250°C; nitrogen carrier-gas flow rate, 55 ml/min), the retention times for the internal standard (phenanthrene) and 1-(3,5-dimethylpyrazole)phthalazine were about 2.00 and 3.68 min, respectively.

Comparison of results obtained for tablets claimed to contain 50 mg by a U.S.P. titrimetric method [22] and the present GC procedure yielded average values (n = 4) of 49.0 ± 1.3 and 48.6 ± 0.6 mg, respectively. On the other hand, assay results for decomposed hydralazine tablets using GC, U.S.P., and ultraviolet [23] methods were 36.0, 40.2, and 37.8 mg, respectively.

B. Guanethidine and Other Guanido-Containing Drugs [24-27]

In 1974, Hengstmann et al. [24] described a general method for the analysis of the guanido-containing drugs used in the treatment of hypertension. As outlined below, the method involves addition of an internal standard (debrisoquin, 1 mg/ml, for guanethidine determination), adjustment of the pH to 10, and preliminary extraction with toluene to remove all potentially interfering amines. After discarding the toluene, the sample is adjusted to pH 13.5 to permit extraction of guanethidine into chloroform followed by its back-extraction into acid. The guanido group is then removed by hydrolysis under strongly alkaline conditions, and the resulting amine, N-(2-aminoethyl)octahydroazocine (OHA), is isolated by extraction with cyclohexane which is subsequently transferred to another silanized vial fitted with a Teflon-coated septum. After addition of 20 µl of formic acid, the solvent is is removed by evaporation at room temperature with a stream of nitrogen.

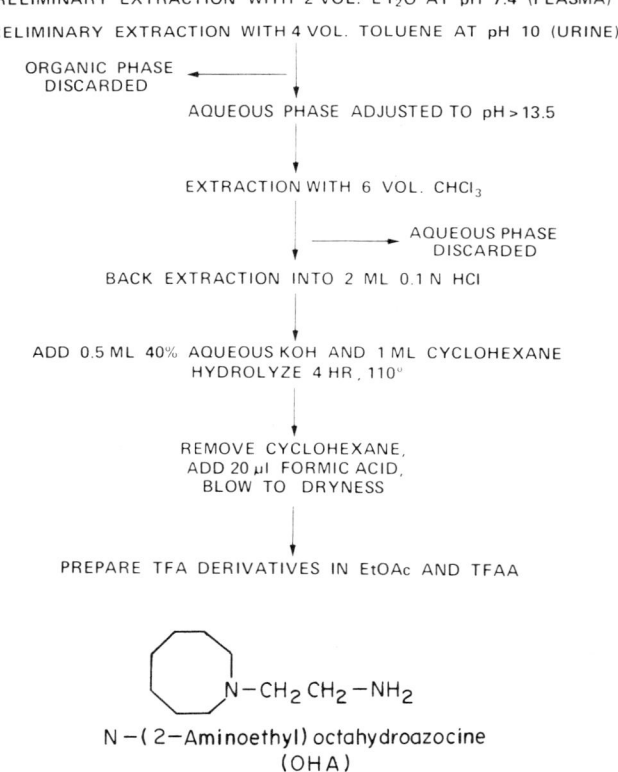

Derivatization of the extract for subsequent GC or GC-MS analysis is carried out in the following manner:

> After addition of 0.2 ml of ethyl acetate and 0.2 ml of trifluroroacetic anhydride, the vial is left at room temperature for 20 min before the solvent and excess reagent are removed with a stream of nitrogen. The residue is dissolved in 50 to 100 μl of ethyl acetate and 1 to 5 μl are injected into the gas chromatograph. The amount of guanethidine present in the original sample is calculated from the area ratio (peak height times peak width at half height) of guanethidine to internal standard using a standard curve.

For GC-MS analysis, modifications were necessary to extract the drug from plasma. This was accomplished as follows:

> To 5 mls of plasma are added 500 ng of debrisoquin and 20 ml of diethyl ether. The tube is shaken for 10 min and centrifuged. The organic layer is discarded. Then 0.5 ml of 50% NaOH are added and the contents thoroughly mixed on a Vortex-type mixer until a homogeneous suspension results. The subsequent steps are the same as those described above except that 20 to 40 μl of ethyl acetate are used for the final solution.

The GC studies were performed with a Varian model 2100 gas chromatograph equipped with a flame ionization detector and one of three column systems: column A, 1.8-m by 4-mm-i.d. glass packed with 3% OV-101 on 100-120 mesh Gas Chrom Q; column B, 1.8-m by 2-mm-i.d. glass packed with 3% OV-17 on 100-120 mesh Gas Chrom Q; column C, 1.8-m by 2-mm-i.d. glass packed with 3% Poly I-110 on 80-100 mesh Gas Chrom Q. Using a nitrogen carrier-gas flow rate of 60 ml/min and injector and detector temperatures of 220 and 200°C, respectively, the retention times of the TFA-derivatives of the hydrolysis products for guanethidine, debrisoquin, and bethanidine are listed in Table 2.5 at the column temperatures specified.

MS determinations were carried out with a LKB 9000 integrated GC-MS instrument equipped with a multiple ion detector, a 0.4-m by 2-mm 3% Poly I-110 or an 0.8-m by 4-mm 3% OV-101 glass column which was held isothermally at 125 or 120°C, respectively. The other GC-MS conditions were injector temperature, 210°C; ion source temperature, 250°C; trap current, 60 μA; electron energy, 70 eV. Noting that guanethidine could be detected at levels greater than 100 ng/ml with the GC-FID instrument whereas urine and plasma containing 1 to 100 ng/ml were readily amenable to analysis by GC-MS via MID detection, the m/e ions that could be used to monitor the TFA-derivatives of the hydrolysis products of guanethidine,

TABLE 2.5

Retention Times for TFA Derivatives of Hydrolysis Products
Derived from Guanido-Type Compounds[a]

TFA derivative of hydrolysis product	Retention time (min)		
	Column A (150°C)	Column B (130°C)	Column C (130°C)
N-(2-Aminoethyl)octahydroazocine (guanethidine)	4.2	3.8	4.6
1,2,3,4-Tetrahydroisoquinoline (debrisoquin)	4.2	5.1	6.7
2-(Aminomethyl)benzo-1,4-dioxane (guanoxan)	6.3	11.8	3.0 (180°C)
Benzylamine (bethanidine)	1.3	1.4	2.3

[a] Adapted from Hengstmann et al. [24].

guanoxan, bethanidine, and debrisoquin are shown by an asterisk in their respective mass spectra illustrated in Figure 2.3.

Erdtmansky and Goehl [25] developed a GC method with electron-capture detection for the determination of the monosubstituted guanido metabolite, 3,4-dihydro-1-methyl-2(1H)-isoquinolinecarboxamidine, of the potential antihypertensive agent, 3,4-dihydro-1-methyl-2(1H)-isoquinoline-carboxamidoxime. Combining extraction and derivatization steps into a single procedure, sample preparation for the determination of the metabolite in plasma or urine consisted of the following:

To a 130- by 15-mm test tube fashioned with a 12/18 ground-glass joint was added 0.1 ml of plasma (urine) and 5 µl of 0.01 N HCl containing the internal standard (debrisoquin, 200 ng/ml). The plasma (urine) was buffered with 50 µl of 1 M NaHCO$_3$, followed by the

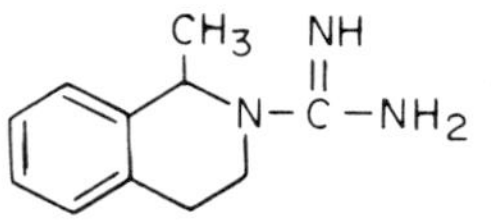

3,4-Dihydro-1-methyl-2(1H)-isoquinolinecarboxamidine

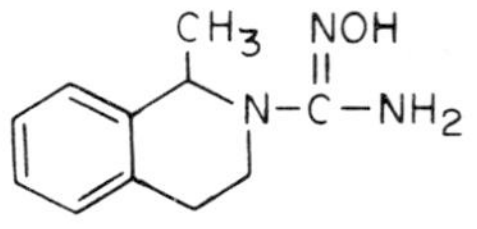

3,4-Dihydro-1-methyl-2(1H)-isoquinolinecarboxamidoxime

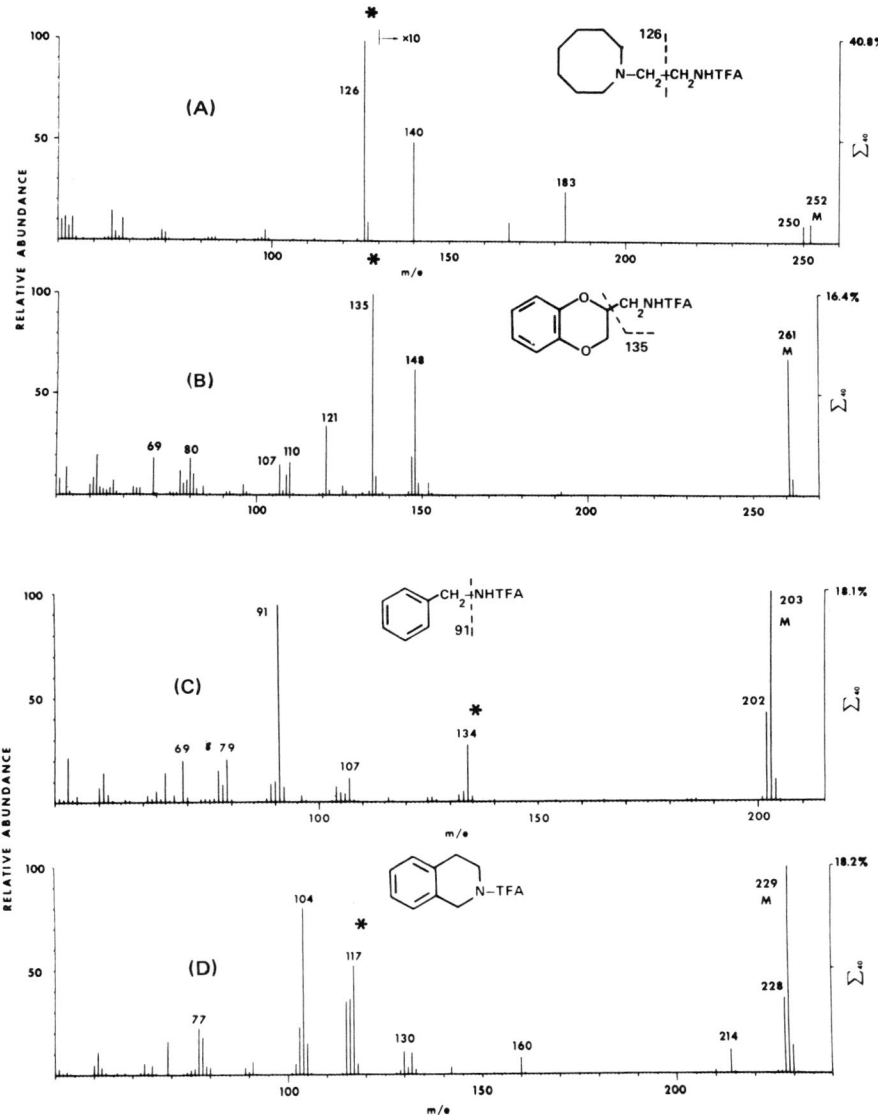

Figure 2.3. Mass spectra of TFA derivatives of N-(2-aminoethyl)-octahydroazocine (A), 2-aminomethyl-1,4-benzodioxane (B), benzylamine (C), and 1,2,3,4-tetrahydroisoquinoline (D). Adapted from Hengstmann et al. [24].

addition of 0.5 ml of benzene and 50 µl of hexafluoroacetylacetone. A 140- by 10-mm open-ended tube with a 12/18 ground-glass joint was connected to the test tube. This acted as a condenser during the heating process. The test tube-condenser assembly was then heated in an aluminum heating block at 100°C for 2 hr. They were then taken from the heating block and the condensers removed. Five milliliters of 3 N NaOH was added to hydrolyze the excess hexafluoroacetylacetone. The samples were vortexed, centrifuged, and 2 µl of the benzene phase was then injected into the gas chromatograph.

Erdtmansky and Goehl quantitated these derivatives in the nanogram/milliliter range using a Hewlett-Packard model 402 gas chromatograph equipped with a tritium electron-capture detector (200 mCi) and 1.8-m by 2-mm-i.d. glass columns packed with 3% OV-17 on 100-120 mesh Gas Chrom Q. To obtain retention times for the derivatives of debrisoquin and 3,4-dihydro-1-methyl-2(1H)-isoquinolinecarboxamidine of approximately 1.84 and 1.58 min, respectively, the following GC conditions were maintained: injector temperature, 200°C; column temperature, 160°C; detector temperature, 200°C; carrier-gas (7% methane in argon) flow rate, 75 ml/min. Using an integrated GC-MS instrument, the structure of the derivative of 3,4-dihydro-1-methyl-2(1H)-isoquinolinecarboxamidine based on MS data was shown to be

As noted by the authors, the lower limit of sensitivity of the procedure was 25 ng/ml of biological fluid. A nonlinear curve was found in the range 25 to 400 ng/ml with a relative standard deviation of 5% throughout this range.

Shortly thereafter, Malcolm and Marten [26] developed an analysis of debrisoquin and its 4-hydroxy metabolite in plasma. After forming derivatives with hexafluoroacetylacetone, samples, containing a deuterated internal standard (d_{10}-decadeuteriodebrisoquin, 10 ng in 10 µl of saturated sodium bicarbonate solution), were examined with a Finnigan 1015D GC-quadrupole MS equipped with a 1.5-m by 2-mm-i.d. glass column packed with 3% OV-17 coated on Gas Chrom Q. Using the specified instrument conditions (helium carrier-gas flow rate, 20 ml/min; column temperature, programmed from 150 to 190°C at 4°C/min; manifold temperature, 60°C;

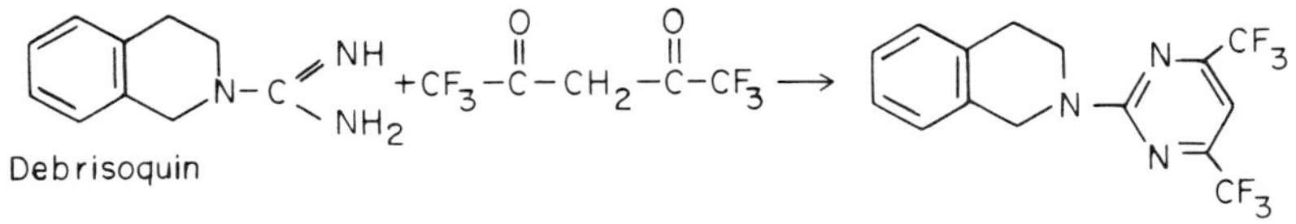

Debrisoquin

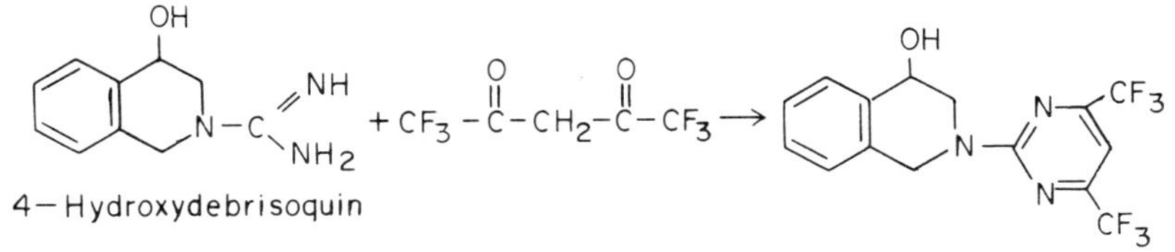

Debrisoquin + CF₃-CO-CH₂-CO-CF₃ → [pyrimidine derivative]

4-Hydroxydebrisoquin + CF₃-CO-CH₂-CO-CF₃ → [hydroxy pyrimidine derivative]

jet separator temperature, 210°C; ionization voltage, 70 eV; ion currents monitored: m/e 344, 347, and 356), a typical mass fragmentographic GC trace after derivatization of plasma containing debrisoquin sulfate (2 ng), 4-hydroxydebrisoquin sulfate (2 ng), and d_{10}-debrisoquin sulfate (10 ng) is shown in Figure 2.4, whereas the mass spectra of the hexafluoroacetylacetone derivatives of debrisoquin and its 4-hydroxy metabolite formed by the reactions given above are indicated in Figure 2.5.

For plasma derivatization and analysis, the procedure recommended was as follows:

Centrifuge tubes (10 ml) fitted with air condensers were used for the derivatization. A solution of the d_{10}-debrisoquin sulfate internal standard (10 ng) in water (10 µl) and saturated sodium bicarbonate solution (50 µl) was added to plasma (100 µl) containing the drug and metabolite (0.1 to 10.0 ng). Hexafluoroacetylacetone (50 µl) in toluene (500 µl) was then introduced and the samples were heated at 100°C for 2 hr. The organic layer was removed with a Pasteur pipette and blown to dryness with a stream of argon. A solution of this material in toluene (7 µl) was then injected onto the GC column.

Deuterated standard (10 ng) was added to plasma samples (100 µl), collected from a previously untreated hypertensive patient after receiving an oral dose of debrisoquin sulfate (20 mg). These were then analyzed for the drug and 4-hydroxy metabolite as described above [Fig. 2.6].

As noted by the authors, although levels of 4-hydroxydebrisoquin are higher than the parent compound (Fig. 2.6), it is more rapidly eliminated and is not detectable 24 hr after drug administration.

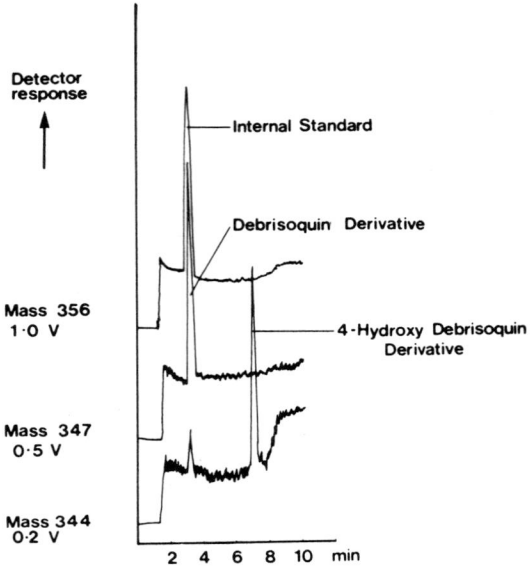

Figure 2.4. Mass fragmentographic GC trace after derivatization of plasma containing debrisoquin sulfate (2 ng), 4-hydroxydebrisoquin sulfate (2 ng), and D_{10}-debrisoquin sulfate (10 ng). From Malcolm and Marten [26], courtesy of Analytical Chemistry.

With the described procedure, the lower limit for quantitative estimation was found to be 1 ng/ml plasma for debrisoquin and 5 ng/ml plasma for the metabolite. Lower levels were detectable, but the accuracy was reduced.

In 1977, Lennard et al. [27] devised similar methods for the simultaneous determination of debrisoquin and its 4-hydroxy metabolite in human urine, involving in situ derivatization with acetylacetone, extraction of the resulting pyrimidines, and gas chromatography using a flame ionization detector or a nitrogen-specific detector. Using one of four sample extraction/derivatization procedures given in detail in the text (method 1, assay for debrisoquin and 4-hydroxydebrisoquin in urine with guanoxan as internal standard and the FID detector; method 2, the same as method 1 except that the GC used was fitted with a nitrogen detector; method 3, assay for debrisoquin in saliva using 3,4-dihydro-1-methyl-2(1H)isoquinolinecarboxamidine as internal standard and the nitrogen-selective detector; method 4, assay for debrisoquin in plasma and whole blood using the

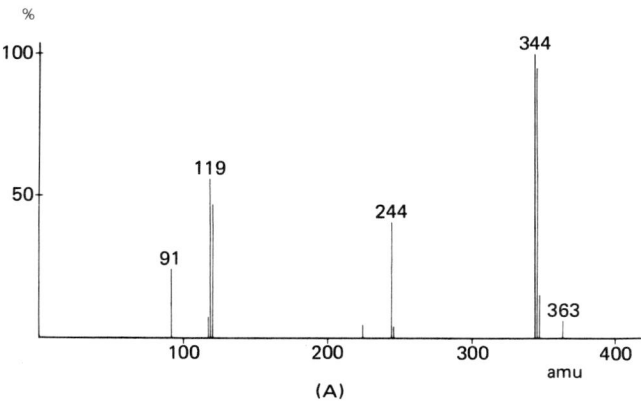

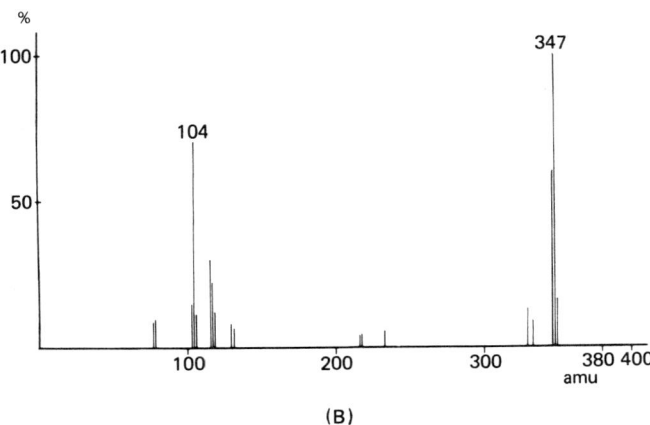

Figure 2.5. Mass spectra of hexafluoroacetylacetone derivatives of (A) 4-hydroxydebrisoquin and (B) debrisoquin. Adapted from Malcolm and Marten [26], courtesy of Analytical Chemistry.

internal standard and detection system of method 3), the gas chromatograph equipped with a flame ionization detector and a 1.8-m by 4-mm-i.d. glass column packed with 3% OV-225 on 100-120 mesh Gas Chrom Q was a Hewlett-Packard model 5700 instrument whose operating conditions were

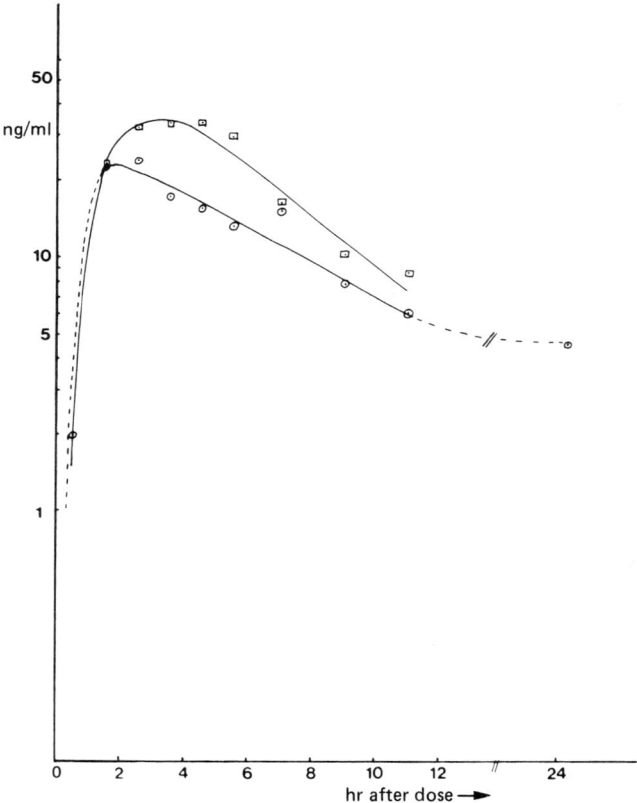

Figure 2.6. Levels of debrisoquin (☉) and 4-hydroxydebrisoquin (□) in plasma after a single oral dose of the drug (20 mg). From Malcolm and Marten [26], courtesy of Analytical Chemistry.

as follows: nitrogen carrier-gas flow rate, 50 ml/min; column temperature, 250°C; detector temperature, 250°C.

For nitrogen-selective detection, a Perkin-Elmer model F-17 gas chromatograph equipped with a nitrogen-phosphorus detector and 1.8-m by 2-mm-i.d. glass column packed with 3% OV-225 on 100-120 Gas Chrom Q was used. The GC unit was operated as follows: column temperature, 245°C (for method 2) or 230°C (for methods 3 and 4); injection temperature, 275°C; detector temperature, 275°C; helium carrier-gas flow rate, 30 ml/min; hydrogen flow rate, 1.5 ml/min; air flow rate, 100 ml/min.

Under the chromatographic conditions of method 1 (FID detection), the retention times of the derivatives of debrisoquin, guanoxan, and 4-hydroxydebrisoquin were 1.2, 2.8, and 3.2 min, respectively. On the other hand, the retention times of 3,4-dihydro-1-methyl-2(1H)-isoquinolinecarboxamidine and debrisoquin derivatives using the chromatographic conditions of methods 3 and 4 were 1.58 and 1.85 min, respectively; the 4-hydroxy compound being eluted in 5.2 min. Capable of accurately measuring concentrations down to 3 ng/ml using a 1.0-ml sample, the methods were applied to the analysis of samples collected after a single 20-mg oral dose of debrisoquin hemisulfate.

C. Clonidine [28-32]

In 1976, Dollery et al. [29] studied the clinical pharmacology and pharmacokinetics of clonidine, a very antihypertensive agent closely related chemically to tolazoline (peripheral vasodilator and α-adrenergic blocking agent), naphazoline, and antazoline (antihistamine).

The determination of clonidine in plasma was performed by selective-ion monitoring using an integrated GC-MS instrument [28]. Deuterated clonidine (clonidine-d_4), 2-(2,6-dichlorophenylamino)-2-imidazoline-4,4,5,5-^{2}H, was used as an internal standard. In the procedure described, clonidine was recovered from plasma (4 ml) following the addition of clonidine-d_4 (400 ng). The pH was adjusted to nearly 10-11 with 1 ml of 10% aqueous Na_2CO_3 and then extracted with ethyl acetate. Clonidine was back-extracted into 0.1 M HCl (1 ml) and, after readjustment of the aqueous phase pH to 10, recovered into ether (5 ml). The extracts containing clonidine and clonidine-d_4 were analyzed with an integrated GC-MS instrument equipped with a 1.0-m glass column packed with 3% OV-17 and operated isothermally at 200°C. The AEI MS-12 mass spectrometer was employed as a multiple-ion detector; the conditions established for analysis being ion source temperature, 210°C; ionizing voltage, 24 eV; trap current, 250 µA; accelerating voltage, 8 kV. In the electron-impact mode, the MS unit was set to monitor m/e 229 (molecular ion of clonidine) and m/e 235 (second isotope peak of the molecular ion of clonidine-d_4). The unlabeled clonidine calibration curve was linear when added to plasma (4 ml) in the range of 0 to 4.0 ng/ml. For this method, the precision was reported to be ±13% at the 1.0 ng/ml level and ±16.5% at 0.5 ng/ml.

In their investigation, a 300-µg oral dose of clonidine was administered to five normal volunteers and measurements of plasma concentration effects on blood pressure, heart rate, circulatory reflexes, sedation, and dry mouth were made for the following 8 hr. Their data indicated that "the plasma concentration rose to a peak of 1.02 ± 0.52 ng/ml at 90 min and fell with a mean half-life of 12.7 hr. Blood pressure of the group fell from 111.0/77.0 to 87.2/60.4 after 3 hr and was 95.2/62.2 mm Hg at 8 hr. Heart rate in recumbency was slowed. Marked sedation and a fall in salivary flow followed the same time course as the plasma concentration. The cold pressor response was reduced but the Valsalva overshoot was little affected."

Davies et al. [30] determined the kinetics of the disposition of intravenous and oral clonidine in five normotensive subjects based on data obtained from GC-MS measurements of the drug in plasma or urine. In their study, sample preparation for subsequent GC-MS analysis consisted of adding 400 ng of 2-(2,6-dichlorophenylamino)-2-imidazoline-4,4,5,5-^{2}H (clonidine-d_4) in 100 µl of methanol as an internal standard to 4-ml aliquots of plasma (or urine). Clonidine was extracted from alkalinized plasma (or diluted urine, 1:4) (pH 10 to 11) with ethyl acetate and, following back-extraction into 0.1 M HCl, the aqueous phase was adjusted to pH 11 and extracted with diethyl ether—a procedure very similar to that described by Draffan et al. [28]. After the evaporation of the solvent to dryness under nitrogen, the residue was dissolved in 20 µl of trimethyllanilinium hydroxide for flash methylation in a Finnigan integrated GC-MS instrument equipped with a 5-ft glass column packed with 3% OV-17 on 100-120 mesh Gas Chrom Q and operated under the following conditions: injector temperature, 260°C; column temperature, 195°C; helium carrier-gas flow rate, 30 ml/min; ionization voltage, 25 eV; electron multiplier voltage, 2 kV. By monitoring in the electron-impact mode m/e 228 for clonidine-d_4 and m/e 257 for clonidine, the retention times for both compounds were 3.5 min; the response ratios for clonidine and its deuterated form determined using peak heights with an interactive model 6000 data system.

With the clonidine calibration curve showing linearity over the 0- to 25-ng/ml range, the limit of detection was 0.15 ng/ml ± 10% (SD).

To describe the disposition of the drug, a two-compartment model was proposed such as that shown below:

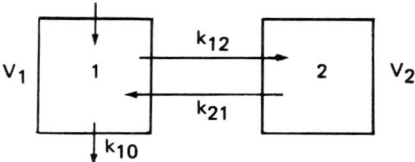

In their analysis of data, the observed postinfusion clonidine concentration were fitted to a biexponential decay curve such as that given by:

$$C_{p(p)} = A'e^{-\alpha t'} + B'e^{-\beta t'} \qquad (2.1)$$

where $C_{p(p)}$ is the postinfusion plasma concentration of clonidine at time t' after termination of the infusion (that is, $t' = t - \tau$, where τ = infusion time) and α and β are first-order hybrid rate constants for the fast and slow disposition processes, respectively. In turn, A' and B' are the ordinate intercepts of the exponential terms at t' = 0; these being related to A and B by the expressions

$$A' = \frac{A(1 - e^{-\alpha\tau})}{\alpha\tau} \tag{2.2}$$

$$B' = \frac{B(1 - e^{-\beta\tau})}{\beta\tau} \tag{2.3}$$

where A and B are the ordinate intercepts of the two exponential terms when t = 0 (equivalent to giving the dose as a bolus injection so that τ = 0).

The amount of clonidine absorbed after an oral dose was calculated was determined by

$$\frac{A_{cum}}{V_1(tn)} = C_{p(tn)} + C_{e(tn)} + C(2)_{tn} \tag{2.4}$$

where A_{cum} is the cumulative amount of clonidine absorbed, V_1 is the volume of compartment 1, C_e is the amount of drug eliminated from compartment 1 divided by V_1, and C(2) is the amount of drug in compartment 2 divided by V_1. By progressively evaluating A_{cum}/V_1 until a maximum value representing the estimated total amount of drug absorbed was determined (A_{max}), the bioavailability of oral clonidine could be calculated from

$$\text{Bioavailability} = \frac{A_{max}}{\text{oral dose}} \tag{2.5}$$

whereas the average renal clearance (Cl_{ren}) of the drug was determined by

$$Cl_{ren} = \frac{\text{total amount of drug excreted unchanged in urine}}{\text{total AUC}} \tag{2.6}$$

where AUC (area under plasma concentration-time curve) after oral dosing was calculated from t = 0 to t = $t_{(fin)}$ [the time of the final or last measured plasma concentration $Ct_{(fin)}$] and from $t_{(fin)}$ to infinity (∞) from the expression

$$(AUC)\, t_{(fin)} \to \infty = \frac{Ct_{(fin)}}{k} \tag{2.7}$$

where k is the first-order elimination rate constant.

Furthermore, after intravenous dosing, AUC was determined from

$$AUC = \frac{A}{\alpha} + \frac{B}{\beta} \tag{2.8}$$

From their GC-MS analyses of plasma and urine and the equations given above, the average two-compartment disposition constants for clonidine following intravenous administration, the average half-lives and bioavailability of clonidine after oral dosing, and the average urinary excretion values of clonidine (based on data obtained from five subjects) are shown in Tables 2.6, 2.7, and 2.8, respectively.

Davies et al. summarized their findings by stating that "the drug is rapidly distributed ($t_{1/2\alpha}$ = 10.8 ± 4.7 min) but slowly eliminated ($t_{1/2\beta}$ = 8.5 ± 0.9 hr). The bioavailability of oral clonidine in the tablets tested averaged 75.2% and 40 to 50% of the bioavailable dose is secreted unchanged in urine. Renal clearances of the drug showed considerable intersubject variation (1.82 ± 0.34 ml/min/kg) and exceed the calculated glomerular filtration rate in some subjects. Oral and intravenous clonidine induced significant falls in blood pressure (> 20/15 mm Hg) in our normotensive subjects and consistently caused marked sedation and dryness of the mouth. Sedation and salivary flow correlated with plasma clonidine concentration over the range 0 to 4 ng/ml. Falls in blood pressure were related to plasma concentration to 1.5 to 2.0 ng/ml but at higher concentrations the hypertensive effect was attenuated."

In 1977, Reid et al. [31] conducted studies in tetraplegic subjects to establish the central hypotensive effect of clonidine. Using also the procedure (GC-MS) developed by Draffan et al. [28], clonidine plasma results showed that, after oral administration of 300 µg in tetraplegic and control subjects, the peak plasma clonidine were similar in tetraplegic (1.36 ± 0.19 ng/ml) and control subjects (1.39 ± 0.14 ng/ml) and occurred approximately 90 min after dosing in both groups. Elimination half-lives were also nearly the same; the mean $t_{1/2}$ from plasma in control subjects being 8.6 ± 1.5 hr (range, 5.2 to 13.0 hr) whereas that for tetraplegics was 9.4 ± 1.4 hr (range, 5.6 to 12.0 hr).

Their investigation revealed that "a single oral dose of 300 µg of clonidine lowered systolic blood pressure by 20 ± 4 mm Hg and diastolic blood pressure by 13 ± 4 mm Hg in five healthy normotensive subjects (controls). Heart rate fell from 56 ± 2 to 52 ± 2 beats/min. In six tetraplegic patients with physiologically complete chronic cerivcal spinal cord transection above the level of the sympathetic outflow, the same dose of clonidine did

ANTIHYPERTENSIVE DRUGS 281

not significantly lower either systolic or diastolic blood pressure. Heart rate fell from 67 ± 4 to 53 ± 2 beats/min. Peak plasma concentrations and elimination of clonidine were similar in tetraplegic and control subjects and there was no difference in the incidence of the principal side effects of clonidine sedation and dry mouth. Although the number of subjects studied is small, the absence of a fall in blood pressure after clonidine in the tetraplegic subjects suggests that the hypotensive action of clonidine in man is dependent on intact descending bulbospinal pathways and is mediated by withdrawal of sympathetic tone and provides direct evidence that some antihypertensive drugs may lower blood pressure in man by a direct action on the brain."

Hodges [32] described in 1976 the identification of 2,6-dichlorophenyl-guanidine as a metabolite of clonidine in urine from the rat and the dog. Following the administration of dose levels of 5 mg/kg and 0.5 mg/kg to two rats and a dog, respectively, isolation of the drug and metabolite in urine collected for 24 hr after drug administration was carried out in the following manner:

> The urines were adjusted to pH 9 with saturated aqueous sodium carbonate solution and extracted with ethyl acetate (3X, equal volume). The extracts were evaporated under vacuum and the residue dissolved in methanol for application to TLC plates. After development in the solvent system chloroform-methanol-ammonium hydroxide (80:30:1) the plates were viewed under ultraviolet light (254 nm). Urine from rats which had been treated with clonidine contained two substances (R_f values of 0.42 and 0.82) which were not present in predose urine. Urine collected from the dog after treatment with clonidine showed one substance (R_f 0.42) which was not present in predose urine.

Subjecting the R_f 0.42 component in rat and dog urine to MS analysis with a LKB 9000S instrument, the compound was identified as 2,6-dichlorophenylguanidine with molecular ions at m/e 203, 205, 207 (RI 9:6:1), and fragment ions at m/e 161, 163, 165 (RI 9:6:1); the pattern of the three ions at 2 mass unit intervals with RI 9:6:1 being characteristic of compounds containing two chlorine atoms. The material from rat urine with a R_f of 0.82 was identified as unchanged clonidine.

D. Diazoxide [33,34]

In 1973, Sadee and co-workers [34] developed a GC-MS method for the determination of diazoxide urine and plasma levels with C-3-trideuteromethyl-diazoxide (diazoxide-d_3) as an internal standard (synthesis given

TABLE 2.6

Average Two-Compartment Disposition Constants Following Intravenous Administration[a]

α (min^{-1})	$t_{1/2\alpha}$ (min)	β (hr^{-1})	$t_{1/2\beta}$ (hr)	k_{12} (min^{-1})
0.134 ± 0.053	10.8 ± 4.7	0.084 ± 0.009	8.5 ± 0.9	0.105 ± 0.047

[a] Adapted from Davies et al. [30].
[b] Vd_{ss} = volume of distribution at steady state.
[c] Cl = plasma clearance of clonidine.

TABLE 2.7

Average Plasma Half-Lives and Bioavailability of Clonidine After Oral Dosing[a]

$t_{1/2}$ (hr)	Bioavailability (%)
8.6 ± 1.5	75.2 ± 1.8

[a] Adapted from Davies et al. [30]

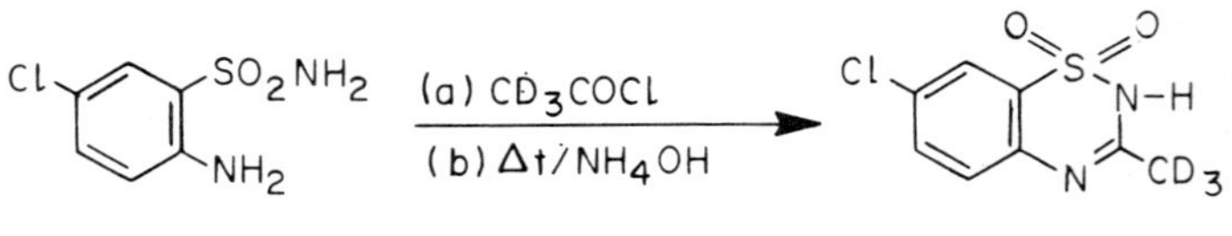

above). Drug isolation from plasma or urine for subsequent GC-MS analysis via mass fragmentography was carried out as follows:

Plasma or urine (0.1 ml) was added to 0.5 ml of 0.1 M phosphate buffer (pH 7) containing diazoxide-d_3 internal standard (1 μg) suitable for measurement of 0.1 to 100 μg/ml of diazoxide. The sample was

k_{21} (min^{-1})	k_{10} (min^{-1})	V_1 (L/kg)	Vd_{ss}^{b} (L/kg)	Cl^c (ml/min/kg)
0.022 ± 0.004	0.008 ± 0.003	0.51 ± 0.11	2.09 ± 0.19	3.05 ± 0.54

extracted in glass-stoppered tubes with 2.5 ml of ethyl ether for 1 min. Two milliliters of ether extract was transferred to a small disposable tube and evaporated to dryness. One milliliter of ethereal diazomethane was added to the tube and left for 30 min at room temperature. The ether was evaporated to dryness, the residue was dissolved in 50 µl of ether for GC, and 1 to 2 µl was injected onto the column.

Assays of diazoxide in human urine and plasma were performed with an integrated GC-MS instrument (a Varian-Mat CH7 mass spectrometer coupled via a two-stage Watson-Biemann-type separator to a Varian 2740 gas chromatograph) equipped with a 6-ft by 1/4-in. glass column packed with 3% SE-30 on 100-120 mesh Gas Chrom Q and operated as follows: injector temperature, 220°C; column temperature, 200°C; separator temperature, 220°C; helium carrier-gas flow rate, 25 ml/min; ion source temperature, 250°C; inlet line temperature, 230°C; accelerating voltage, 3 kV; emission current, 300 µa; multiplier gain, 2×10^5; mass range, m/e 243 to 248, scanned repetitively at two scans per second.

By monitoring the molecular ions of nondeuterated and deuterated diazoxide of m/e 244 and 247, respectively, and using the GC-MS conditions given above, the retention time of N-methylated diazoxide was 1.3 min; this being 3 sec longer than the retention time of the deuterated internal standard.

Based on GC-MS data, Sadee et al. concluded that:

Plasma elimination half-lives of diazoxide ranged from 20 to 53 hr in four severely hypertensive patients, which did not correlate with

TABLE 2.8

Average Urinary Excretion Data for Clonidine[a]

Percent dose in 24 hr urine		Renal clearance (ml/min/kg)	Nonrenal clearance[b] (ml/min/kg)
Intravenous	Oral		
48.9 ± 2.5	38.0 ± 1.4	1.82 ± 0.34	1.24 ± 0.30

[a] Adapted from Davies et al. [30].
[b] Nonrenal clearance = total body plasma clearance - average renal clearance.

endogenous plasma creatinine levels. A rapid infusion over 10 to 15 sec of an antihypertensive dose presumably resulted in a very transient precipitation of diazoxide due to its limited solubility of approximately 380 μg/ml of plasma. Urinary excretion accounted for 4 to 6% of the dose within 24 hr after administration in the four patients studied and totaled 19 and 22% in two patients. Renal clearance of diazoxide was below 1 ml/min on the first day following administration and increased to 2 to 3 ml/min on consecutive days. It was concluded that renal excretion of diazoxide is self-limited by antihypertensive doses in severely hypertensive patients. The major route of elimination in these patients may be due to metabolism.

E. Reserpine and Rescinnamine [35]

In 1976, Settimj et al. [35] described a GC method in which, under the conditions used for alkaline hydrolysis of reserpine and rescinnamine in absolute and aqueous methanol, and after esterification (with diazomethane) of the resulting acid fraction, methyl 3,4,5-trimethoxybenzoate was quantitatively recovered, whereas methyl trans-3,4,5-trimethoxycinnamate, in normal lighting conditions, was either partly isomerized to methyl cis-trimethoxycinnamate or formed an adduct with a molecule of methanol, yielding methyl 3-methoxy-3-(3,4,5-trimethoxyphenyl)propionate.

The resulting methyl esters were separated and quantitated using a Perkin-Elmer 900 GC instrument equipped with a flame ionization detector and a 240-cm by 0.2-cm-i.d. glass column packed with 15% Apiezon L on acid-washed, 80-100 mesh Chromosorb W; the other GC conditions were sample size, 5 μl; injector temperature, 260°C; column temperature, 230°C; detector temperature, 200°C; nitrogen carrier-gas flow rate, 30 ml/min.

Using the above GC conditions and methyl stearate as internal standard, the retention times of methyl 3,4,5-trimethoxybenzoate, methyl 3-methoxy-3-(3,4,5-trimethoxyphenyl)propionate, methyl cis-3,4,5-trimethoxycinnamate, methyl trans-3,4,5-trimethoxycinnamate, and methyl stearate (I. S.) were approximately 4.38, 6.85, 8.41, 13.30, and 21.90 min, respectively. Although the method was reported to be reliable for reserpine determinations down to 500 µg, for rescinnamine it was satisfactory only for quantities down to 2000 µg. The structures of the methyl derivatives derived from alkaline hydrolysis are illustrated below:

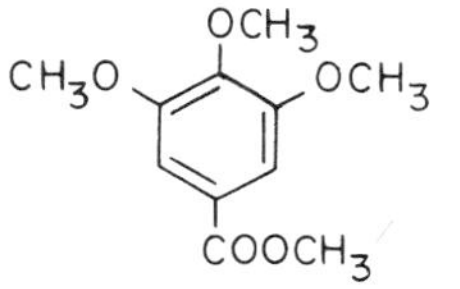

Methyl 3,4,5− trimethoxybenzoate

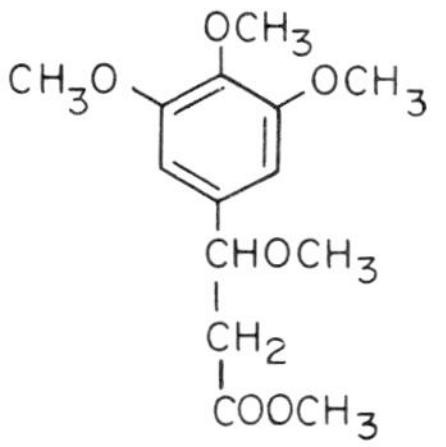

Methyl 3−methoxy−3−(3,4,5−tri−methoxyphenyl) propionate

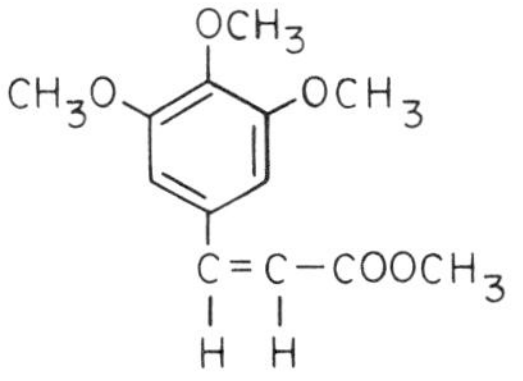

Methyl cis−3,4,5−trimethoxy−cinnamate

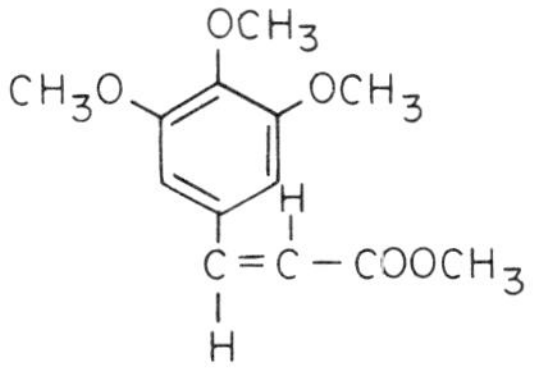

Methyl trans−3,4,5−trimethoxy−cinnamate

F. (6,7-Dichloro-2-methyl-1-oxo-2-phenyl-5-indanyloxy)acetic Acid [36]

Zacchei and Wishousky [36] developed highly specific and sensitive GC methods for the determination of (6,7-dichloro-2-methyl-1-oxo-2-phenyl-5-indanyloxy)acetic acid in biological fluids. The procedures involve the addition of an internal standard, (6,7-dichloro-2-cyclopentyl-2-methyl-1-oxo-5-indanyloxy)acetic acid (10.0 µg), to the biological specimens (1.0 ml of plasma or an appropriate aliquot of urine) followed by extraction of the acids into 25 ml of benzene at pH 1. The indanones are back-extracted into NaOH and reextracted into 5 ml of methylene chloride under acidic conditions. After the conversion of the acids to methyl esters with diazomethane, the derivatives were analyzed using one of three GC instruments: (1) a Hewlett-Packard model 5750 equipped with a flame ionization detector and a 122-cm by 4-mm-i.d. glass column packed with 3% OV-210 on 100-120 mesh Gas Chrom Q (helium carrier-gas flow rate, 48 ml/min), (2) a Packard model 7400 equipped with a ^{63}Ni electron-capture detector and a 122-cm by 4-mm-i.d. glass column packed with 3% OV-210 on 100-120 mesh Gas Chrom Q operated isothermally for the determination of (6,7-dichloro-2-methyl-1-oxo-2-phenyl-5-indanyloxy) acetic acid and [6,7-dichloro-2-(4-hydroxyphenyl)-2-methyl-1-oxo-5-indanyloxy]acetic acid (a metabolite of the parent compound) following derivatization with diazomethane and N,O-bis(trimethylsilyl)acetamide (nitrogen carrier-gas flow rate, 80 ml/min), and (3) a Hewlett-Packard model 5830A equipped with a flame ionization detector and a ^{63}Ni electron-capture detector. Using any of the three instruments, the injector and detector temperatures were maintained about 10 to 30°C higher than the column temperatures. In addition to the above analytical equipment, Zacchei and Wishousky used for mass spectral studies a LKB 9000S equipped with a 122-cm by 3-mm-i.d. glass column packed with 3% OV-210 on 100-120 mesh Gas Chrom Q; the integrated GC-MS unit being operated as follows: column temperature, 250°C; injector temperature, 260°C; ion source temperature, 270°C; separator temperature, 265°C; helium carrier-gas flow rate, 30 ml/min; ionizing voltage, 70 eV; accelerating voltage, 3.5 kV.

Using the FID chromatographic instrument with a column temperature of 250°C, the retention time of the methyl esters of the parent drug and the internal standard were 2.8 and 2.0 min, respectively.

When increased sensitivity was required, the electron-capture detector was used with minor changes noted in the procedure: (1) 25 ng of internal standard was added and (2) pesticide-grade benzene was used to dissolve the esters prior to injection.

With regard to the analysis of the metabolite, either the FID or ECD gas chromatograph was used, depending on its concentration.

[6,7-Dichlohloro-2-(4 hyroxyphenyl)-2-methyl-1-oxo-5- indanyloxy] acetic Acid

Using the procedures described, Zacchei and Wishousky reported that (1) when the derivatives are analyzed by FID or ECD, the limits of

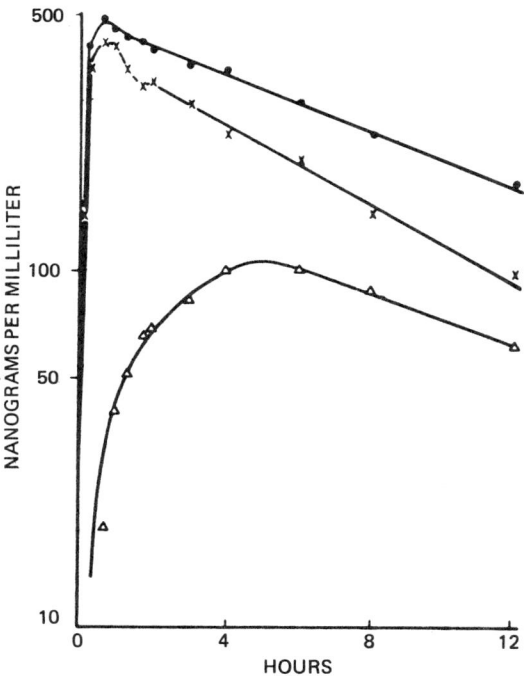

Figure 2.7. Human plasma levels of the parent drug (x), the metabolite (Δ), and total radioactivity (●) (calculated as parent drug equivalents). Adapted from Zacchei and Wishousky [36].

detection were approximately 1 μg/ml and 2.5 ng/ml of plasma, respectively; (2) a recovery of 98.8 ± 11.9% was obtained using ECD detection from plasma (n = 322); and (3) the recoveries with FID detection were 99.1 ± 4.4% (plasma, n = 207) and 99.8 ± 4.9% (urine, n = 163).

Applying the procedure to the determination of human plasma levels of the parent drug and its metabolite (Fig. 2.7), their GC values showed that the plasma half-life of total radioactivity (calculated as nanogram equivalents of parent drug per milliliter) was about 7 hr. The initial phase of the parent drug elimination curve indicated an apparent $t_{1/2\alpha}$ of 5.5 hr; the metabolite value yielding an apparent plasma half-life of 8.4 hr. About 1 hr after drug administration, peak levels of drug and radioactivity occurred.

II. HYPOGLYCEMIC AGENTS

In the management of diabetes, the most common oral antidiabetic drugs fall into either of two compound types; (1) sulfonylureas or (2) biguanides, as indicated in Figure 2.8.

A. Sulfonylurea Drugs [2, 3, 10, 13, 37-52]

In 1970, Sabih and Sabih [37] developed GC methods for the measurement of tolbutamide and chlorpropamide in blood and urine and in pharmaceutical preparations. The extraction of the drugs from biological media (plasma or urine) and their subsequent conversion to methyl derivatives with dimethyl sulfate in the presence of base was performed in the following manner:

One-milliliter plasma samples containing either of the sulfonylurea drugs were acidified with 1 ml of a saturated solution of NaH_2PO_4 and extracted with five volumes of chloroform by shaking carefully for 2 min. Layers were separated by centrifugation (2000 rpm for 5 to 10 min); emulsions were broken by stirring with a wooden stick and recentrifuged for another 5 to 10 min. The aqueous layer was aspirated and four-fifths of the chloroform layer was placed in a second centrifuge tube. Solvent was removed under a stream of air, and the sulfonylurea residue was dissolved in 1 ml of methanolic potassium carbonate followed by 0.1 ml of dimethyl sulfate. The resulting mixture was heated on a water bath at 70°C for 5 min. Following removal of the methanol at that temperature by a steady stream of air, 1 ml of 0.2 M acetate buffer, pH 5.6, was added and followed by 5 ml of heptane. Extraction was aided by the use of a Vortex mixer. After centrifugation, 4 ml of the heptane extract from the tube was transferred to a 5-ml flask from which the heptane was evaporated with a stream of air. The resulting residue was dissolved in 100 μl of chloroform. One- to five-microliter aliquots were injected onto the GC column.

[For pharmaceutical preparations]; one tablet of tolbutamide or chlorpropamide was pulverized in a mortar to a fine powder and triturated with 50 ml of ethanol. The mixture was then filtered and the filtrate transferred to a 100-ml volumetric flask and made to volume with ethanol. Aliquots were placed in separate centrifuge tubes and the ethanol was removed under a stream of air. The residues were than converted to the methyl derivatives and chromatographed.

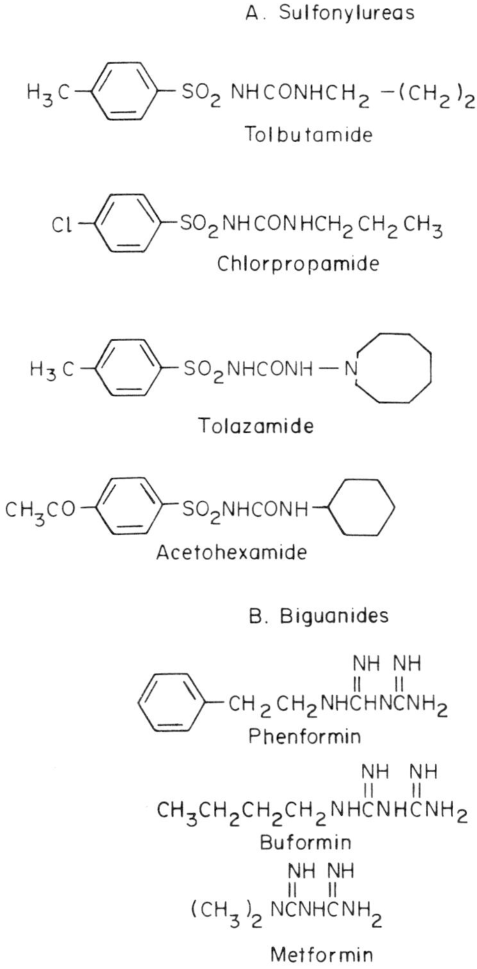

HYPOGLYCEMIC AGENTS

A. Sulfonylureas

$H_3C\text{-}\bigcirc\text{-}SO_2\text{ NHCONHCH}_2-(CH_2)_2-CH_3$
Tolbutamide

$Cl\text{-}\bigcirc\text{-}SO_2\text{NHCONHCH}_2CH_2CH_3$
Chlorpropamide

$H_3C\text{-}\bigcirc\text{-}SO_2\text{NHCONH}-N\bigcirc$
Tolazamide

$CH_3CO\text{-}\bigcirc\text{-}SO_2\text{NHCONH}\text{-}\bigcirc$
Acetohexamide

B. Biguanides

$\bigcirc\text{-}CH_2CH_2\text{NH}\overset{\text{NH}}{\overset{\|}{C}}\text{NH}\overset{\text{NH}}{\overset{\|}{C}}NH_2$
Phenformin

$CH_3CH_2CH_2CH_2\text{NH}\overset{\text{NH}}{\overset{\|}{C}}\text{NH}\overset{\text{NH}}{\overset{\|}{C}}NH_2$
Buformin

$(CH_3)_2\text{N}\overset{\text{NH}}{\overset{\|}{C}}\text{NH}\overset{\text{NH}}{\overset{\|}{C}}NH_2$
Metformin

Figure 2.8. Structure of commonly used hypoglycemic drugs.

GC analyses were performed with a F&M model 5755B gas chromatograph equipped with a flame ionization detector and 1.37-m by 0.33-cm stainless steel columns packed with 5% DC-200 on 80-100 mesh Gas Chrom Q. For the determination of tolbutamide, the GC conditions used were injector temperature, 330°C; column temperature, 205 to 210°C; detector temperature, 320°C; helium carrier-gas flow rate, 50 ml/min.

TABLE 2.9

Recoveries of Tolbutamide and Chlorpropamide from Plasma[a]

Amount added (μg)	Percent recovery	
	Tolbutamide	Chlorpropamide
5	96	94
10	98	97
20	97	100
30	100	96
40	102	94
60	96	—
Average:	98.2 ± 1.9	96.2 ± 1.8

[a] Adapted from Sabih and Sabih [37].

For chlorpropamide analysis, the injector and detector temperatures were as noted above, but the column was operated at 180°C with a helium flow rate of 40 ml/min. With these GC conditions, the retention times of the methyl derivatives of tolbutamide (column = 205 to 210°C, helium flow = 50 ml/min) and chlorpropamide (column = 180°C, helium flow = 40 ml/min) were 2.0 and 3.8 min, respectively.

In Table 2.9 are shown the recoveries obtained for plasma samples to which had been added varying amounts of tolbutamide and chlorpropamide. As described, the method was capable of measuring as little as 0.1 μg of these drugs.

In 1971, Wickramasinghe and Shaw [38] described a GC method for the determination of tolazamide in plasma of drug-treated guinea pigs. The drug from plasma specimens from dosed guinea pigs was extracted for subsequent thin-layer chromatographic analysis by placing a 1-ml plasma sample in a 15-ml centrifuge tube, adjusting the pH to 2.5 using 1 N HCl and then extracting with 5 ml of chloroform. Emulsions which formed were broken up by centrifugation at 1000 rpm. A measured volume of the chloroform extract (4 ml) was transferred by pipette to a second centrifuge tube and evaporated to dryness under nitrogen. These extracts were subjected to TLC analysis using precoated plates of silica gel F-254 of 250-μm thickness and a solvent system composed of chloroform-methanol-formic acid (98.5:1.0:0.5). After locating the tolazamide zone using a UV lamp (254 nm), the tolazamide zone was removed and extracted out twice

Cl—⟨C₆H₄⟩—SO₂NHCONH—(CH₂)₃—CH₃

1-(n-Butyl)-3-p-chlorobenzenesulfonyl-
urea (Internal Standard)

with 1 ml of methanol. To this 2-ml methanol extract was added 0.1 ml of an internal standard solution containing 12 μg of 1-(n-butyl)-3-p-chlorobenzenesulfonylurea, and the total solution was then evaporated to dryness under nitrogen. The residue was redissolved in 20 μl of chloroform and analyzed by GC.

In their investigation, Wickramasinghe and Shaw performed the GC separations and analyses using a F&M model 402 gas chromatograph equipped with a flame ionization detector and 70-cm by 3-mm-i.d. U-shaped glass columns packed with 0.5% Carbowax 20M coated on 80-100 mesh Chromosorb G and operated isothermally at 190°. The other GC settings maintained were injector temperature, 236°C; detector temperature, 220°C; helium carrier-gas flow rate, 80 ml/min. Using these conditions, the underivatized drug and internal standard were quantitatively degraded (either thermally or catalytically) to p-toluenesulfonamide and p-chlorobenzenesulfonamide, respectively; with retention times being approximately 2.0 and 3.2 min, respectively.

H₃C—⟨C₆H₄⟩—SO₂NH₂   Cl—⟨C₆H₄⟩—SO₂NH₂

p-Toluenesulfonamide   p-Chlorobenzenesulfonamide

Using a calibration curve prepared by plotting tolazamide concentration (μg/ml of plasma) versus the peak height ratio of p-toluenesulfonamide to p-chlorobenzenesulfonamide, the average recovery (mean ± S.D.) of tolazamide added to guinea pig plasma over a 0.77- to 9.25-μg/ml range was 99.6 ± 7.64% (n = 8).

With a lower limit of detection reported to be 0.70 μg/ml of plasma, plasma concentrations of tolazamide versus time in guinea pigs after single-dose oral administration of 15 mg/kg body weight were determined. They noted that a peak plasma tolazamide concentration of 12.5 μg/ml was observed at 1 hr after oral drug administration and, by using the data between 1 and 14 hr, the plasma drug elimination half-life was estimated to be 2.7 hr.

Using a LKB 9000 integrated GC-MS instrument equipped with a column (length not specified) packed with 3% OV-17 on 80-120 mesh Gas Chrom Q and operated isothermally at 200°C with the injector temperature and helium carrier-gas flow rate maintained at 220°C and 45 ml/min, respectively, three peaks were observed for tolazamide, which were identified as follows:

Peak	Prominent m/e ions	Component
1	140, 112 (M-28), 84 (M-56)	Isocyanate fragment
2	171, 155 (M-16), 139 (M-32), 123 (M-48)	p-Toluenesulfonamide
3	256, 171, 156, 139	Unknown

On the other hand, the internal standard yielded only one peak when subjected to GC-MS analysis, which was attributed to p-chlorobenzenesulfonamide, having a molecular ion at m/e 191 and other prominent peaks at m/e 175 (M-16), 127 (M-64), and 111 (M-80).

When subjecting tolazamide to mass spectral analysis via direct probe insertion at two different probe inlet temperatures (70 eV), different mass spectra were obtained as evidenced by the m/e ions listed below:

Inlet Probe Temperature (°C)	Prominent m/e ions
145	311 (M), 197 (M-114), 171 (M-140), 155 (M-156), 140 (M-171), 113 (M-198), 98 (M-213), 91 (M-220)
220	171 (M-140), 155 (M-156), 140 (M-171)

Prescott and Redman [39] described in 1972 an improved method for the GC estimation of tolbutamide and chlorpropamide in which the drugs are extracted into toluene, back-extracted into alkali, and methylated with dimethylsulfate. The methylated derivatives are extracted into n-hexane, concentrated by evaporation, and chromatographed with a Hewlett-Packard model 402 gas chromatograph equipped with flame ionization detectors and two 4-ft by 1/4-in.-o.d. glass columns packed with either 3.8% W98 on 80-100 mesh Diatoport S (column temperature, 220°C; nitrogen carrier-gas flow rate, 25 ml/min) or 1% Carbowax 20 M on 80-100 mesh Gas Chrom Q (column temperature, 220°C; nitrogen flow rate, 60 ml/min). With these columns, the injector and detector temperatures were 235 and 260°C, respectively.

In the procedure outlined above, tolbutamide (5 µg/ml) was used as internal standard for the determination of chlorpropamide, whereas chlorpropamide (20 µg/ml) acted as I.S. for tolbutamide analyses.

With the 3.8% W98 column and the GC conditions specified, the retention times of the methylated derivatives of both drugs and some of their metabolites were as follows: p-chlorobenzenesulfonamide, 0.7 min; tolbutamide, 2.2 min; chlorpropamide, 1.7 min; carboxytolbutamide, 4.8 min; and hydroxymethyltolbutamide, 4.2 min. On the other hand, the recovery of tolbutamide from aqueous solutions was only 88 to 91% of that from human plasma, whereas the opposite effect was seen with chlorpropamide (104 to 114%).

Simmons et al. [40] developed a GC method using a flame ionization detector for the determination of tolbutamide in serum in which the drug is extracted from acidified serum (pH 5.4), methylated with dimethyl sulfate, and the resulting N-methyltolbutamide determined using N-propyl-p-chlorobenzenesulfonamide as internal standard. Under suitable GC conditions, N-methyltolbutamide is quantitatively pyrolyzed to N-methyl-p-toluenesulfonamide. As noted by Simmons et al., peak areas for

H_3C-⟨⟩-$SO_2N(CH_3)$-$CONH$-$(CH_2)_3$-CH_3 H_3C-⟨⟩-SO_2-$NHCH_3$

N-Methyltolbutamide   N-Methyl-p-toluenesulfonamide

Cl-⟨⟩-SO_2NH-$(CH_2)_2$-CH_3

N-Propyl-p-chlorobenzenesulfonamide

equimolar concentrations of these two compounds were similar and linear with respect to the internal standard over a range of 10 to 50 μg of tolbutamide equivalents per 100 μl. Overall recoveries from human and beagle serum were 80.8 ± 3.5% and 82.0 ± 3.0%, respectively, based on the N-methyltolbutamide external standard curve.

Simmons et al. emphatically noted that, contrary to claims made by other investigators [37], methylation of tolbutamide does not stabilize the molecule and prevent its decomposition on the column under high inlet temperatures. In the present study, the instrument and conditions used, which gave retention times of 4.5 and 6.8 min for N-methyl-p-toluenesulfonamide and N-propyl-p-chlorobenzenesulfonamide, respectively, are listed below:

GC instrument: Mikro-Tek model MT-220 equipped with a flame ionization detector

Column: 6-ft by 1/4-in.-o.d. U-shaped glass packed with 3% OV-17 on 100-120 mesh Chromosorb W-HP

Injector temperature (°C): 285

Column temperature (°C): 190

Detector temperature (°C): 285

Nitrogen carrier-gas flow rate (ml/min): 20

Oxygen and hydrogen flow rate adjusted to give maximum response.

In 1972, Taylor [41] reported his findings on the pharmacokinetics and biotransformation of chlorpropamide in man in which GC and high-pressure liquid chromatography were used to identify and quantify its various metabolites as shown in Figure 2.9.

Taylor measured chlorpropamide concentrations in plasma and urine using a modified version of the procedure of Sabih and Sabih [37]. The methyl derivative was prepared by use of at least a tenfold excess of diazomethane and analyzed with a Barber-Colman model 5000 gas chromatograph equipped with an electron-capture detector and a 6-ft by 3.5-mm-i.d. glass column packed with 5% DC-200 and operated at 210°C with a nitrogen carrier-gas flow rate of 80 ml/min. The same conditions were used to determine urinary p-chlorobenzenesulfonylurea excretion, whereas

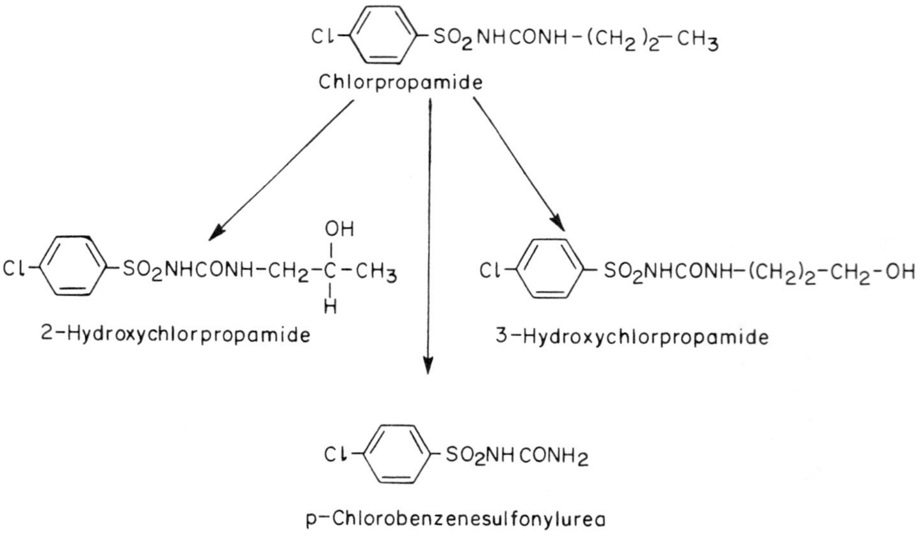

$Cl-\langle\ \rangle-SO_2NHCONH-(CH_2)_2-CH_3$

Chlorpropamide

$Cl-\langle\ \rangle-SO_2NHCONH-CH_2-\overset{OH}{\underset{H}{C}}-CH_3$

2-Hydroxychlorpropamide

$Cl-\langle\ \rangle-SO_2NHCONH-(CH_2)_2-CH_2-OH$

3-Hydroxychlorpropamide

$Cl-\langle\ \rangle-SO_2NHCONH_2$

p-Chlorobenzenesulfonylurea

Figure 2.9. Chlorpropamide metabolites identified and recovered in human urine of four diabetic subjects.

the hydrolysis product of chlorpropamide (p-chlorobenzenesulfonamide) was chromatographed at a lower column temperature (192°C).

With regard to HPLC separations, the drug-related compounds were eluted from TLC plates, combined, and concentrated to a final volume of 1.0 ml in methanol. Using UV detection and a du Pont model 830 high-pressure liquid chromatograph, separations were achieved at 130 psi with a pH 4.0 citric acid buffer-mobile phase on a 1-m by 3-mm-i.d. stainless steel column packed with Permaphase ETH. With these conditions, the retention times of 2-hydroxytolbutamide, p-chlorobenzenesulfonylurea, p-chlorobenzenesulfonamide, and chlorpropamide were 15.94, 21.50, 26.1, and 39.6 min, respectively.

Taylor summarized his findings relative to the chlorpropamide pharmacokinetics determined in six normal adult volunteers after a single oral 250-mg dose as follows:

> Drug absorption half-lifes varied from 0.1 to 1.5 hr with a calculated mean of 0.5 hr. Half-life for drug in plasma ranged from 25 to 42 hr with a calculated mean of 33 hr while the half-life estimated from urinary excretion data averaged 36 hr. In addition to drug, p-chlorobenzenesulfonylurea, 2-hydroxychlorpropamide, and 3-hydroxychlorpropamide were recovered from urine of four diabetic subjects receiving 250 to 500 mg of chlorpropamide daily. Approximately 2% of the daily dose was recovered from urine as p-chlorobenzenesulfonamide, a degradation product of p-chlorobenzenesulfonylurea, and a similar amount was excreted as 3-hydroxychlorpropamide. Drug, p-chlorobenzenesulfonylurea, and 2-hydroxychlorpropamide excretion quantitated in 24-hr urine samples of these diabetic subjects by high-pressure liquid chromatography averaged 18, 21, and 55% of dose, respectively. Two hours after chlorpropamide administration, unchanged drug accounted for 95% of total drug and metabolite concentrations in plasma, indicating that p-chlorobenzenesulfonylurea and 2-hydroxychlorpropamide have significantly shorter elimination half-lifes than unchanged drug.

In 1973, Matin and Rowland described GC methods for the determination of tolbutamide and chlorpropamide [42] and the simultaneous analysis of tolbutamide and its metabolites [43] in biological fluids.

For the determination of tolbutamide and chlorpropamide [42], Matin and Rowland proposed the following procedure for the extraction of the drugs from plasma or blood prior to GC analysis:

> To 0.5 ml of plasma or blood, add 1 ml of phosphate buffer and 0.1 ml of the aqueous internal standard solution. For the determination of tolbutamide, use chlorpropamide and vice versa, adjusting the

amount of internal standard to the anticipated concentrations of the respective sulfonylurea. Extract the buffered sample containing the I.S. with 10 ml of hexane containing 0.5% isoamyl alcohol, centrifuge, and pipette 7 ml of the hexane extract into another tube to which 1 ml of 1 N NaOH had been added. After shaking and removal of the hexane layer, add 1 ml of 2 N HCl and 2 ml of pentyl acetate to the basic layer, shake for 2 min, and centrifuge. Pipette 1 ml of the pentyl acetate extract into a third tube containing 1 ml of 0.05% dinitrofluorobenzene solution, lightly stopper, and heat for 1 hr at 125°C, on a constant-temperature oil bath. After cooling, 1 to 5 μl are withdrawn and injected into the gas chromatograph.

The propyl and butyl 2,4-dinitroanilines, formed from chlorpropamide and tolbutamide, respectively, were analyzed with a Varian 1200 gas chromatograph equipped with a ^{63}Ni electron-capture detector and a 6-ft by 1/8-in.-o.d. glass column packed with 3% OV-17 on 100-120 mesh, acid-washed, DMCS-treated Chromosorb W. The other GC conditions recommended were carrier-gas (5% methane in argon) flow rate, 30 ml/min; injector temperature, 225°C; column temperature, 210°C; detector temperature, 310°C.

For the simultaneous determination of tolbutamide and its metabolites, Matin and Rowland [43] used essentially the same procedure, GC instrument, and operating conditions described above. For their determination in biological fluids, some slight procedural changes were made as noted below:

To the biological sample (0.5 ml) were added aqueous solutions (0.1 ml each) of internal standard, chlorpropamide and T-isoprop (1-isopropyl-3-p-carboxyphenylsulfonylurea), for tolbutamide and

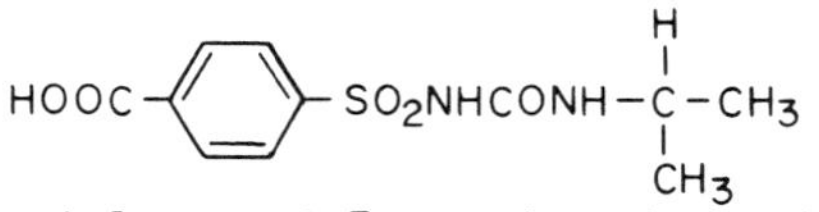

HOOC—⟨C$_6$H$_4$⟩—SO$_2$NHCONH—CH(CH$_3$)$_2$

1-Isopropyl-3-p-carboxyphenylsulfonylurea (T-isoprop)

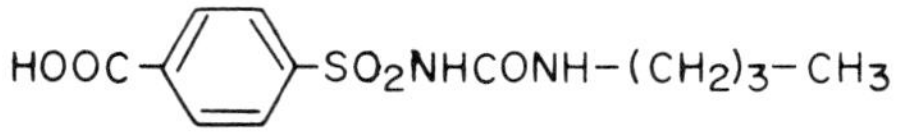

HOOC—⟨C$_6$H$_4$⟩—SO$_2$NHCONH—(CH$_2$)$_3$—CH$_3$

1-Butyl-3-p-carboxyphenylsulfonylurea (T-COOH)

T-COOH (1-butyl-3-p-carboxyphenylsulfonylurea). The amounts of internal standard were adjusted to the anticipated concentration of the compounds.

In general, 10 µg of chlorpropamide and 2.5 µg of T-isoprop were found satisfactory. The mixture was then acidified with 0.5 N HCl (1 ml), extracted with ether (10 ml), and centrifuged. The ether layer was transferred into another screw-capped tube containing 0.5 N NaOH (0.5 ml); it being important to transfer as much ether as possible since the internal standard for T-OH (1-butyl-3-p-hydroxymethylphenylsulfonylurea) had not yet been added. The tube

$$HO-CH_2-\underset{}{\underset{}{\bigcirc}}-SO_2NHCONH-(CH_2)_3-CH_3$$

1-Butyl-3-p-hydroxymethylphenylsulfonylurea
(T-OH)

was capped, shaken, and centrifuged to separate the phases. The ether was aspirated off and discarded and the basic aqueous layer containing the compounds was acidified by adding phosphate buffer (1 ml). Tolbutamide and the internal standard chlorpropamide were selectively extracted out of the aqueous mixture with 0.5% isoamyl alcohol in hexane (10 ml), and tolbutamide determined as reported previously [42]. The aqueous layer was rewashed with 5 ml of 0.5% isoamyl alcohol in hexane.

After removing hexane by aspiration, chlorpropamide (2 µg) in aqueous solution was again added as the internal standard for the metabolite T-OH. This mixture was then acidified with 2 N HCl (0.3 ml), extracted with 0.5% isoamyl alcohol in CH_2Cl_2 (10 ml), centrifuged, and the aqueous layer removed by suction. The CH_2Cl_2 layer was transferred into a separatory tube (a 15-ml screw-cap culture tube fitted at the bottom with a size 22/24 Teflon stopcock) containing citrate buffer (1 ml). After phase separation the lower CH_2Cl_2 layer (containing T-OH and chlorpropamide) was transferred into another tube containing 1 N NaOH (1 ml), shaken, centrifuged, and an aliquot of the basic layer (0.8 ml) was transferred into another test tube. An aliquot (0.8 ml) of the remaining citrate buffer layer (containing the T-COOH metabolite and the corresponding internal standard) was transferred to another test tube. The separated aqueous solutions of T-OH and T-COOH were then acidified with 2 N HCl (1 ml), extracted with pentyl acetate (1 to 2 ml), centrifuged, and an aliquot of pentyl acetate (0.5 to 1.0 ml) was transferred to tubes containing 0.025 ml of 0.5% 2,4-dinitrofluorobenzene solution in pentyl acetate. The tubes were lightly stoppered, heated for 1 hr at 125°C and after cooling, 1 to 5 µl of pentyl acetate were injected into the chromatograph. The peak height ratio of the metabolite to the internal standard was measured and the concentration of the metabolite was calculated by reference to a calibration curve of peak height ratio versus concentration, obtained by taking 0 to 25 µg of individual metabolite and several mixtures of the two metabolites in 0.5 ml of plasma or urine through the assay procedure.

As further noted by Matin and Rowland:

The method reported is based on the selective extraction properties of tolbutamide and its two metabolites, T-OH and T-COOH, at different pH values and molarity of the solution. The selective extraction of tolbutamide into hexane is essentially quantitative at the pH of the phosphate buffer and the selective extraction of the two metabolites is 98% at the pH of the citrate buffer used. There is a small carryover of T-OH (<5%) into the T-COOH layer and an even smaller crossover (<1%) of T-COOH into the T-OH layer. This carryover is corrected for by using appropriately prepared calibration curves.

The recovery of T-OH and T-COOH from plasma and urine was identical to the recovery from aqueous solutions. When the already extracted plasma samples of varying concentrations were subjected to the assay procedures no discernible GC peaks were observed. Moreover, when the plasma samples or aqueous solutions containing 0, 10, 25, 50, 75, and 100 µg/ml of either metabolite were analyzed, the GC peak height ratio observed between the metabolite and the internal standard from the aqueous solution or the plasma samples were identical. The recovery was also determined by adding tritiated metabolites to plasma and urine samples. After equilibration the samples were processed as described and aliquots of the pentyl acetate layer were counted. The recovery of the metabolites was found to be 98% complete.

The day-to-day coefficients of variation of the GC assay for the T-OH metabolite at 2.5 (n = 5), 5.0 (n = 5), 10.0 (n = 6), 20.0 (n = 4), and 25.0 (n = 5) µg/ml were 3.4, 2.9, 3.1, 4.5, and 5.2%, respectively, and that for the T-COOH metabolite at the same concentrations were 1.5, 3.5, 2.2, 3.0, and 3.7%, respectively.

The GC procedure was used for the determination of metabolites in plasma and urine when the concentration was less than 10 µg/ml. This assay utilizes the electron-capture properties of the resulting N-substituted 2,4-dinitroanilines. One can readily determine 1 µg of sulfonylurea/ml of sample with this procedure. If necessary the sensitivity can be increased by concentrating the pentyl acetate layer before chromatographic assay. Samples assayed colorimetrically and by GC after appropriate dilutions gave similar results indicating good correlation between the two methods.

The N-propyl, isopropyl, and butyl-2,4-dinitroanilines formed from chlorpropamide, 1-isopropyl-3-p-carboxyphenylsulfonylurea, and the two metabolites, respectively, are well resolved by GC, as shown in Figures [2.10 and 2.11]. The retention time for isopropyl, propyl, and butyl-2,4-dinitroanilines were 4, 5, and 6 min, respectively. The similarity of the pH-dependent extraction characteristics between T-isoprop and T-COOH and between chlorpropamide

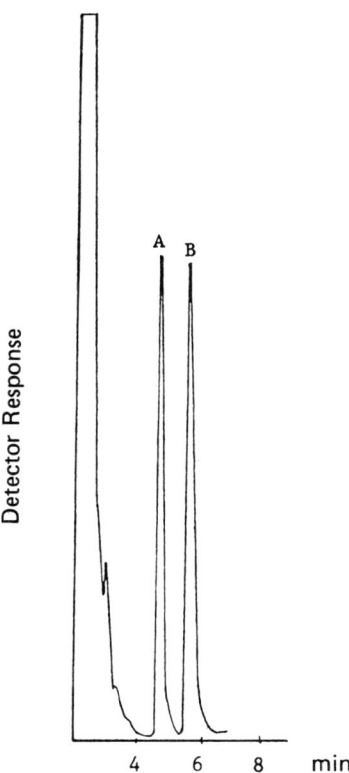

Figure 2.10. Chromatogram of plasma extract, showing propyl-2,4-dinitroaniline (A) and butyl-2,4-dinitroaniline (B) formed from chlorpropamide (2 μg/ml) and T-OH (2.5 μg/ml). From Matin and Rowland [43], courtesy of Marcel Dekker, Inc.

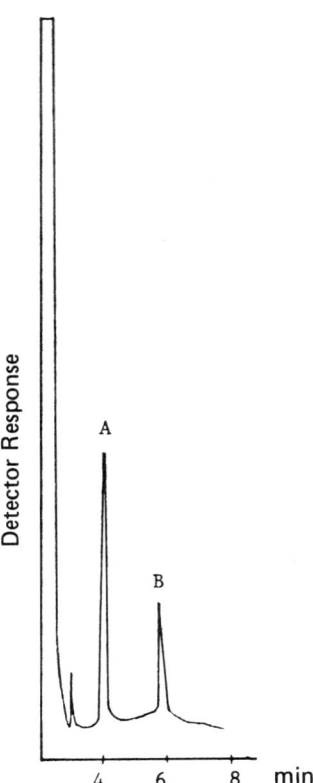

Figure 2.11. Chromatogram of plasma extract, showing isopropyl-2,4-dinitroaniline (A) and butyl-2,4-dinitroaniline (B) formed from 1-isopropyl-3-p-carboxyphenylsulfonyl urea (2.5 µg/ml) and T-COOH (1 µg/ml). From Matin and Rowland [43], courtesy of Marcel Dekker, Inc.

and T-OH makes them suitable internal standards in the respective metabolite assays. The ideal standard for T-OH is either 1-propyl or 1-isopropyl-3-p-hydroxymethylsulfonylurea. However, the general availability of chlorpropamide and its partition similarity to T-OH at the employed pH values makes it a suitable internal standard. Calibration curves were prepared by taking 0 to 25 µg of individual metabolites/ml of biological fluid through the GC procedure. The detector response was found to be linear in this concentration range. No detectable peaks at the same retention time as the substituted anilines were observed when plasma or urine from subjects not receiving tolbutamide were analyzed. Using the GC procedure as little as 1 µg of sulfonylurea/ml of sample can be measured without difficulty. However, if increased sensitivity is desired, smaller volumes (50 µl) of pentyl acetate can be used to carry out the derivatization reaction.

Plasma concentrations and urinary excretion rates of tolbutamide and its metabolites achieved in a human volunteer after the intravenous administration of 1 g of tolbutamide are shown in Figures [2.12 and 2.13].

The maximum blood concentrations achieved were 1.5 µg/ml for T-OH and 3.0 µg/ml for T-COOH. The two metabolites decay with the same half-life as that of tolbutamide.

The urinary excretion rates were maximum between 2 and 2.5 hr after administration of the drug with a value of 24 mg/hr for T-OH and 90 mg/hr for T-COOH. Practically all of the administered dose could be accounted for in urine as the two metabolites.

Shortly thereafter, in 1974, Knight and Matin [45] reported on the utilization of a solid sampler as a means of introducing extracts of biological samples into the ion source for the quantification of some compounds which are unstable under GC conditions. The method, illustrated by the quantitation of tolbutamide (T) in biological samples, is based on the extraction of the sulfonylurea from biological fluids, followed by methylation with diazomethane and the introduction of the sample into the mass spectrometer with a solid sampler. Methane was used as the chemical ionization reactant gas, which permitted the quasimolecular ions formed from the protonated N-1 methylated sulfonylureas to be measured quantitatively.

The mass spectrometer used for this study was a Finnigan model 1015D, operated in the chemical ionization mode. The sample was placed in a disposable glass capillary tube, which can be attached to the probe. The probe containing the glass capillary was inserted into the ion source and heated until the sample evaporates. The evaporation profile was continuously scanned every 2 sec for the ions formed.

With regard to extraction and analysis, Knight and Matin performed these separate functions as follows:

To the plasma sample (0.1 to 0.2 ml) an aqueous solution (0.05 ml) containing 5 µg of the internal standard T-D_2 [N-(p-methylbenzene-sulfonyl)-N'-n-dideuterobutylsulfonylurea] was added. The mixture was acidified with 3 N HCl (0.5 ml) and extracted with ether (10 ml) and, after centrifugation, the ether layer was transferred into another screw-capped tube. An ethereal solution of diazomethane (CH_2N_2,

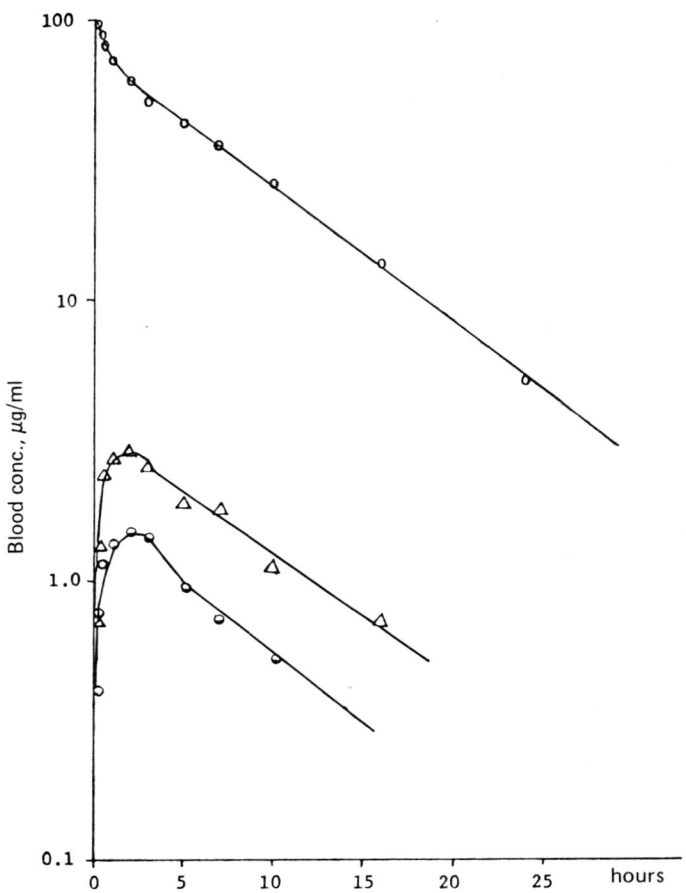

Figure 2.12. Blood concentrations of tolbutamide (O-O), T-COOH (△-△), and T-OH (●-●) following the intravenous administration of 1 g of tolbutamide to man. From Matin and Rowland [43], courtesy of Marcel Dekker, Inc.

1 to 1.5 ml) was added to each tube. After standing at room temperature for 10 min, the ether was evaporated by placing the tubes in a water bath at 50°C and under a light stream of nitrogen. The residue was taken up to 50 μl of methanol and 1 to 2 μl were transferred into a disposable glass capillary tube. The capillary tube was attached to

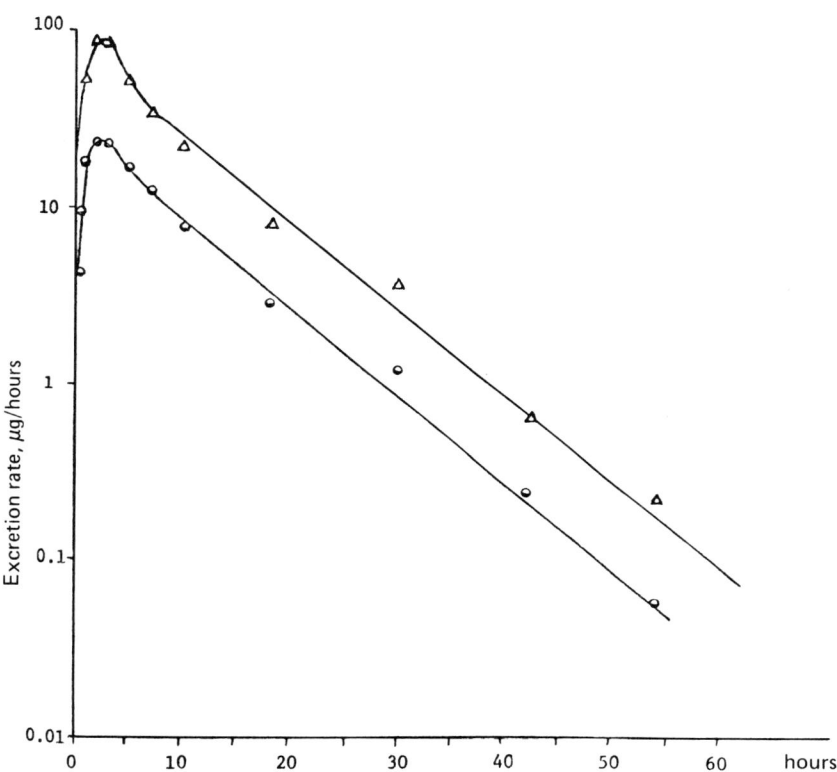

Figure 2.13. The urinary excretion rates for T-COOH (△-△) and T-OH (●-●) observed after the intravenous administration of 1 g of tolbutamide to man. From Matin and Rowland [43], courtesy of Marcel Dekker, Inc.

the solid probe and was introduced into the ionizer. The probe was then heated from 50 to 150°C. This process aids in the complete removal of sulfonylurea from the glass capillary tube. During evaporation, the spectrum was scanned for the specific quasimolecular ions formed from the protonated sulfonylurea. The specific ions scanned repetitively were T at 285, $T-D_2$ at 287 amu. A ratio of the ion peak areas for the proteo and deutero compounds were obtained. The concentration of the compound was obtained by reference to a calibration curve prepared by plotting the ratio of proteo to deutero peak areas versus the concentration of proteo compound added.

Relative to their unique method, which measures the intact sulfonylurea molecule and is based on the use of chemical ionization mass spectrometry (CI-MS), they further noted that:

> The CI-MS system is high-pressure mass spectrometry where ionization of the substance under study is effected by reactant ions. The reactant ions are formed by submitting a reactant gas to electron bombardment at a pressure of about 1 mm Hg. Because of the high pressure the extensively ionized gas undergoes ion molecule reaction with itself and with sample molecules. The latter are present at a relatively low concentration. In this study methane was used as the reactant gas. Upon evaporation from the solid probe, the N-1 methylsulfonylurea molecule undergoes ion molecule reaction with methane to form protonated quasimolecular ions $(M+1)^+$. The quasimolecular ions are separated using a quadrupole mass filter and then measured quantitatively using a computer program. Deuterium-substituted compound T-D_2 was used as the internal standard. The use of a stable isotope-substituted molecule reduces experimental errors during extraction or evaporation. The deuterium-substituted compound possesses an evaporation profile very similar to the proteo compound [Fig. 2.14]. Even though the proteo and deutero compounds evaporate simultaneously, they can be specifically measured due to the difference in molecular weights and hence in the m/e

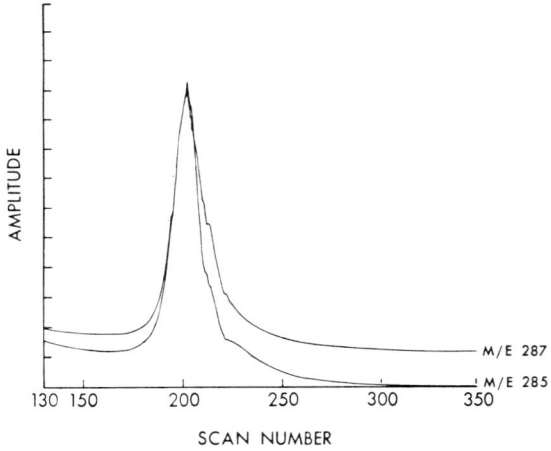

Figure 2.14. The computer reconstructed evaporation profile of T (m/e = 285) and TD_2 (m/e = 287) from the solid sampler. From Knight and Matin [45], courtesy of Marcel Dekker, Inc.

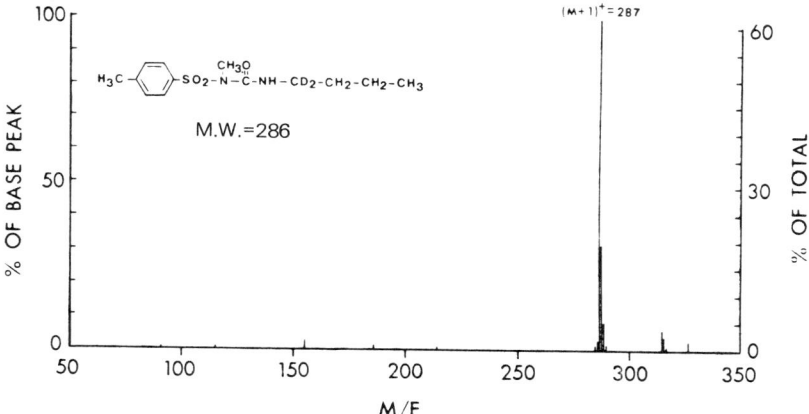

Figure 2.15. The chemical ionization mass spectrum of TD$_2$ obtained by introducing the sample in the ionizer via solid sampler. From Knight and Matin [45], courtesy of Marcel Dekker, Inc.

value of the ion formed. Since methane was used as the chemical ionization reactant gas, only abundant molecular-ions were formed [Fig. 2.15]. The intensity ratio of the proteo and deutero compounds in a single scan taken at the apex of the evaporation profile provided the basis for quantitative measurement. Similar results were obtained when total area under the entire evaporation curve were measured. When blank plasma samples from rabbit were subjected to the analysis procedure, minimal signals were observed in the region of interest.

The data was collected in the form of ion evaporation profiles and was stored on disc. The collected data was simultaneously displayed on the cathode ray tube (CRT) unit provided with the data system. Another program available with the Finnigan data system was later used to read the data and integrate selected ion intensities from the evaporation profile. The CRT unit enables the area of integration to be easily defined. Mass spectrometric calibration curves were prepared by taking 0 to 25 μg of tolbutamide through the assay procedure. The ratio of the area of proteo and deutero compounds was plotted against the concentration of proteo compound added. By reference to this calibration curve, the concentration of tolbutamide in plasma samples of a rabbit after the intravenous administration of tolbutamide was calculated. The plasma level-time profile of tolbutamide following the intravenous administration of 100 mg of tolbutamide to

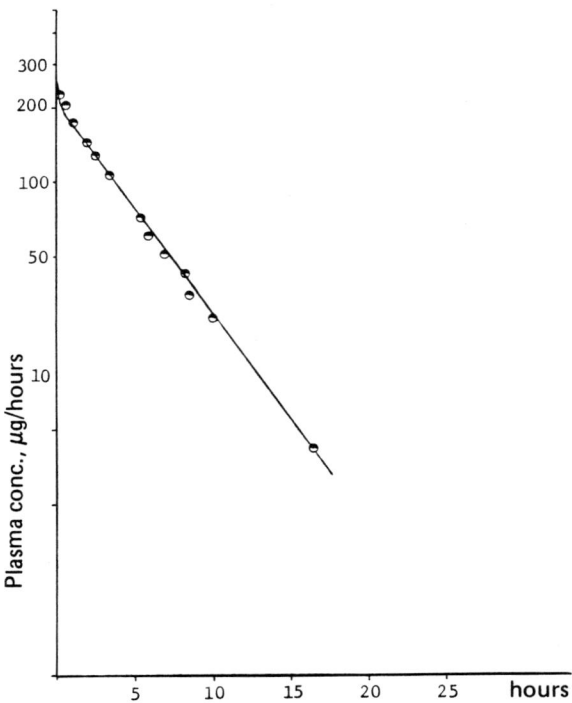

Figure 2.16. Plasma concentration of tolbutamide (O-O), following the intravenous administration of 100 mg of tolbutamide to rabbit. From Knight and Matin [45], courtesy of Marcel Dekker, Inc.

a rabbit is shown in Figure [2.16]. Tolbutamide exhibits an initial rapid distribution phase followed by a slower elimination phase with a half-life of 3.5 hr.

Matin et al. [46] in 1974 also described the excretion of tolbutamide in saliva of diabetic patients receiving single intravenous doses of 1 g of tolbutamide. Using gas chromatography with electron-capture detection [42], pharmacokinetic parameters could be obtained from either saliva or plasma tolbutamide levels. The decline in concentration of tolbutamide (which appeared promptly in saliva after intravenous administration) in saliva and plasma was biphasic, and could be described by an equation similar to that depicted by Eq. (2.1); the biexponential decay curve suggesting that the body behaves as two distinct pools with regard to tolbutamide; that is, a

HYPOGLYCEMIC AGENTS

two-compartment model such as that proposed for the disposition of clonidine and described earlier in this chapter.

Matin et al. also noted that, in the case of lipid-soluble acidic compounds, the saliva/plasma drug concentration ratio can be predicted based on the degree of ionization in the two fluids by Eq. (2.9), where R = saliva/plasma concentration of unbound drug, pHs = pH of the saliva, and pHp = pH of the plasma.

$$R = \frac{1 + 10^{(pHs-pKa)}}{1 + 10^{(pHp-pKa)}} \qquad (2.9)$$

On the other hand, if total drug concentration in plasma (i.e., "free" and bound) is measured, then the ratio would be predicted by Eq. (2.10), where fp = fraction of "free" drug in plasma and fs = fraction of "free" drug in saliva (Note: fs = 1 when drug exists totally in the "free" form).

$$R' = \left[\frac{1 + 10^{(pHs-pKa)}}{1 + 10^{(pHp-pKa)}}\right] \times \left[\frac{fp}{fs}\right] \qquad (2.10)$$

Using Eqs. (2.9) and (2.10), the average value of fp (fraction of "free" drug in plasma) over the concentration range of 5 to 150 μg of tolbutamide/ml of plasma was rather constant, 0.093 ± 0.0033 (n = 3).

Furthermore, there was a good linear relationship between tolbutamide concentration in saliva and plasma; salivary levels being 1.2% of plasma levels. Some of the pharmacokinetics parameters obtained from plasma and saliva in three subjects are listed in Table 2.10, where one notes that the terminal half-life values are well within the range of tolbutamide halflifes reported previously in the literature.

Aggarwal and Sunshine [44] developed a simple method for the determination of sulfonylureas that is not susceptible to significant interference from metabolites.

Sample preparation prior to examination of the extract by CG or GC-MS was performed in the following manner:

To 3.0 ml of plasma suspected to contain a sulfonylurea and to several standards in plasma, each contained in a 16- by 125-mm culture tube with a Teflon-lined screw cap, add 1.0 ml of the H_3PO_4 and 5.0 ml of the internal standard solution (0.5 g of aprobarbital in 500 ml of toluene; 10 ml of this stock solution then diluted to 100 ml with toluene). Urine or aqueous samples and standards can be analyzed by the same technique if 1 ml of a 1 mole/liter acetate buffer (pH 5.2) is substituted for the 1 ml of 0.2 mole/liter H_3PO_4. Shake

TABLE 2.10

Pharmacokinetic Data for Tolbutamide Obtained from
Saliva and Plasma in Three Subjects[a]

	Subject		
	A	B	C
α (hr^{-1})	2.01	2.71	0.18
β (hr^{-1})	0.091	0.110	0.089
$t_{1/2}$ (hr)	7.6	6.3	7.8
Vd (liters)	8.21	6.40	7.32
R'	0.012 ± 0.00015	0.012 ± 0.00032	0.013 ± 0.00052

$t_{1/2}$ = terminal half-life of tolbutamide

Vd = volume of distribution of tolbutamide with reference to plasma

R' = ratio of tolbutamide in saliva to plasma

[a] Adapted from Matin et al. [46].

for 2 min and centrifuge to separate the phases. Transfer about 4 ml of the toluene layer to a clean "concentratube" with a Pasteur pipette. Concentratubes are designed to hold about 20 ml, and taper to a sharp tip, which holds about 10 μl. It is desirable to use tubes of this or similar design, because it is difficult to isolate the small TMAnH (trimethylanilinium hydroxide) layer and aspirate it into a syringe with conventional glassware.

Use a Vortex-type mixer to mix the contents of the concentratube and while vortexing slowly add 200 μl of the TMAnH solution. Continue mixing for a total of 15 sec and then centrifuge for 5 min. Withdraw 3 μl of the TMAnH (lower) phase with a 10-μl syringe and inject it into the injection port of the GC over a 10-sec interval. This slow injection is necessary to avoid tailing of the solvent peaks.

GC studies were carried out with a Hewlett-Packard model 7620 gas chromatograph equipped with dual flame ionization detectors and 6-ft by 1/8-in.-o.d. stainless steel columns packed with 10% W98 on 80-100 mesh Chromosorb W-HP. Operating conditions were injector temperature, 260°C; column temperature, 180°C; detector temperature, 290°C; helium carrier-gas flow rate, 30 ml/min.

Identity of GC peaks was via GC-MS analysis using a Perkin-Elmer model 900 gas chromatograph interfaced with a Hitachi RMU-6L mass spectrometer equipped and operated in the following manner: 5-ft by 1/8-in. stainless steel column packed with 3% OV-17 on Gas Chrom Q; injector temperature, 250°C; column temperature, 150°C; ion source and interface temperature, 250°C; ionization energy, 70 eV.

GC-MS studies of peaks revealed the following:

1. Analysis of a mixture of chlorpropamide and TMAnH showed that the mass spectrum of the GC peak was consistent with N,N-dimethyl-p-chlorobenzenesulfonamide.

2. Analysis of a mixture of tolbutamide and TMAnH yielded N,N-dimethyl-p-toluenesulfonamide, which is identical to the product obtained for "on-column" injections of tolazamide/TMAnH mixtures.

3. Chlorpropamide metabolites (2-hydroxychlorpropamide, p-chlorobenzenesulfonamide, p-chlorobenzenesulfonylurea) dissolved in TMAnH and injected under the stated conditions yielded only one GC peak, which had the same retention time as N,N-dimethyl-p-chlorobenzenesulfonamide.

4. Carboxytolbutamide/TMAnH injections onto the GC column gave a peak which was presumed to be the methyl ester of N,N-dimethyl-p-carboxytolbutamide.

5. The retention times of TMAnH derivatives of substances co-extracted with sulfonylureas were amobarbital, 6.81 min; pentobarbital, 7.68 min; N,N-dimethyl-p-toluenesulfonamide, 7.80 min; N,N-dimethyl-p-chlorobenzenesulfonamide, 8.23 min; secobarbital, 8.86 min; phenobarbital, 12.92 min; methyl ester of N,N-dimethyl-p-carboxyphenylsulfonamide, 13.40 min.

6. Over a 0.5- to 100-μg/ml concentration range, the average recoveries of drug added to plasma were tolbutamide, 82 ± 5%; chlorpropamide, 76 ± 6%; tolazamide, 73 ± 4%.

Braselton et al. [47] developed a rapid, sensitive, and specific method for the quantitation of serum levels of two antidiabetic sulfonylureas, chlorpropamide (CP) and tolbutamide (TB). Thermally stable derivatives of CP, TB, and the major products of TB metabolism, hydroxytolbutamide (HTB) and carboxytolbutamide (CTB), were prepared. Serum levels of CP and TB were determined following extraction of acidified serum with ethyl acetate, formation of N-methyl derivatives with diazomethane, and then formation of the N-methyl-N-trifluoroacetyl derivatives with trifluoroacetic anhydride. The derivatized compounds were analyzed by GC with

FID detection and by GC-MS, and quantitated using the internal standard method. Derivatives of the major tolbutamide metabolites, hydroxytolbutamide and carboxytolbutamide, may also be prepared and chromatographed under similar conditions.

For the formation of N-methyl derivatives of sulfonylurea standards, a simple procedure was used: "One hundred nanomoles of a stock solution of each sulfonylurea in 100 μl of methanol were mixed with 0.4 ml of diazomethane in ether in 1-ml conical-tipped reaction vials and allowed to react 5 min at room temperature, then evaporated with a stream of nitrogen."

The formation of trifluoroacetyl derivatives consisted of the following: The N-methyl sulfonylureas prepared above were dissolved in 45 μl of ethyl acetate, 5 μl of pyridine, and reacted with 50 μl of trifluoroacetic anhydride at 65°C for 30 min. The solvents were removed with a stream of nitrogen, and the compounds dissolved in 100 μl of cyclohexane. One- to two-microliter aliquots were injected into the gas chromatograph.

The preparation of human serum standards was straightforward:

Aliquots of a stock solution of tolbutamide or chlorpropamide in methanol containing 12.5, 25.0, 50.0, 100, and 200 nmoles were placed in 15-ml conical centrifuge tubes along with 100 nmoles of the appropriate internal standard. Chlorpropamide was used as the internal standard for tolbutamide measurement, and tolbutamide as the internal standard for chlorpropamide measurement. The samples were dried with a stream of nitrogen, and 1-ml aliquots of human serum added to the centrifuged tubes and mixed well on a Vortex mixer. A control blank was prepared using 1 ml of serum alone. The samples were acidified with 1 ml of 1 N HCl, and extracted three times with 2 ml each of ethyl acetate. The combined ethyl acetate fractions were concentrated and transferred to 1-ml conical-tipped reaction vials and dried with a stream of nitrogen. The N-methyl-TFA derivatives were prepared as described above.

The instrumentation used by Braselton et al. for the separation and quantitation of these sulfonylurea derivatives consisted of both GC and integrated GC-MS equipment:

1. Integrated gas chromatography-mass spectrometry: The compounds were chromatographed on a Finnigan gas chromatograph-mass spectrometer (GC-MS) coupled with a PDP-8 computer (using System 150 software). The injector and separator temperatures were 240°C; spectra were taken at 70 eV. Columns were 1.5-m by 2-mm-i.d. glass, packed with 1% SP2100 on 100-120 mesh Supelcoport, and operated at 170°C, with a helium carrier-gas flow rate of

approximately 30 ml/min. For measurement of peak height ratios, the data were represented as total ion current chromatograms, and reconstructed specific ion chromatograms of ions m/e 91;111 and m/e 195;209.

2. Gas chromatography: The compounds were also chromatographed on a Varian 2100 GC equipped with a flame ionization detector. The columns were 1.8-m by 2-mm-i.d. glass packed with the same packings as the columns used for GC-MS and cured simultaneously with them. GC determinations were made with a column temperature of 165°C, injector temperature of 240°C, detector temperature of 270°C, and a nitrogen carrier-gas flow rate of 30 ml/min.

In a very thorough discussion of their data, Braselton et al. noted that:

The N-methyl-TFA derivatives of chlorpropamide and tolbutamide chromatographed as single symmetrical peaks on SP2100 with retention times of 4.7 and 6.2 min, respectively [Fig. 2.17]. The

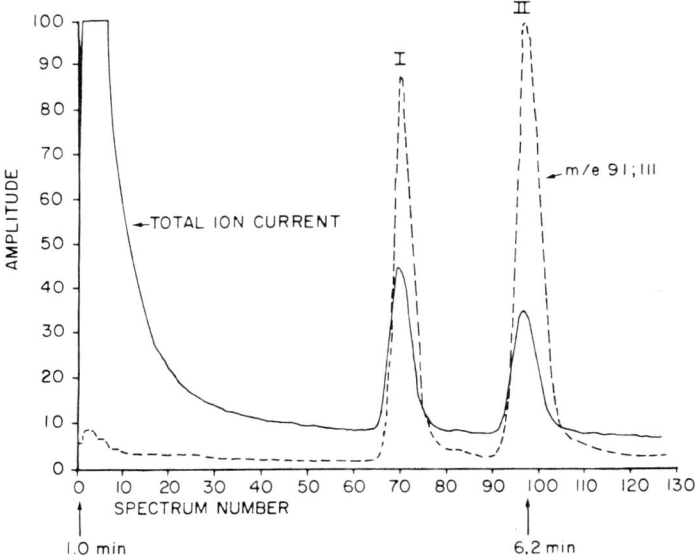

Figure 2.17. Chromatogram of 1 nmole each of chlorpropamide-N-Me-TFA (I) and tolbutamide N-Me-TFA (II) on 1% SP2100 (1.5 m X 2mm-i.d.) at 170°C. The solid line is the total ion current tracing and the broken line the reconstructed gas chromatogram of ions m/e 91 and 111. From Braselton et al. [47], courtesy of Marcel Dekker, Inc.

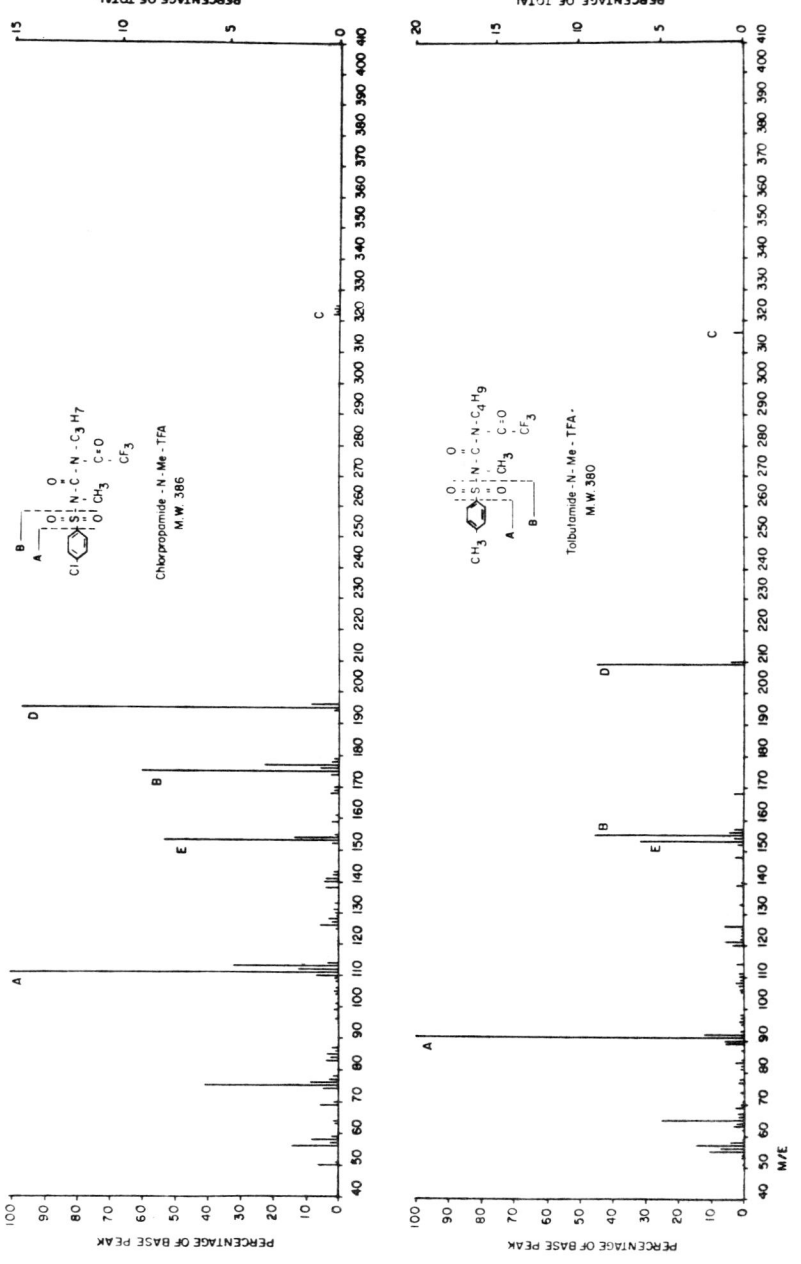

Figure 2.18. Mass spectra at 70 eV of chlorpropamide-N-Me-TFA (upper) and tolbutamide-N-Me-TFA (lower). From Braselton et al. [47], courtesy of Marcel Dekker, Inc.

corresponding mass spectra of these compounds are shown in Figure [2.18]. Fragments A (m/e 91; 111) and B (m/e 155; 175) arise by direct cleavage of the molecule, while fragments C (M-64), D (m/e 195;209) and E (m/e 153) probably arise from a rearrangement involving loss of SO_2, such as has been shown to occur in tolbutamide [53] and N-methyltolbutamide [54].

$$\left[R_1 \underset{}{\bigcirc} \underset{O}{\overset{O}{\underset{\|}{S}}} - \underset{CH_3}{\overset{}{\underset{|}{N}}} - \underset{C=O}{\overset{O}{\underset{\|}{C}}} - N - CH_2 - CH_2 - R_2 \right]^{+\cdot} \xrightarrow{-SO_2} \left[R_1 \underset{}{\bigcirc} - O - \underset{\underset{CH_3}{|}}{\overset{CF_3}{\underset{}{\overset{C \nwarrow O}{\underset{N}{|}}}}} \underset{CH_2 - CH_2 - R_2}{} \right]^{+\cdot}$$

I. $R_1 = Cl$, $R_2 = CH_3$
II. $R_1 = CH_3$, $R_2 = CH_2 CH_3$
III. $R_1 = CF_3\text{-}COOCH_2$, $R_2 = CH_2 CH_3$
IV. $R_1 = CH_3 OOC$, $R_2 = CH_2 CH_3$

C (M-64)

$- R_1 \bigcirc O \cdot$

$CH_3 - \overset{+}{N} = C = N = \underset{\underset{OH}{|}}{C} - CF_3 \quad \xleftarrow{- CH_2 = CHR_2} \quad CH_3 - \overset{+}{N} = C = N \overset{C \nwarrow O}{\underset{CH_2 - \underset{H}{\overset{|}{C}} - R_2}{\underset{}{\overset{CF_3}{}}}}$

$\Updownarrow$

$CH_3 - N = C = \overset{+}{\underset{\underset{H}{|}}{N}} - \underset{O}{\overset{}{\underset{\|}{C}}} - CF_3$

E (m/e 153)

D $\begin{pmatrix} R_2 = CH_3, m/e\ 195 \\ R_2 = CH_2 CH_3,\ m/e\ 209 \end{pmatrix}$

Measurement of relative peak heights for the purpose of quantitation can be made on the total ion current chromatogram or reconstructed gas chromatograms of specific fragment ions, such as m/e 91; 111 [Fig. 2.17]. No interference from serum was seen at the retention time of tolbutamide or chlorpropamide when either the total ion current or specific ion chromatograms were used.

A straight-line relationship of the relative peak height of sulfonylurea to internal standard versus concentration was obtained from 12.5 to 200 nmoles/ml of serum for the chlorpropamide extraction, using tolbutamide as internal standard [Fig. 2.19], when measurements were made on the total ion current or m/e 111; 91 reconstructed gas chromatograms. The difference in slopes of the total ion current and m/e 111; 91 curves is due to ion m/e 91 of the

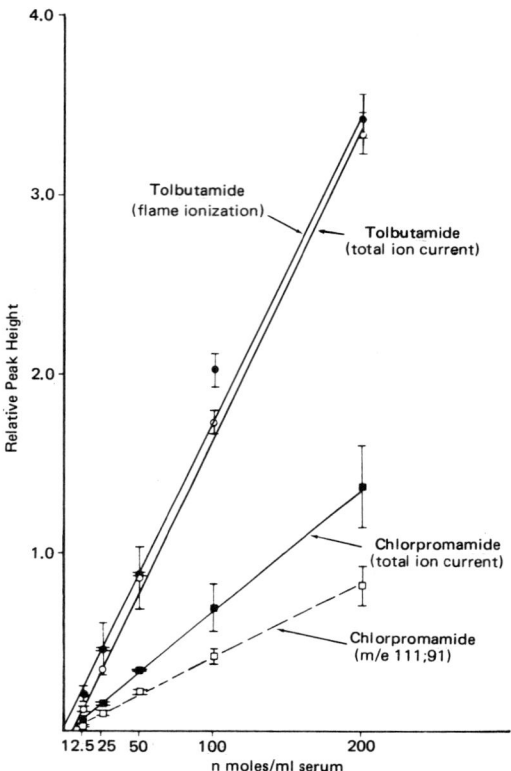

Figure 2.19. Recovery relative to the appropriate internal standard of chlorpropamide and tolbutamide from spiked serum samples. Curves shown are for chlorpropamide recovery determined by GC/MS using the total ion current (■—■) and m/e 111; 91 (□—□) chromatograms for measurement of relative peak height; and for tolbutamide recovery determined by GC/MS using the total ion current (O—O) and by GLC using flame ionization (●—●) for measurement. Data shown are the means of two independent determinations and their range. From Braselton et al. [47], courtesy of Marcel Dekker, Inc.

tolbutamide being a greater percentage of the total ionization of the tolbutamide spectrum (20% Σ_{50}) than ion m/e 111 is of the chlorpropamide spectrum (15% Σ_{50}).

A linear relationship was also observed for tolbutamide extraction from serum, using chlorpropamide as internal standard [Fig. 2.19].

In addition, the curves obtained by GC-MS using the total ion current and GC using flame ionization were virtually superimposable, indicating the less expensive GC method can be used for routine application.

The sensitivity of the method using GC with flame ionization is more than sufficient for studies of tolbutamide and chlorpropamide metabolism under normal therapeutic doses of the drugs, where serum levels in the range of 26 to 740 nmoles/ml have been reported [55-57]. The mass spectra of the N-methyl-TFA derivatives [Fig. 2.18] contain several prominent ions which are suitable for mass fragmentography, and allow one to extend GC-MS sensitivity by several orders of magnitude. By focusing on ions m/e 153 and 209 of tolbutamide, and m/e 153 and 195 of chlorpropamide, we are able to measure as little as 1 pmole of these compounds in serum extracts. Additional time and expense are needed for this type of sensitivity, which in our opinion is usually unnecessary. Thermally stable derivatives of the major tolbutamide metabolites, hydroxytolbutamide and carboxytolbutamide, chromatograph more slowly on SP2100 so that temperature programming is necessary to obtain reasonably short elution times [Fig. 2.20] for measurement of these compounds along with the parent compound. Because of their slower retention times, they do not interfere with measurement of the unmetabolized drug.

The problems encountered with other methods for measurement of the thermally unstable sulfonylureas have been pointed out by others [37, 39]. Colorimetric and spectrophotometric methods can be inaccurate because of extraction and interference by other drugs [57] and metabolites [58]. A solvent extraction procedure for separation of tolbutamide metabolites from parent drug has been described [43] but the method involves a number of time-consuming and cumbersome solvent partitions, followed by GC measurement of the nonspecific butylamine portion of the molecule, and is thus not suitable for long-term studies of pharmacokinetics of these compounds.

The chemical ionization-mass spectrometry method of Knight and Matin [45] appears to be specific for tolbutamide, and probably could be adapted to measurement of metabolites as well, when the stable isotope labeled compounds become available.

The ability to form thermally stable derivatives for GC provides several advantages. The method is rapid, since the total time for formation of stable derivatives is less than an hour after initial extraction from serum and the GC step takes less than 10 min for elution of tolbutamide and metabolites. Since only a GC with flame ionization detection is sufficient instrumentation, large blocks of time on more sophisticated equipment are not necessary.

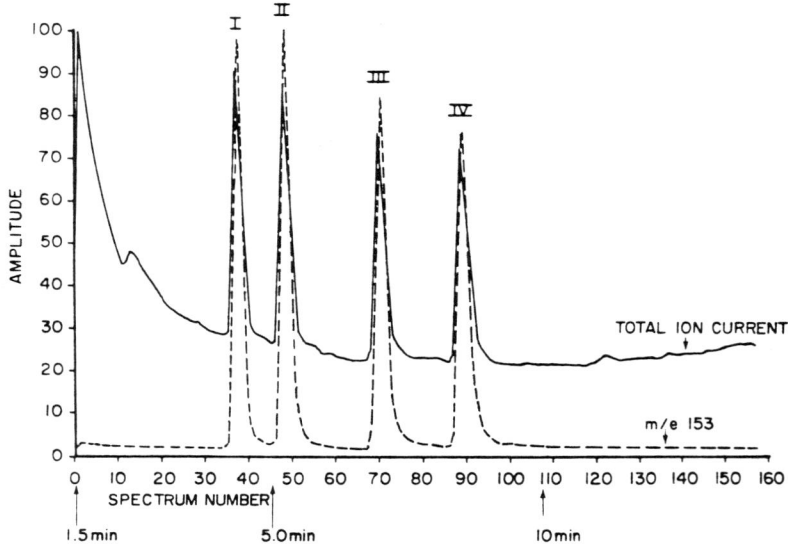

Figure 2.20. Chromatogram of 1 nmole each of chlorpropamide-N-Me-TFA (I), tolbutamide-N-Me-TFA (II), hydroxytolbutamide-N-Me-bis-TFA (III), and carboxytolbutamide-N-Me-TFA-methyl ester (IV). The compounds were chromatographed on 1% SP2100 at 170°C isothermally for 1.5 min, and then programmed to 250 at 6°C/min. The total ion current tracing is shown as a solid line, and reconstructed gas chromatogram of ion m/e 153 as a broken line. From Braselton et al. [47], courtesy of Marcel Dekker, Inc.

Shortly thereafter, Braselton et al. [48] described in detail the mass spectral (electron impact) and GC characteristics of the N-methyl and N-methyltrifluoroacetyl, N-methylpentafluoropropionyl, and N-methyl-heptafluorobutyryl derivatives of the sulfonylureas tolbutamide, hydroxytolbutamide, carboxytolbutamide, chlorpropamide, and tolazamide. The derivatized compounds were thermally stable as shown by mass spectrometry and exhibited excellent GC properties on three liquid phases, 3% OV-1, 3% OV-17, and 3% SP-2401.

The procedures recommended for the formation of N-methyl and N-methylperfluoroacyl derivatives were as follows:

1. Formation of N-methyl derivatives: these were prepared by two different procedures; the first using dimethyl sulfate as reagent by the method of Prescott and Redman [39]. N-Methylsulfonylurea-d_3

derivatives were also synthesized by this procedure, using dimethyl-d_6-sulfate and CH_3OD. The second method used diazomethane to form the methyl derivatives (100 nmoles of each sulfonylurea in 100 μl of methanol was mixed with 0.5 ml of ethereal diazomethane in 1-ml conical-tipped vials and allowed to react for 5 min at room temperature, then evaporated to dryness with a stream of nitrogen).

2. Formation of N-methylperfluoroacyl derivatives: The N-methyl derivatives prepared above were dissolved in 50 μl of ethyl acetate: pyridine (9:1) and reacted with 50 μl of trifluoroacetic anhydride, pentafluoropropionic anhydride, or heptafluorobutyric anhydride for 30 min at 65°C. Following the evaporation of the reagents with a stream of nitrogen, the residues were dissolved in 100 μl of cyclohexane. This solution was now ready for either GC or GC-MS investigations.

The above derivatives were analyzed with a Finnigan 1015D GC-MS instrument interfaced with a Systems Industries 150 data acquisition and control system and equipped with 1.5-m by 2-mm-i.d. glass columns packed with either 3% OV-1 (on 80-100 mesh Suplecoport), 3% OV-17 (on 100-120 mesh Gas Chrom Q), or 3% SP-2401 (on 100-120 mesh Suplecoport). The other GC-MS conditions used were column temperature, 230°C; injector temperature, 240°C; separator temperature, 240°C; ionizing voltage, 70 eV; helium carrier-gas flow rate, 30 ml/min. Straight GC studies were performed with a Varian 2100 gas chromatograph equipped with a ^{63}Ni electron-capture detector and 1.8-m by 2-mm-i.d. glass columns; in this study, the nitrogen carrier-gas flow rate was maintained at 37 ml/min.

With regard to mass spectral investigations of N-methyl and N-methylperfluoroacyl derivatives, Braselton et al. showed that:

1. The mass spectra of the N-methyl derivatives formed by reaction with dimethyl sulfate were identical to the spectra of derivatives formed by diazomethane and the formation of the N-methyl derivative of carboxytolbutamide also resulted in the formation of the methyl ester.

2. The spectra of the N-methyl derivatives of chlorpropamide and tolbutamide metabolites indicated that fragmentation of these compounds involved a rearrangement with a loss of SO_2 in contrast to the tolazamide derivative which did not lose SO_2. Figure 2.21 shows the general structure of the fragment ions a-k described by Sabih [54] for N-methyltolbutamide, whereas in Table 2.11 the corresponding ions obtained by Braselton et al. from N-methylhydroxytolbutamide, N-methylcarboxytolbutamide, and N-methylchlorpropamide are compared.

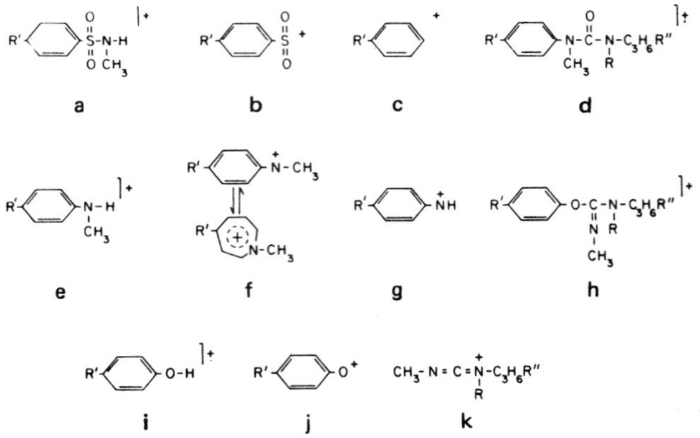

Figure 2.21. Ions a-k described by Sabih [54] for N-Me-tolbutamide. They are shown here as general structures since they appear in the mass spectra of a number of the sulfonylurea derivatives (Table 2.11). Other ions are shown in Figures 2.22 and 2.23. Ion f of Sabih probably exists as shown above (I) R' = CH_3, R" = CH_3; (II) R' = $ROCH_2$, R" = CH_3; (III) R' = CH_3OOC, R" = CH_3; (IV) R' = Cl, R" = H; (TFA) R = $COCF_3$; (PFP) R = COC_2F_5; (HFB) R = COC_3F_7. From Braselton et al. [48], courtesy of Analytical Chemistry.

3. Fragment ions containing the perfluoroacyl groups are readily identified by the 50-amu increases from the TFA to the PFP derivatives and the 100-amu increases from the TFA to the HFB derivatives.

4. Whereas the scheme in Figure 2.22 accounts for the major rearrangement ions of the sulfonylurea-methylperfluoroacyl spectra, other major fragment ions in their spectra may arise from ion h ($M-SO_2$) as shown in Figure 2.23.

With regard to the GC characteristics of the N-methylperfluoroacyl derivatives, Braselton et al. summarized their GC results in the following manner:

Table [2.12] lists the retention times of the methylperfluoroacyl derivatives and those relative to tolbutamide-Me-TFA determined on several different stationary phases.
The compounds within a single perfluoroalkyl series (TFA, PFP, or HFB) were well separated on the 3% OV-1 and OV-17 phases, but

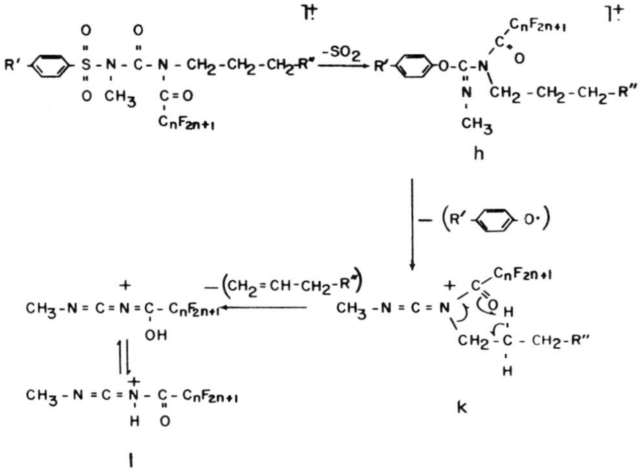

Figure 2.22. Compound I: R' = R" = CH$_3$; II: R' = C$_n$F$_{2n+1}$COOCH$_2$, R" = CH$_3$; III: R' = CH$_3$OOC, R" = CH$_3$; IV: R' = Cl, R" = H. From Braselton et al. [48], courtesy of Analytical Chemistry.

the two tolbutamide metabolites as the Me-TFA derivatives were not separated on 3% SP-2401. A noticeable decrease in retention time for each compound on OV-17 was observed with each additional CF$_2$ increment in the perfluoroalkyl group. The elution time characteristics were more complex on the methyl silicone phase, OV-1, where the Me-PFP derivatives eluted faster than the respective Me-TFAs, but Me-HFB derivatives eluted more slowly. This elution order was also seen with the perfluoroacyl derivatives of carbamate pesticides when chromatographed on methyl silicone liquid phase [59] and probably reflects a combination of molecular size and polarity effects.

It should also be noted that the derivatives showed high sensitivity to electron-capture detection: tolbutamide-N-methyltrifluoroacetate sensitivity = 2.8 X 10^{-16} mole/sec at a 3:1 signal-to-noise ratio.

In 1976, Midha et al. [49] developed a GC procedure for the quantitative estimation of intact chlorpropamide and tolbutamide concentrations in plasma using the drugs as mutual internal standards. After the extraction of plasma containing the drug and internal standard with toluene, the dried residue is treated with ethereal diazomethane to form the methyl derivatives of tolbutamide and chlorpropamide; aliquots of this ethereal solution are then injected into the gas chromatographic unit for analysis.

TABLE 2.11

Significant Fragment Ions of Sulfonylurea N-Me and
Me-Perfluoroacyl Derivatives[a]

Compound	R_1	(Δamu)[c]	R_2 (Δamu)[c]	Mol. wt.	a
I-Me	CH_3		C_4H_9	284	185
I-CD_3	CH_3		C_4H_9	287	188
I-Me-TFA	CH_3		C_4H_9	380	
I-CD_3-TFA	CH_3		C_4H_9	383	
I-Me-PFP	CH_3		C_4H_9	430	
I-Me-HFB	CH_3		C_4H_9	480	
II-Me	CH_2OH	(+16)	C_4H_9	300	201
II-Me-TFA	CH_2OCOCF_3	(+112)	C_4H_9	492	
II-Me-PFP	$CH_2OCOC_2F_5$	(+162)	C_4H_9	592	
II-Me-HFB	$CH_2OCOC_3F_7$	(+212)	C_4H_9	692	397
III-Me	$COOCH_3$	(+44)	C_4H_9	328	229
III-Me-TFA	$COOCH_3$	(+44)	C_4H_9	424	229
III-Me-PFP	$COOCH_3$	(+44)	C_4H_9	474	
III-Me-HFB	$COOCH_3$	(+44)	C_4H_9	524	
IV-Me	Cl	(+20)	C_3H_7(-14)	290	205
IV-CD_3	Cl	(+20)	C_3H_7(-14)	293	208
IV-Me-TFA	Cl	(+20)	C_3H_7(-14)	386	205
IV-CD_3-TFA	Cl	(+20)	C_3H_7(-14)	389	208
IV-Me-PFP	Cl	(+20)	C_3H_7(-14)	436	
IV-Me-HFB	Cl	(+20)	C_3H_7(-14)	486	

[a] From Braselton et al. [48], courtesy of <u>Analytical Chemistry.</u>

[b] Ions a-k correspond to those described in the spectrum of N-Me-tolbutamide by Sabih [54].

[c] Represents the change in mass from the corresponding group of tolbutamide.

[d] Could not be determined because of coincidence with isotope peak of ion l.

[e] Could not be determined because of coincidence with isotope peak of ion b.

					ions[b] (m/e values)							
b	c	d(h)	e	f	g	i	j	k	l	m	n	o
155	91	220	121	120	106	108	107	113				
155	91	223	124	123	106	108	107	116				
155	91	316	121	120		108	107	209	153	148	168	126
155	91	319	124	123		108	107	212	156	151	168	126
155	91	366	121	120		108	107	259	203	148	218	176
155	91	416	121	120		108	107	309	253	148	268	226
171	107	236	137	136		124	123	113				
267	203	428	233	232				209	153	260	168	126
317	253	528	283	282				259	203	310	218	176
367	303	628	333	332				309	253	360	268	226
199	135	264	165	164	150	152		113				
199	135	360	165	164		152		209	153	192	168	126
199	135	410	165	164		152		259	203	192	218	176
199	135	460	165	164		152		309	253	192	268	226
175	111	226	141	140		128	127	99				
175	111	229	144	143		128	127	102				
175	111	322	141	140		128	127	195	153	168	−[d]	126
175	111	325	144	143		128	127	198	156	171	154	126
175	111	372	141	140		128	127	245	203	168	−[d]	−[e]
175	111	422	141	140		128	127	295	253	168	−[d]	226

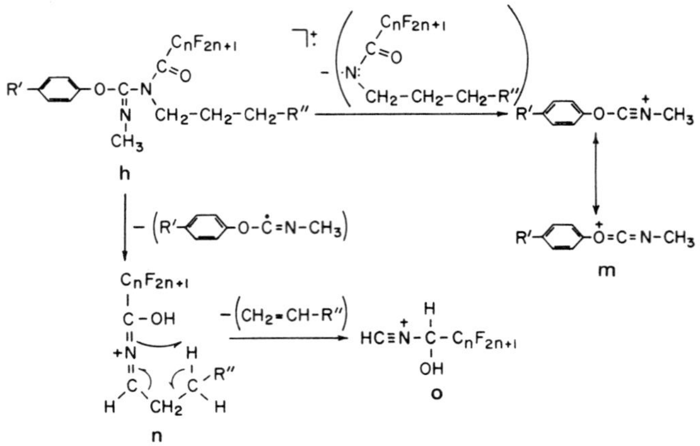

Figure 2.23. R' and R" are identified in the legend to Figure 2.22. From Braselton et al. [48], courtesy of Analytical Chemistry.

The separation of these methyl derivatives was achieved using a Perkin-Elmer model 3920 gas chromatograph equipped with a glass-lined injection port, a flame ionization detector, and a 6-ft by 3-mm-i.d. coiled glass column packed with 5% OV-25 on 80-100 mesh, acid-washed, DMCS-treated Chromosorb W. Operating conditions were injector temperature, 200°C; column temperature, 220°C; detector temperature, 285°C; nitrogen carrier-gas flow rate, 60 ml/min. Using these conditions, the retention times of methylated chlorpropamide and tolbutamide were 4.50 and 5.90 min, respectively.

Methylation of chlorpropamide with diazomethane yielded three GC peaks with retention times of 2.2, 4.5, and 10.5 when the temperature of the injection port was set at 275°C. GC-MS analysis of the eluted peaks identified them as: first peak, N-methyl-p-chlorobenzensulfonamide (major fragment ions at m/e 205-207, 175-177, and 111-113); second eluted peak, N-methylchlopropamide (diagnostic ions at m/e 261-263, 232-234, 226-228, 175-177, and 111-113); third peak, the methyl enol ether of chlorpropamide (prominent ions at m/e 290-292, 258-260, 175-177, and 111-113). It was noted that at an injection temperature of 200°C or slightly less, peaks 1 and 3 decreased dramatically whereas the N-methyl derivative of chlorpropamide increased at the expense of the other two degradation products.

Similarly, methylation of tolbutamide with diazomethane gave three peaks with retention times of 2.0, 5.9, and 13.9 min. By GC-MS, peak 1 was identified as N-methyl-p-toluenesulfonamide (m/e ions at 185, 155,

TABLE 2.12

GC-MS RRT and Retention Time Data of Sulfonylurea Methylperfluoroalkyl Derivatives[a]

Compound	3% OV-1		3% OV-17		3% SP-2401	
	RRT	RT (min)	RRT	RT (min)	RRT	RT (min)
Chlorpropamide-Me-TFA	0.80	1.50	0.86	1.84	0.81	1.86
Chlorpropamide-Me-PFP	0.79	1.48	0.66	1.40		
Chlorpropamide-Me-HFB	0.81	1.52	0.62	1.33		
Tolbutamide-Me-TFA	1.00	1.88	1.00	2.14	1.00	2.30
Tolbutamide-Me-PFP	0.94	1.77	0.78	1.67		
Tolbutamide-Me-HFB	0.94	1.77	0.73	1.56		
Hydroxytolbutamide-Me-TFA	1.39	2.62	1.26	2.70	1.97	4.53
Hydroxytolbutamide-Me-PFP	1.30	2.44	0.92	1.97		
Hydroxytolbutamide-Me-HFB	1.50	2.82	0.89	1.90		
Carboxytolbutamide-Me-TFA	1.97	3.70	2.06	4.42	1.97	4.53
Carboxytolbutamide-Me-PFP	1.79	3.36	1.73	3.70		
Carboxytolbutamide-Me-HFB	1.83	3.44	1.62	3.46		
Tolazamide-Me-TFA	2.88	5.42	3.51	7.50	2.22	5.10
Tolazamide-Me-PFP	2.61	4.90	3.08	6.60		
Tolazamide-Me-HFB	2.62	4.93	2.81	6.00		

[a] Adapted from Braselton et al. [48], courtesy of Analytical Chemistry.

141, 121, and 91), whereas peaks 2 and 3 were N-methyltolbutamide (m/e 241, 220, 212, 185, 155, 121, and 91) and the methyl enol ether of tolbutamide (m/e 284, 269, 255, 241, 184, 155, 121, and 91). As the injection port temperature was dropped from 275 to 200°C, peak 1, due to N-methyl-p-toluenesulfonamide (see Fig. 2.24) decreased, and peak 2, due to N-methyltolbutamide, increased.

Based on the above injection port temperature studies, Midha et al. recommended the use of an injector temperature of 200°C for quantitative analyses since thermal breakdown of the methylated drugs was minimal.

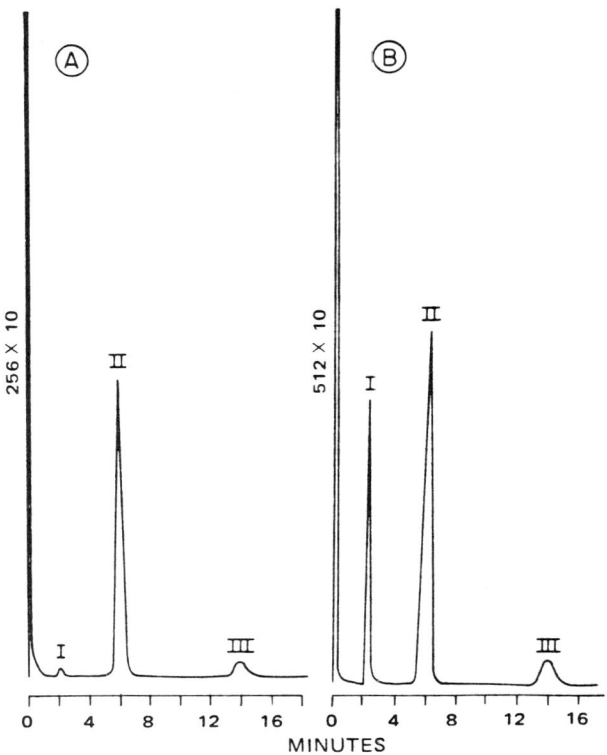

Figure 2.24. Typical chromatograms of methylated tolbutamide. Key: A, injection port temperature 200°C; and B, injection port temperature 275°C. From Midha et al. [49], courtesy of the Journal of Pharmaceutical Sciences.

They also reported that "the response of the flame ionization detector to chlorpropamide and tolbutamide was linear with concentrations over the 0.20 to 25.00 µg/ml range. The ratio of the peak heights of chlorpropamide or tolbutamide and their respective internal standard (tolbutamide or chlorpropamide) plotted against concentration in the 0.20- to 25.00-µg/ml range gave straight lines passing through the origin (r = 1.0). Mean slope values of 0.146 ± 0.002 and 0.290 ± 0.003 were obtained for chlorpropamide and tolbutamide, respectively. The overall coefficients of variation were 3.4% and 3.1%, respectively. The overall recoveries of chlorpropamide and tolbutamide from plasma were of the order of 72.1 ± 3.3 and 83.9 ± 1.5%, respectively.

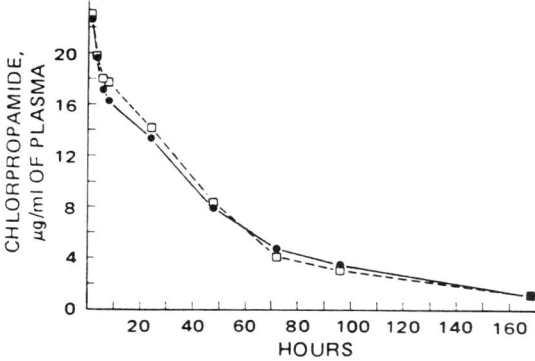

Figure 2.25. Comparison of plasma chlorpropamide levels by GC method with that of an HPLC method following a single oral dose of a 125-mg tablet of chlorpropamide to a human volunteer (73 kg). Key: ●, GC method; and □, HPLC method. From Midha et al. [49], courtesy of the Journal of Pharmaceutical Sciences.

Methylation of the major metabolites of tolbutamide showed two peaks using the GC conditions specified: methylated p-toluenesulfonylurea, 2.0 and 2.45 min; methylated hydroxytolbutamide, 9.7 and 23.6 min; methylated carboxytolbutamide, 10.8 and 12.9 min.

On the other hand, methylated 2-hydroxychlorpropamide and 3-hydroxychlorpropamide broke down to give N-methyl-p-chlorobenzenesulfonamide, with major peaks for intact methylated derivatives of alcohols observed at 7.84 and 10.4 min.

In Figures 2.25 and 2.26 are shown comparisons of plasma levels of chlorpropamide and tolbutamide, respectively, obtained by this GC procedure and values derived using a recently developed high-pressure liquid chromatographic method [60].

In 1977, Williams et al. [50] measured tolbutamide plasma protein binding and pharmacokinetic parameters after intravenous administration of the drug to five subjects during and after apparent recovery from acute viral hepatitis in order to study the influence of acute hepatic disease on the disposition of tolbutamide. Using the GC procedure of Matin and Rowland [42] for the determination of tolbutamide in plasma, Williams et al. noted that:

> Although during the acute phase of illness protein binding decreased in all, volume of distribution of tolbutamide (0.15 ± 0.03 liter/kg) did not change [see Table 2.13]. Clearance based on total concentration of tolbutamide in plasma increased in all subjects during the

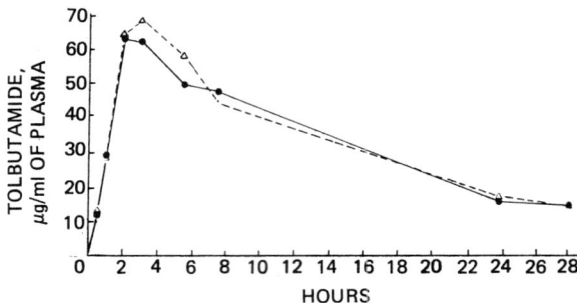

Figure 2.26. Comparison of plasma tolbutamide levels by GC methods with that of an HPLC method following a single oral dose of a 500-mg tablet of tolbutamide to a human volunteer (73 kg). Key: ●, GC method; and △, HPLC method. From Midha et al. [49], courtesy of the Journal of Pharmaceutical Sciences.

acute phase of study (26 ± 5.4 ml/hr/kg) in comparison to the recovery phase (18 ± 2.8 ml/hr/kg, $p < 0.02$). Protein binding decreased after unconjugated bilirubin was added to plasma from the recovery phase, but not to the extent observed during the acute phase of illness at comparable levels of bilirubin. Clearance based on unbound drug concentration, calculated by dividing the observed plasma clearance by the fraction of unbound drug in plasma, did not differ significantly between the two study phases (300 ± 47 and 260 ± 39 ml/hr/kg). These observations suggest that the increase in clearance based on total drug concentration in plasma during hepatitis can be attributed solely to decreased plasma binding. This decrease in binding may be attributed in part, but not entirely, to increased concentration of bilirubin during illness. The concentration of unbound drug in plasma at steady state is determined by the rate of drug administration and the clearance based on unbound drug. If this clearance does not change during hepatic disease, no dosage alterations for tolbutamide and other comparable drugs are necessary to maintain a constant concentration of unbound drug.

In Table 2.14 can be found averaged biochemical measures of hepatic disease as well as the percent change noted in the fraction of unbound drug (f) and clearance based on unbound concentration of drug (Cl_u) during and after apparent recovery from acute viral hepatitis.

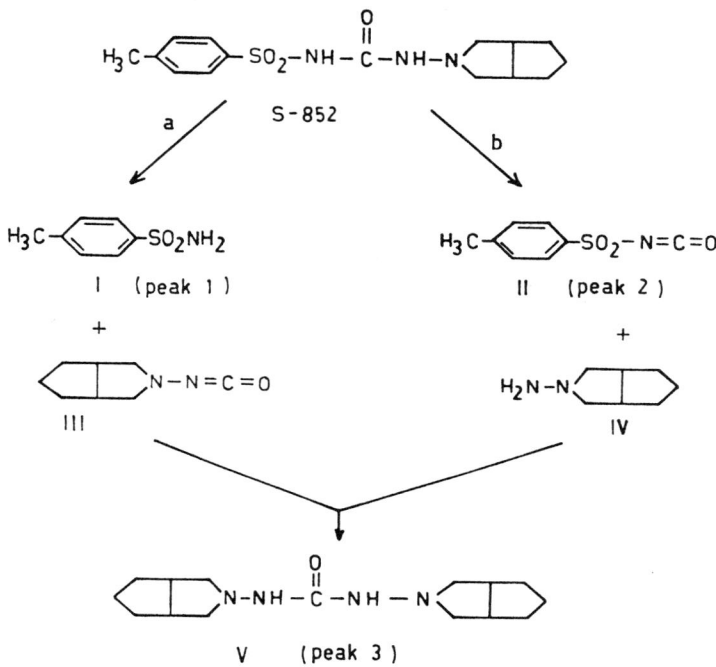

Figure 2.27. Thermal degradation pathway of S-852. From Belvedere et al. [51], courtesy of the Journal of Chromatographic Science.

Belvedere et al. [51] investigated by integrated GC-MS the thermal decomposition products of S-852, N-(p-toluenesulfonyl)-N'-[aza-bicyclo-(3.3.0)octyl] urea, a hypoglycemic drug which also inhibits platelet aggregation.

An acetone solution of the drug (1 mg/1 ml) was examined chromatographically using the following instrumentation:

1. Gas chromatography: A Carlo Erba Fractovap gas chromatograph equipped with flame ionization detector and a 1-m by 4-mm-i.d. glass column packed with 3% OV-17 on 100-120 mesh Gas Chrom Q and operated as follows: injector temperature, 300°C; column tem-

perature, programmed from 90 to 280°C at 10°C/min; nitrogen carrier-gas flow rate, 60 ml/min.

2. Gas chromatography-mass spectrometry: A LKB 9000 integrated GC-MS instrument using the GC conditions and column described above with one exception—the carrier gas was helium maintained at a flow rate of 30 ml/min. The MS conditions were electron energy, 70 ev; ion source temperature, 290°C; accelerating voltage, 3.5 kV; trap current, 60 µA.

Using the above GC-MS conditions, three peaks were observed; peaks 1, 2, and 3 separated by temperature programming having elution temperatures of 200, 210, and 270°C, respectively. In Figure 2.27, which depicts two possible degradation pathways for the drug, the identity and structures of the three peaks are shown.

As noted by Belvedere et al., "the thermal degradation of the drug, according to pathway (a), leads to the formation of compound I, which corresponds to the first GC peak, and to the isocyanate III that is not detectable. Pathway (b) also gives rise to two products: compound II, which corresponds to the second GC peak, and the amine IV, which did not give any peak in the programmed gas chromatogram. From these data, it is possible to deduce that the isocyanate and the amine IV reacted together in the injection port of the gas chromatograph, giving rise to the N,N'-substituted urea, corresponding to the third peak of the gas chromatogram.

The structures and prominent fragment ions of the parent drug and its degradation products are given in Figure 2.28.

Finally, in 1977, Kleber et al. [52] developed a sensitive and specific GC assay for acetohexamide and its major metabolite, hydroxyhexamide, in plasma and urine. Using tolbutamide as internal standard, the compounds are extracted from acidified plasma or urine with toluene, converted to methyl derivatives with dimethyl sulfate, and measured by GC using flame ionization detection. With GC-MS, the compounds measured are the

$$CH_3-\overset{OH}{\underset{H}{C}}-\langle\ \rangle-SO_2NHCONH-\langle\ \rangle$$

Hydroxyhexamide

N-methylsulfonamides resulting from GC pyrolysis of tolbutamide, acetohexamide, and hydroxyhexamide.

Compound	Prominent m/e ions
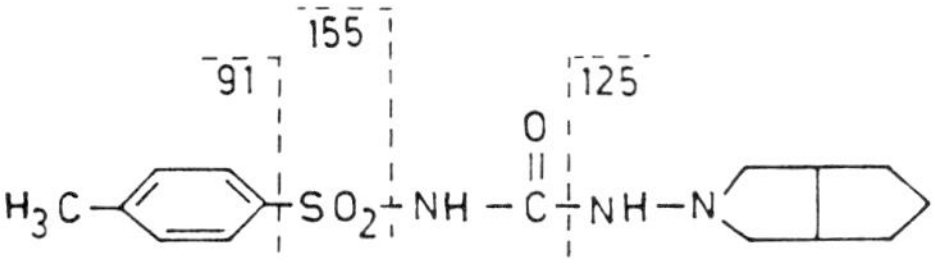 **Parent Drug (S-852)** H₃C–⟨C₆H₄⟩–SO₂–NH–C(=O)–NH–N⟨ring⟩ fragments: 91, 155, 125 S-852 M.W. 323	323 (5), 197 (19), 155 (37), 125 (25), 91 (100)
Peak 1 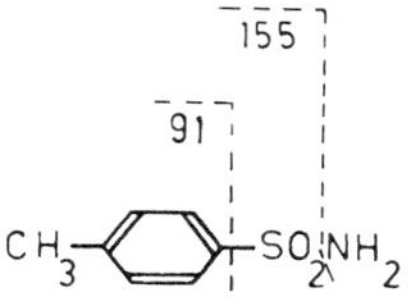 CH₃–⟨C₆H₄⟩–SO₂NH₂ fragments: 91, 155 M.W. 171	171 (28), 155 (28), 91 (100), 65 (28)
Peak 2 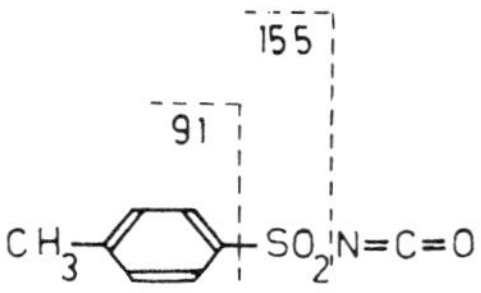 CH₃–⟨C₆H₄⟩–SO₂N=C=O fragments: 91, 155 M.W. 197	197 (10), 171 (30), 155 (41), 91 (100)
Peak 3 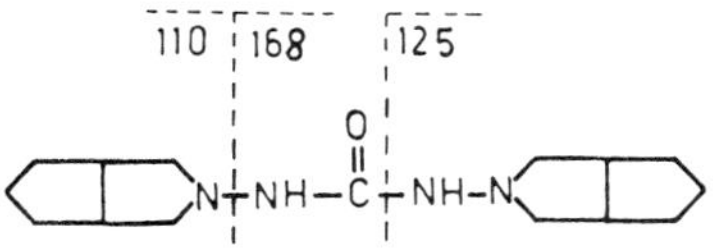 ⟨ring⟩N–NH–C(=O)–NH–N⟨ring⟩ fragments: 110, 168, 125 M.W. 278	278 (12), 168 (84), 151 (48), 126 (73), 110 (100)

Figure 2.28. Mass spectral data for S-852 and its major thermal degradation products.

TABLE 2.13

Averaged Pharmacokinetic Parameters for Tolbutamide and Total Bilirubin in Five Subjects During and After Apparent Recovery from Hepatitis[a]

V_d		k_d		$t_{1/2}$		Cl_p		Total bilirubin (mg/100 ml)	
During	After	During	After	During	After	During	After	During	After
0.15 ± 0.03	0.15 ± 0.03	0.18 ± 0.04	0.12 ± 0.03^b	4.0 ± 0.9	5.9 ± 1.4^b	26 ± 5.4	18 ± 2.8^c	6.7 ± 1.2	0.8 ± 0.2

[a] Adapted from Williams et al. [50].
[b] Difference between means is significant, $p < 0.01$.
[c] Difference between means is significant, $p < 0.02$.

V_d = volume of distribution (liter/kg); k_d = rate of elimination (hr^{-1}); $t_{1/2}$ = half-life (hr); Cl_p = plasma clearance (ml/hr/kg)

TABLE 2.14

Averaged Biochemical Measures of Hepatic Disease, Percent Change in Unbound Fraction of Drug, and Clearance Based on Unbound Drug Concentration During and After Apparent Recovery from Acute Viral Hepatitis[a]

SGOT (I.U./liter)		LDH (I.U./liter)		Alkaline Phosphatase (I.U./liter)		Albumin (g/100 ml)		Percent change in unbound fraction		Cl_u	
During	After	During	After	During	After	During	After	During	After	During	After
703 ± 475	38 ± 6	265 ± 101	113 ± 8	206 ± 62	89 ± 31	3.9 ± 0.1	4.1 ± 0.3	28.0 ± 6.5	13.0 ± 6.2	300 ± 47	260 ± 39[b]

[a] Adapted from Williams et al. [50].
[b] Difference is not significant.

For this analytical study, Kleber et al. used a Hewlett-Packard model 402 gas chromatograph equipped with dual flame ionization detectors and 0.61-m by 3-mm-i.d. glass columns packed with 0.5% PEG 20M on 80-100 mesh Gas Chrom Q. With the GC conditions recommended (column temperature, programmed from 190 to 240°C at a heating rate of 5°C/min; detector temperature, 260°C; helium carrier-gas flow rate, 90 ml/min), the retention times of N-methyl-p-toluenesulfonamide (from tolbutamide), N-methyl-p-acetylbenzenesulfonamide (from acetohexamide), and p-(1-hydroxyethyl)-N-methylbenzenesulfonamide were 1.50, 5.00, and 8.00 min, respectively. Using this GC assay procedure, the average recoveries of acetohexamide and its hydroxy metabolite added to plasma were $98.8 \pm 0.2\%$ and $110.7 \pm 20.2\%$, respectively.

The method was applied to a bioavailability investigation which was conducted to compare acetohexamide tablets and to demonstrate the utility of the GC procedure. Tablets from three different lots, plus a placebo tablet to estimate basal response, were administered to eight subjects in a four-way crossover study. Each subject fasted for 8 hr before receiving a therapeutic dose of 1.5 tablets, 750 mg, of acetohexamide. Blood samples were drawn at -1, 0, 1, 2, 3, 4, 6, and 8 hr after administration. In addition to the determination of acetohexamide and hydroxyhexamide in blood, blood glucose and serum insulin were determined; the results of these four different analyses are illustrated in Figure 2.29.

As further noted by Kleber et al.:

> The physiological responses (elevation of serum insulin and lowering of blood glucose) may more truly reflect the bioavailability of acetohexamide from the three tablet formations, because the metabolite, hydroxyhexamide, is not only physiologically active but also has a more prolonged effect than the parent drug. Since no substantial differences were found in the plasma concentrations of hydroxyhexamide from these tablet lots, the physiological responses may more closely reflect the plasma metabolite concentrations or a combination of the plasma concentrations of drug and metabolite.

B. Biguanide Drugs [61-65]

In 1972, Wickramasinghe and Shaw [61] studied the GC behavior of several biguanides: buformin, phenformin, and phenylbiguanide (the latter compound used as an internal standard).

The GC instrumentation used for this investigation was a F&M model 402 gas chromatograph equipped with a flame ionization detector and a 70-cm

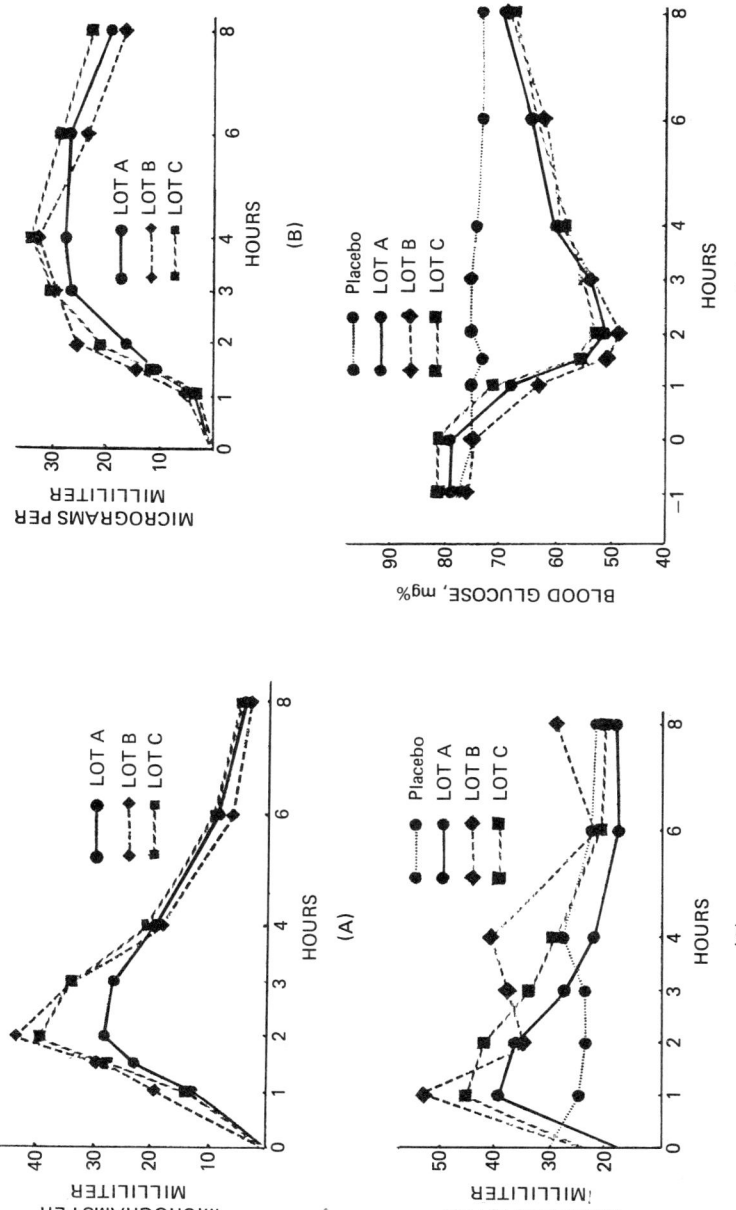

Figure 2.29. Comparison of analytical data after administration of 750 mg of acetohexamide to eight subjects; A, mean plasma concentrations of acetohexamide; B, mean plasma levels of hydroxyhexamide; C, mean insulin levels in serum; D, mean blood glucose responses. Adapted from Kleber et al. [52], courtesy of the Journal of Pharmaceutical Sciences.

Phenylbiguanide: phenyl–NHC(=NH)NHC(=NH)NH₂

by 3-mm-i.d. U-shaped glass colum packed with 0.5% Carbowax 20M on 80-100 mesh glass beads. To obtain retention times of 1.1 and 2.4 min for buformin and phenylbiguanide, respectively, the following operating conditions were maintained: helium carrier-gas flow rate, 80 ml/min; injector temperature, 276°C; column temperature, 225°C; detector temperature, 235°C. Capable of detecting 0.1 µg of buformin hydrochloride "on column," quantitative results were obtained with a calibration curve prepared by plotting the peak height ratios calculated by dividing the buformin peak height (2.4 min) by that of the phenylbiguanide (1.1 min) versus the buformin concentration.

GC-MS studies were performed with a LKB 9000 integrated instrument equipped with a 70-cm by 3-mm-i.d. U-shaped glass column packed with 0.5% Carbowax 20M on 80-100 mesh glass beads; the other operating parameters were injector temperature, about 250°C; column temperature, 230°C; helium carrier-gas flow rate, about 45 ml/min (Note: no MS parameters given in the text).

With the GC-MS instrument, several interesting discoveries were noted when mass spectra of the GC peaks due to buformin, phenylbiguanide, and phenformin were examined, their findings were summarized as follows:

1. Buformin: The mass spectrum of its single GC peak showed prominent m/e ions at 238, 223, 209, 196, 195, 182, 153, 140, 139, and 126; this being totally unexpected in view of the fact that the molecular weight of buformin is 157. Subsequent studies of the 2.2-min peak attributed to buformin revealed that the GC peak consisted of two buformin pyrolytic products which were isolated and identified

2,4-Di-(n-butylamino)-6-amino-1,3,5-triazine

2-n-Butylamino-4,6-diamino-1,3,5-triazine

as 2,4-di-(n-butylamino)-6-amino-1,3,5-triazine and 2-n-butyl-4,6-diamino-1,3,5-triazine. The mass spectrum of 2,4-di-(n-butylamino)-6-amino-1,3,5-trizine showed a molecular ion at m/e 238 and other prominent peaks at 223 (M-15), 209 (M-29), 195 (M-43), 182 (M-52), 167 (M-71), 153 (M-85), 139 (M-99), 126 (M-112), 111 (M-127), 97 (M-141), 85 (M-153), 76 (M-162), 72 (M-166), and 68 (M-170). On the other hand, the 2-n-butyl-4,6-diamino-1,3,5-triazine product yielded a molecular ion at m/e 182 as well as prominent m/e ions at 167 (M-15), 153 (M-29), 139 (M-43), 126 (M-56), 111 (M-127), 97 (M-85), 85 (M-97), and 68 (M-114).

2. Phenylbiguanide: When phenylbiguanide was chromatographed, two peaks were observed; the first, with a retention time of about 1 min, had a molecular ion of m/e 135 and was judged to be phenylguanidine, whereas the second peak, eluting in approximately 18 min, showed a molecular ion at m/e 201 which indicated that its tructure might be 2-phenylamino-4,6-diamino-1,3,5-triazine. These structures are illustrated below:

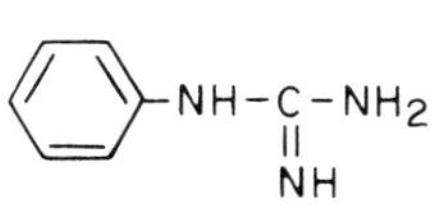

Phenylguanidine

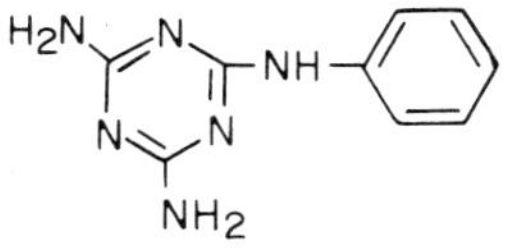

2-Phenylamino-4,6-diamino-1,3,5-triazine

3. Phenformin: When phenformin was chromatographed, the mass spectrum of its single GC peak (retention time about 22 min) showed a molecular ion at m/e 230 and several other prominent m/e ions; 139 (M-91), 110 (M-120), 91 (M-139), 68 (M-162). Its structure was postulated to be 2-(β-phenethylamino)-4,6-diamino-1,3,5-triazine.

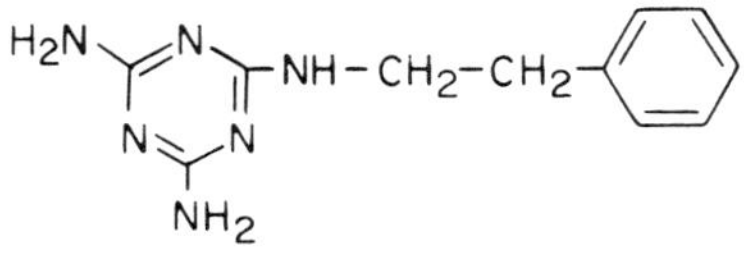

2-(β-Phenethylamino)-4,6-diamino-1,3,5-triazine

When applied to the determination of buformin in biological specimens, the utility of the GC method could not be demonstrated because the procedure was insensitive at the low concentrations of buformin being considered. However, the method could be conveniently adapted for the determination of the drug in pharmaceutical preparations.

Matin et al. [62] described a general GC method for the quantitation of biguanides using electron-capture detection. The method is based on the cyclization of biguanides (phenformin, buformin, and metformin) to the corresponding 2-substituted 4-monochlorodifluoromethyl-2,6-diamino-1,3,5-s-triazine when acylated with monochlorodifluoroacetic anhydride.

The acetylation reaction of biguanides with monochlorodifluoroacetic anhydride to form 2,6-disubstituted-4-monochlorodifluoromethyl-1,3,5-triazines is illustrated below.

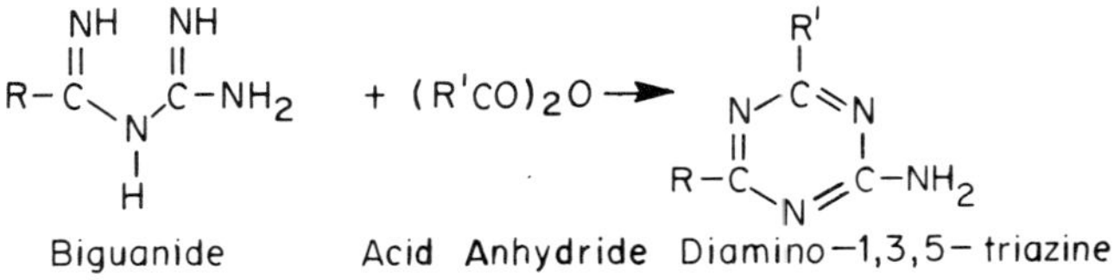

```
         NH   NH                                    R'
         ||   ||                                    |
     R-C     C-NH2   + (R'CO)2O  →          N     C     N
         \ N /                                ||         |
           |                               R-C         C-NH2
           H                                   \ N /
      Biguanide         Acid Anhydride    Diamino-1,3,5-triazine
```

where R = ⟨phenyl⟩-CH$_2$CH$_2$NH- (phenformin), H$_9$C$_4$NH- (buformin),

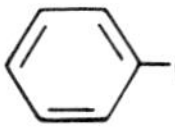

(H$_3$C)-N-(metformin), H$_7$C$_3$NH- (propylbiguanide), or ⟨phenyl⟩-CH$_2$NH-

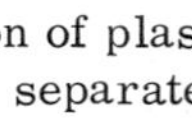

(benzylbiguanide) and R' = ClF$_2$C-.

The method employed by Matin et al. involves "the addition of the appropriate internal standards, benzylbiguanide for phenformin and propylbiguanide for buformin and metformin, and precipitation of plasma proteins by trichloroacetic acid in 1 N HCl. The supernatant is separated, made alkaline with 10 N NaOH, and the compounds are extracted into 10 ml of CH$_2$Cl$_2$. In the case of metformin, the alkaline layer is saturated with sodium chloride (0.5 g) before extraction with CH$_2$Cl$_2$. Monochlorodifluoroacetic anhydride is added to the CH$_2$Cl$_2$ fraction and the tubes are placed in a water bath at 50°C. When the evaporation of CH$_2$Cl$_2$ is complete, the excess anhydride is destroyed by adding 1 N NaOH and the cyclized product is extracted into 50 μl of pentyl acetate and 1 to 2 μl are injected into the gas chromatograph."

For this investigation, the chromatographic separations were performed with a Varian model 1200 gas chromatograph equipped with a ^{63}Ni electron-capture detector and a 2.12-m by 0.3-cm glass column packed with 3% OV-17 on 100-120 mesh Chromosorb W-HP (acid-washed and DMCS-treated). With the specified GC conditions maintained (injector temperature, 250°C; column temperatures, 210, 165 and 180°C for phenformin, metformin, and buformin, respectively; detector temperature, 310°C; mixed carrier-gas (5% CH_4 in argon) flow rate, 30 ml/min), the retention times of the 2,6-disubstituted-4-monochlorodifluoromethyl-1,3,5-triazines were as follows:

1. At 210°C: benzylbiguanide, 4.4 min; phenformin, 5.6 min

2. At 165°C: metformin, 3.7 min; propylbiguanide, 5.3 min

3. At 180°C: propylbiguanide, 2.7 min; buformin, 5.3 min

Using the GC method for quantitative analysis, it was reported that the calibration curves for all three drugs were linear between the range of 0 to 100 ng/ml of biological fluid, the lower limit of detection was less than 1 ng/ml of plasma, and the recovery using ^{14}C-labeled phenformin was approximately 97% when two 10-ml CH_2Cl_2 extractions were performed.

Confirmation of the structure of the eluted peaks was obtained by subjecting the processed samples to analysis by integrated GC-MS. This phase of their study was carried out with an AEI/MS-12 gas chromatograph-mass spectrometer equipped with a 2.12-m by 0.31-cm glass column packed with 3% OV-1 on 100-120 mesh, acid-washed, DMCS-treated Chromosorb W-HP. The operating temperature of the ion source was 250°C, whereas the trap current and the electron energy were 500 μA and 70 eV, respectively. Figure 2.30 shows the mass spectra obtained by GC-MS of phenformin (A), buformin (B), and metformin (C) after extraction from plasma and derivatization.

As noted by Matin et al.:

To show the clinical usefulness of the developed method, a diabetic patient was administered a therapeutic dose of 100 mg sustained release preparation of phenformin orally. The plasma levels achieved are shown in Figure [2.31]. The curve shows that it took 2 to 3 hr to achieve the peak plasma level of 150 ng/ml. Plasma concentrations then declined with an initial half-life of 4.5 hr (i.e., rate constant = 0.15) followed by a terminal half-life of 13 hr (rate constant = 0.05 hr). The urinary excretion rate plot for the same patient is shown in Figure [2.32]. The cumulative excretion of unchanged phenformin at 36 hr was 48% of the dose and excretion into urine could be detected up to 60 hr after the administration of the dose.

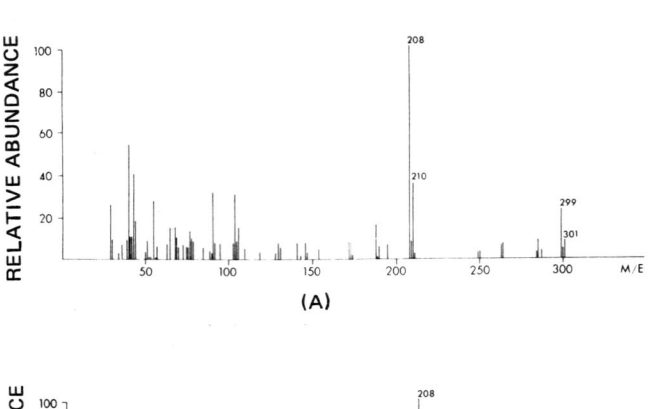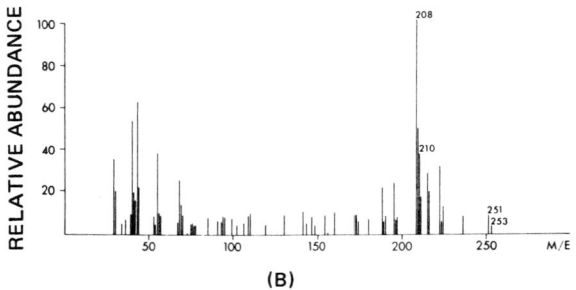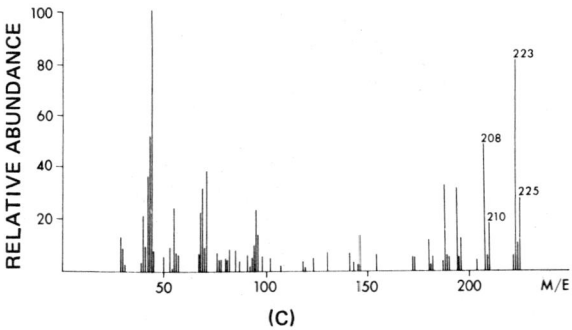

Figure 2.30. Mass spectra of phenformin (A), buformin (B), and metformin (C) after extraction and derivatization. Adapted from Matin et al. [62], courtesy of Analytical Chemistry.

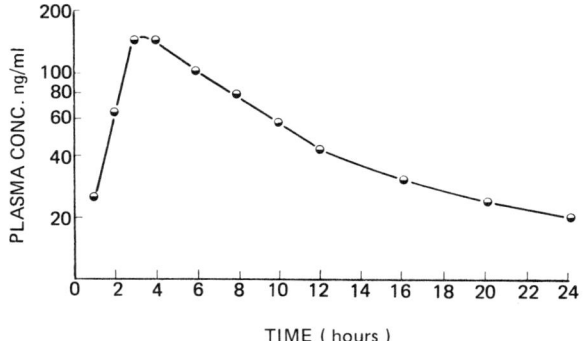

Figure 2.31. Plasma level-time profile of phenformin in a diabetic patient after the oral administration of a single 100-mg sustained release dose of phenformin. From Matin et al. [62], courtesy of Analytical Chemistry.

Mottale and Stewart [63] presented a GC method in 1975 for the detection of β-phenethylbiguanide (phenformin) and its p-hydroxy urinary metabolite. Sample preparation for subsequent GC analysis consisted of the following:

Serum preparation: A solution containing 20 μl of 0.5 N acetic acid and 2 ml of absolute ethanol was added to 0.2 ml of serum in a 12-ml

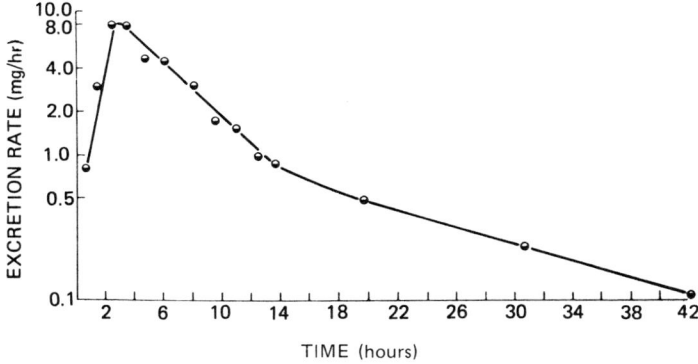

Figure 2.32. Urinary excretion rate-time profile of phenformin observed in the patient whose plasma levels are shown in Figure 2.31. From Matin et al. [62], courtesy of Analytical Chemistry.

conical centrifuge tube. The mixture was shaken with a vortex mixer for 5 min to ensure extraction of phenformin or possible metabolites, centrifuged for 10 min at 400 g, and the precipitated material discarded. The supernatant solution was collected in a clean conical centrifuge tube and taken to dryness in vacuo, at 30°C. Standard naphthylamine solution (50 µl prepared by dissolving 2.0 mg/ml of naphthylamine in absolute ethanol) was then added and the contents of the tube were again taken to complete dryness on the Buchler Rotary Evapo-mix. Trifluoroacetic anhydride (100 µl) was added to the dried residue. The centrifuge tube was covered with parafilm and then shaken with a vortex mixer for approximately 5 sec. The excess reagent was evaporated under vacuum. The residue was dissolved in 100 µl of anhydrous acetone; 1 µl of this solution was then analyzed for the presence of phenformin or its p-hydroxy metabolite by GC.

Urine preparation: Urine, 0.2 ml, was pipetted into a conical centrifuge tube and taken to dryness in vacuo at 30°C. Standard naphthylamine solution, 50 µl, was added and the drying step repeated. Ethanol, 2 ml, was added and the procedure continued as described for the serum preparation.

p−Hydroxy Metabolite of Phenformin

The products resulting from the TFA reaction, 2-amino-4-trifluoromethyl-6-(2-phenethyl)-amino-1,3,5-triazine (structure A) and the trifluoroacetyl ester of p-hydroxyphenformin (structure B), were analyzed with a Beckman model 45 gas chromatograph equipped with a dual flame ionization detector and a 6-ft by 1/8-in.-o.d. U-shaped stainless steel column packed with 10% SE-30 coated on 80-100 mesh Chromosorb W-HT. The retention times reported for naphthylamine, the triazine derivative of phenformin, and the TFA ester of p-hydroxyphenformin were 1.00, 4.83, and 7.83 min, respectively. These values were obtained using the

Structure A   Structure B

following GC settings: injector temperature, 275°C; column temperature, 208°C; detector temperature, 280°C; detector line, 300°C; helium carrier-gas flow rate, 25 ml/min; hydrogen flow rate, 40 ml/min; air flow rate, 290 ml/min.

Using calibration curves prepared by plotting the ratio of the peak area of phenformin or its metabolite to the peak height of naphthylamine (internal standard) versus concentration (phenformin or p-hydroxyphenformin), the practical limit of sensitivity for the method as described was about 0.2 μg for phenformin and 0.5 μg for its metabolite per milliliter of serum or urine.

Mottale and Stewart noted that "a time course study of blood concentration and elimination rate following intraperitoneal injection of 100 mg/kg of phenformin to normal rats was performed. Phenformin was found to be present in the blood and urine, p-hydroxyphenformin was only detected in the urine. Twenty-four hours following intraperitoneal injection, the urine contained 32% of the administered dose, 20% as unaltered phenformin and 12% as p-hydroxyphenformin."

In 1975, Alkalay et al. [65] obtained information about the pharmacokinetics of phenformin in two adult male volunteers based on the conversion of the biguanide into a s-triazine which then could be assayed by means of gas chromatography or mass fragmentography [64]. Cumulative excretion of phenformin in urine, following oral administration of four 25-mg tablets to each of two human subjects, showed that most of the drug elimination occurs during the first 24 hr, as illustrated in Figure 2.33, which also includes time profiles for urinary excretion rates and for plasma and saliva concentrations of phenformin for the same volunteer. As indicated, the terminal exponential declines in all three curves suggest a drug half-life of approximately 11 hr, whereas the β phase in the urinary profile requires about 1 day before becoming apparent. Using the equilibrium dialysis method at 37°C to assess drug binding to plasma proteins by keeping the drug concentration in plasma at about 130 ng/ml, Alkalay et al. reported drug binding values amounting to 18.7 ± 0.7% of added phenformin.

In 1976, Alkalay et al. [64] prepared substituted s-triazines by the treatment of biguanides with various organic acid anhydrides, which permitted the ready conversion of the hypoglycemic drugs phenformin, buformin, and metformin, and of other analogous biguanides, into compounds suitable for GC and mass fragmentographic determination with a high degree of sensitivity. As reported by these investigators, two acylation methods were employed for the conversion of biguanides into substituted s-triazines:

Method A: Aqueous solutions of biguanide salts were made strongly alkaline with 10 N KOH and extracted with methylene chloride. Solvent evaporation gave the free bases. To 250-mg amounts of these bases, placed in 40-ml test tubes equipped with screw caps (lined

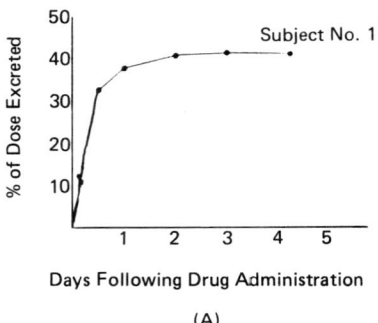

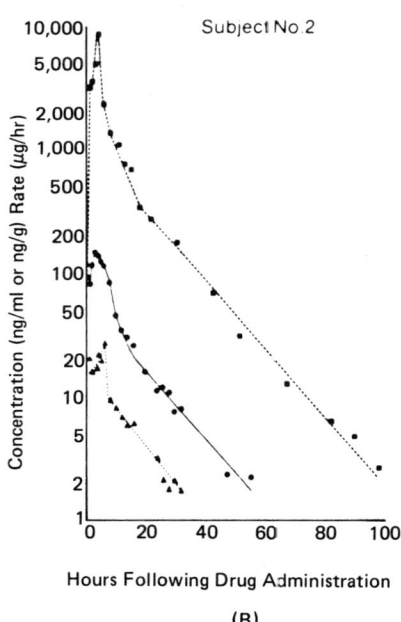

Figure 2.33. (A) Cumulative excretion of phenformin in urine, following oral administration of four 25-mg phenformin tablets. (B) Time profiles for urinary excretion rates and for plasma and saliva concentrations of phenformin in the same subject after drug administration. (■–■), urinary excretion (µg/ml); (●–●), plasma concentration (ng/ml); (▲–▲), saliva concentration (ng/ml). Adapted from Alkalay et al. [65].

with Teflon), was added 15 ml of a 3% solution of the appropriate organic acid anhydride (chlorodifluoroacetic anhydride, dichlorofluoroacetic anhydride, heptafluorobutyric anhydride, pentafluoropropionic anhydride or trifluoroacetic anhydride) in methylene chloride. The stoppered test tubes were heated at 50°C for 10 min. After cooling, each sample was washed with 3 ml of 2 N NaOH. The organic phase was dried over anhydrous magnesium sulfate, filtered, and evaporated to dryness. The residues were recrystallized from solvent mixtures of ether and n-hexane.

Method B: One gram of biguanide salt and 1 ml of triethylamine were placed in a 5-ml acylation tube and cooled to approximately -40°C. Four milliliters of the appropriate organic acid anhydride was added to the mixture, and the tube was promptly sealed. Following the exothermic reaction, the tube was heated at 130°C for 30 min. After cooling, the reaction mixture was partitioned between 25 ml of cold water and 100 ml of ether. The organic extract was washed consecutively with 1 N KOH, 1 N HCl, and water. It was dried over anhydrous magnesium sulfate, filtered, and evaporated to dryness. The residue was recrystallized from an ether and n-hexane solvent mixture.

The substituted s-triazines formed with phenformin, buformin, and metformin and other biguanides selected for use as possible internal standards [amformin, 1-ethyl-1-phenethylbiguanide, 1-(p-methoxyphenethyl)biguanide, d-1(α-methylphenethyl)biguanide, and 1-(p-methylphenethyl)biguanide] were reacted with the organic acid anhydrides listed above) and were examined chromatographically using gas chromatographs equipped with flame ionization detectors and electron capture (^{63}Ni or Sc^{3}H foils) detectors and 6-ft by 2-mm-i.d. glass columns packed with 3% OV-1 or OV-17 on 80-100 mesh Chromosorb W-HP. The determination of Kovats retention indices for these products (see Table 2.15) were obtained using the following GC conditions: injector temperature, 250°C; column temperature, 210°C; detector temperature, 280°C; argon carrier-gas flow rate, 35 ml/min. Also included in Table 2.15 are mass spectral data for these substituted s-triazines.

III. THYROID HORMONES AND DRUGS

As early as 1966, the accurate determination of thyroid hormones in biomedical as well as pharmaceutical investigations was of such great importance that over the ensuing years many excellent GC and GC-MS procedures were developed [66-86] for the analysis of the parent compounds and their precursors or metabolites illustrated in Figure 2.34. To make them amenable to GC or GC-MS analysis, several derivatization procedures were proposed which will be discussed in this section. The biosynthesis of the thyroid hormones (iodinated derivatives of thyronine) involves essentially five principal steps: (1) the active uptake and concentration of inorganic iodide in the thyroid, (2) the iodination of tyrosine residues in thyroglobin, (3) the coupling of two appropriate iodotyrosine molecules to form thyroxine or triiodotyrosine, (4) the cleavage of thyroxine from thyroglobin and, finally, (5) the removal of iodide from the iodotyrosines for subsequent synthesis by the gland [87].

As noted by Searcy [87]:

One of the most striking properties of thyroid hormones is their effect on metabolic rate. They also play an important role in temperature regulation by controlling heat production. The lipid-lowering properties have been well established, particularly with respect to cholesterol metabolism. Although changes in carbohydrate metabolism are vague, hyperthyroid patients usually exhibit diabetic-like glucose tolerances. Widespread protein catabolism is associated with an overabundance of thyroid hormone, but this is brought about indirectly by the simultaneous secretion of pituitary somatotropin and cortical glucocorticoids. Thyroid secretion may, however, regulate the formation and destruction rate of certain plasma proteins.

Thyroid hormones govern the responsiveness to sympathetic stimulation and support adult brain function. This accounts for the dull mental reactions noted in many myxedema patients. Water and electrolyte balance appears to be responsive to thyroid activity, since a defect in function is characterized by the accumulation of subcutaneous body fluid. The hydrodynamic effects are probably not entirely direct, but are secondary to changes in cardiac and renal functions. Thyroid hormone apparently affects calcium and phosphorous homeostasis by affecting osteoclasts.

The influence of thyroid activity on liver function is evidenced by the impairment in the hepatic conversion of carotene to vitamin A associated with myxedema. This accounts for apparent jaundice exhibited by some patients that actually stems from hypercarotenemia. Thyroid hormone has also been implicated in hematopoiesis and the maintenance of bone marrow.

Latest GC and/or GC-MS literature references for the analysis of thyroid hormones and precursors/metabolites shown in Figure 2.34 are listed in Table 2.16.

A. Derivatization of Thyroid Hormones and Precursors

Depending on the investigator(s), thyroid hormones and precursors/metabolites have been determined by GC or GC-MS using several types of derivatives; namely, (1) methyl/methoxy, (2) methyl/ditrifluoroacetyl, (3) methyl/diheptafluorobutyryl, (4) methyl/dipivalyl, and (5) trimethylsilyl.

1. Methyl Ester/Methoxy Derivative

In 1971, Zimmerer and Grady [66] developed a GC method for the assay of sodium thyroxine in which sample preparation consisted of the following:

> Weigh 8 mg of undried d- or l-thyroxine into a narrow tube (small centrifuge tube or screw-cap vial) and add 0.1 ml of dimethyl sulfoxide containing aqueous HCl, 5% by volume. Solution is rapid. Add 1.0 ml of chromatographic-grade methylene chloride containing 1.00 mg of estradiol benzoate, NF reference standard as the assay internal standard. At this point, fine droplets may appear which consist of sodium chloride and any water present. In a hood, add 1.0 ml of diazomethane reagent, about 0.6 M in 2:1 ether-methylene chloride prepared by distillation of ethereal diazomethane into methylene chloride. Mix and allow to stand for 30 min using a polyethylene stopper. Uncover and evaporate the solution to a volume of about 0.2 ml in a stream of nitrogen. The tube may be placed in warm water to speed the evaporation. Add 1 ml of methylene chloride and mix. A clear, colorless solution is obtained, containing a fine precipitate of salt.

From the above solution, 1.5 µl or about 12 µg of derivative are withdrawn and injected on-column into a gas chromatograph (model not specified) equipped with a 0.6-m by 4-mm-i.d. glass column packed with 3% OV-1 coated on acid-washed, silanized, 80-100 mesh Gas Chrom Q and a flame ionization detector. Using the specified conditions (injector temperature, 260°C; column temperature, 250°C; detector temperature, 260°C; helium carrier-gas flow rate, 80 ml/min), the retention times relative to that of estradiol benzoate of the pair of methylated peaks obtained for T_4 were 1.82 and 2.07 with quantitative data derived from peak area measurements.

TABLE 2.15

GC and Mass Spectral Data for Substituted s-Triazines Derived from Biguanides[a]

Name	Method
2-Amino-4-phenethylamino-6-trifluoromethyl-s-triazine	B
2-Amino-4-pentafluoroethyl-6-phenethylamino-s-triazine	A
2-Amino-4-heptafluoropropyl-6-phenethylamino-s-triazine	A
2-Amino-4-chlorodifluoromethyl-6-phenethylamino-s-triazine	A
2-Amino-4-dichlorofluoromethyl-6-phenethylamino-s-triazine	A
2-Amino-4-(p-methylphenethyl)amino-6-trifluoromethyl-s-triazine	A
2-Amino-4-(p-methylphenethyl)amino-6-pentafluoroethyl-s-triazine	A
2-Amino-4-heptafluoropropyl-6-(p-methylphenethyl)amino-s-triazine	A
2-Amino-4-chlorodifluoromethyl-6-(p-methylphenethyl)amino-s-triazine	A
2-Amino-4-(p-methoxyphenethyl)amino-6-trifluoromethyl-s-triazine	B
2-Amino-4-(α-methylphenethyl)amino-6-trifluoromethyl-s-triazine	A
2-Amino-4-(α-methylphenethyl)amino-6-pentafluoroethyl-s-triazine	A
2-Amino-4-heptafluoropropyl-6-(α-methylphenethyl)amino-s-triazine	A
2-Amino-4-chlorodifluoromethyl-6-(α-methylphenethyl)amino-s-triazine	A
2-Amino-4-(N-ethyl-N-phenethyl)amino-6-trifluoromethyl-s-triazine	B
2-Amino-4-(N-ethyl-N-phenethyl)amino-6-pentafluoroethyl-s-triazine	A
2-Amino-4-(N-ethyl-N-phenethyl)amino-6-heptafluoropropyl-s-triazine	A
2-Amino-4-chlorodifluoromethyl-6-(N-ethyl-N-phenethyl)amino-s-triazine	A
2-Amino-4-butylamino-6-trifluoromethyl-s-triazine	B
2-Amino-4-butylamino-6-pentafluoroethyl-s-triazine	A
2-Amino-4-butylamino-6-heptafluoropropyl-s-triazine	A
2-Amino-4-butylamino-6-chlorodifluoromethyl-s-triazine	A
2-Amino-4-pentylamino-6-trifluoromethyl-s-triazine	B
2-Amino-4-pentafluoroethyl-6-pentylamino-s-triazine	A
2-Amino-4-heptafluoropropyl-6-pentylamino-s-triazine	A
2-Amino-4-chlorodifluoromethyl-6-pentylamino-s-triazine	A
2-Amino-4-dimethylamino-6-trifluoromethyl-s-triazine	B

[a] Adapted from Alkalay et al. [64], courtesy of the Journal of Pharmaceutical Sciences.
[b] The mass spectral data were obtained on an AEI model MS 902 magnetic instrument at 70 eV.
[c] The relative intensity of each ion is shown in parentheses as percent of base peak value.

Kovats indices		Molecular ions[b]		Most abundant ions[b] m/e > 60				
3% OV-1	3% OV-17							
2008	2430	283	(30)[c]	192 (100)	91 (38)	104 (38)	193 (20)	
1989	2360	333	(27)	242 (100)	91 (35)	104 (27)	243 (9)	
2007	2339	383	(32)	292 (100)	91 (41)	104 (27)	293 (10)	
2209	2667	299	(31)	208 (100)	91 (40)	210 (33)	104 (28)	
2359	2881	315	(32)	244 (100)	226 (65)	91 (34)	104 (34)	317 (21)
2118	2518	297	(40)	118 (100)	192 (70)	105 (29)	180 (19)	117 (18)	119 (11)
2097	2448	347	(33)	118 (100)	242 (71)	105 (31)	230 (18)	119 (16)	117 (9)
2112	2425	397	(27)	118 (100)	292 (47)	105 (30)	117 (18)	119 (15)	280 (14)
2295	2741	313	(20)	118 (100)	208 (49)	105 (34)	117 (22)	196 (17)	210 (16)
2243	2715	313	(7)	134 (100)	121 (50)	192 (11)	135 (10)	
1988	2386	297	(3)	206 (100)	91 (24)	207 (10)	138 (8)	
1972	2312	347	(5)	256 (100)	69 (13)	275 (11)	91 (10)	
1995	2318	397	(7)	306 (100)	69 (18)	91 (13)	307 (12)	
2171	2601	313	(2)	222 (100)	224 (31)	91 (17)	223 (9)	
2014	2365	311	(25)	220 (100)	192 (50)	221 (16)	91 (11)	
2025	2305	361	(16)	270 (100)	242 (40)	271 (13)	91 (8)	
2037	2276	411	(17)	320 (100)	292 (31)	91 (17)	321 (13)	
2212	2583	327	(14)	236 (100)	238 (34)	208 (23)	91 (18)	237 (10)
1590	1871	235	(32)	192 (100)	193 (41)	206 (21)	179 (21)	138 (9)
1575	1824	285	(30)	242 (100)	243 (52)	256 (40)	229 (22)	188 (11)
1590	1803	335	(33)	292 (100)	293 (46)	306 (32)	279 (18)	316 (11)
1757	2047	251	(26)	208 (100)	209 (55)	210 (36)	222 (32)	195 (28)	216 (18)
1672	1960	249	(31)	192 (100)	193 (43)	206 (22)	179 (18)	220 (14)	138 (9)
1672	1915	299	(34)	242 (100)	243 (50)	256 (30)	270 (19)	229 (17)	280 (10)
1686	1894	349	(35)	292 (100)	293 (56)	306 (38)	320 (21)	279 (19)	330 (11)
1850	2150	265	(27)	208 (100)	209 (60)	210 (35)	222 (32)	195 (23)	236 (21)
1378	1628	207 (100)		192 (73)	178 (20)	188 (13)		

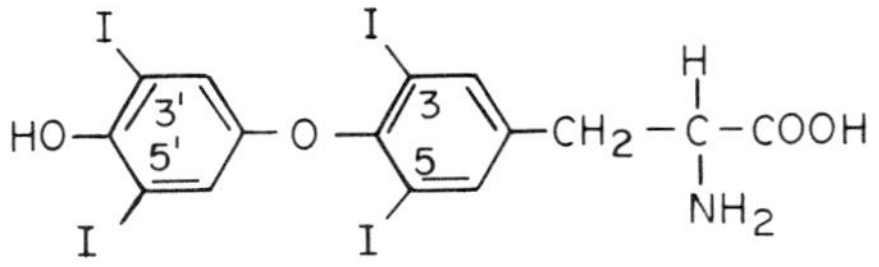

Thyroxine (T_4)
($3,3',5,5'$ – Tetraiodothyronine)

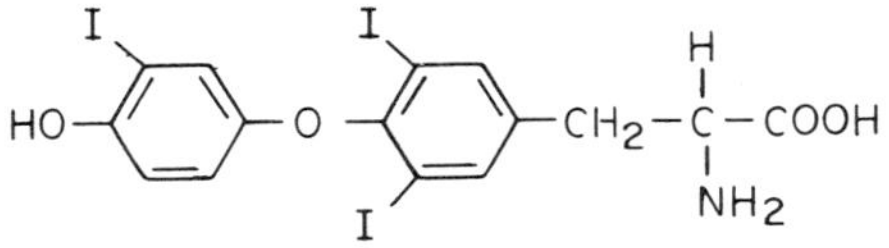

$3,3',5$–Triiodothyronine (T_3 or $3,3',5-T_3$)

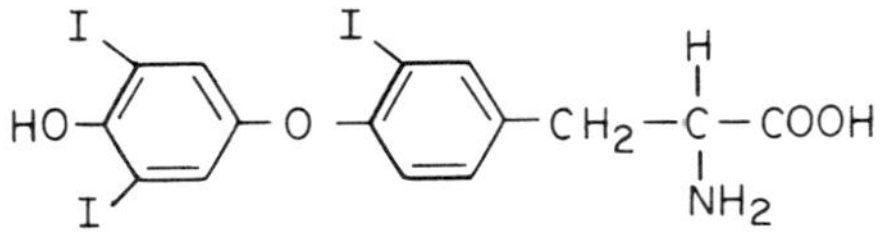

$3,3',5'$–Triiodothyronine ($3,3',5'-T_3$ or reverse T_3)

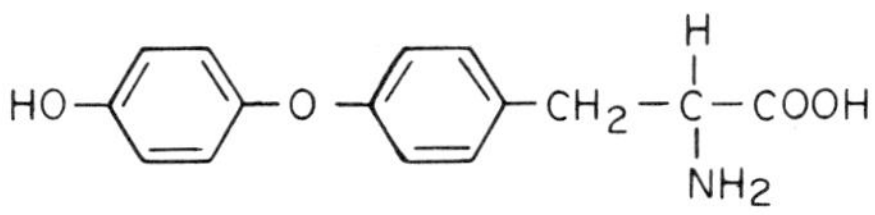

Thyronine (T_1)

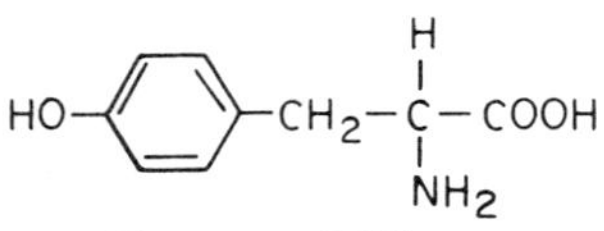

Tyrosine (TY)

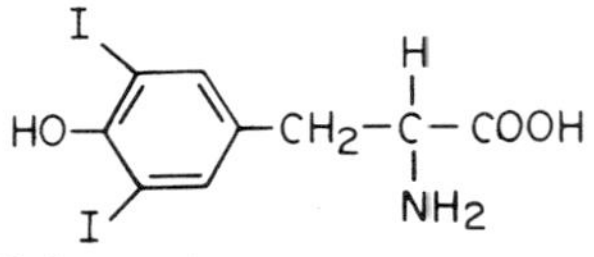

3,5-Diiodotyrosine
(3,5–DITY)

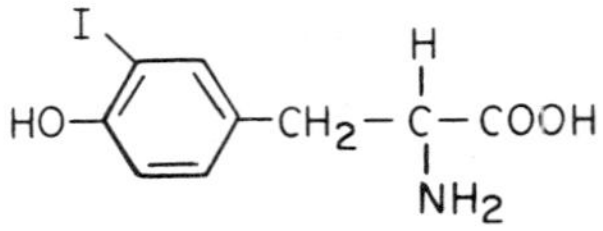

3–Iodotyrosine
(3–MITY)

Figure 2.34. Thyroid hormones and precursors/metabolites.

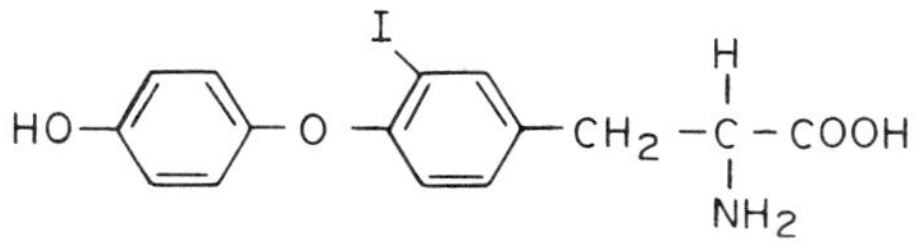

3-Monoiodothyronine (3-T_1)

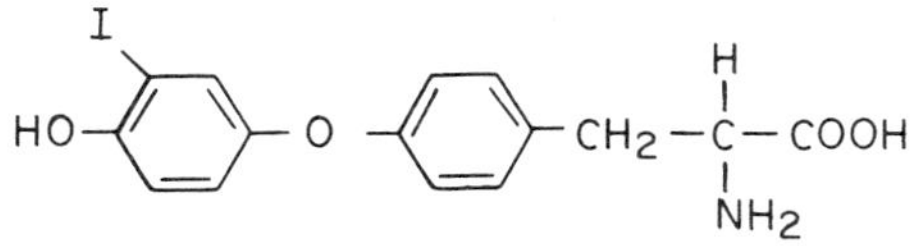

3'-Monoiodothyronine (3'-T_1)

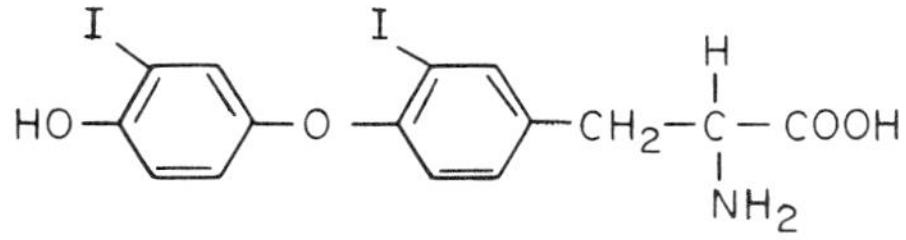

3,3'-Diiodothyronine (3,3'-T_2)

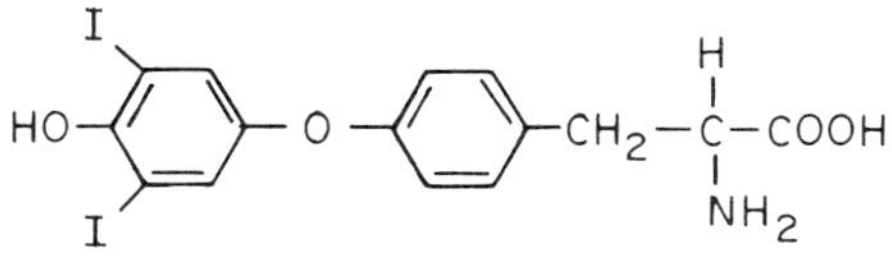

3',5'-Diiodothyronine (3',5'-T_2)

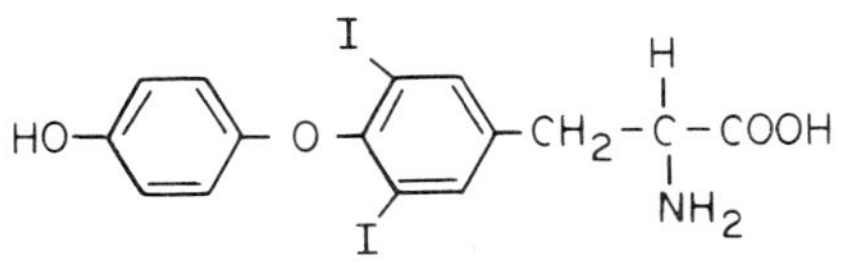

3,5-Diiodothyronine (3,5-T_2)

Figure 2.34. (continued)

TABLE 2.16

Literature References for GC and/or GC-MS Analysis of Thyroid Hormones and Their Precursors/Metabolites

Compound	References
Thyroxine (T_4)	66-72, 75-82
3,3',5-Triiodothyronine (T_3)	66-72, 75-83, 85, 86
3,3',5'-Triiodothyronine (3,3',5'-T_3 or reverse T_3)	68-70, 77, 83, 85, 86
Thyronine (T_1)	75, 80, 83, 85
Tyrosine (TY)	71, 75, 79, 80, 82, 83
3,5-Diiodotyrosine (3,5-DITY)	66, 67, 71, 72, 75, 79-83
3-Iodotyrosine (3-MITY)	67, 71, 72, 75, 80-83
3-Monoiodothyronine (3-T_1)	83, 85
3'-Monoiodothyronine (3'-T_1)	85
3,3'-Diiodothyronine (3,3'-T_2)	66, 83, 85
3',5'-Diiodothyronine (3',5'-T_2)	66, 85
3,5-Diiodothyronine (3,5-T_2)	66-69, 75, 76, 79, 82, 83, 85

With regard to the chromatographic characteristics of compounds investigated by Zimmerer and Grady, they noted that:

> For chromatographic purity, an internal standard is not added and suitable changes in electrometer attenuation are made to allow calculations of area percent of all peaks. Liothyronine (T_3) elutes as a pair of peaks at relative retention of 0.82 and 0.93; diiodothyronine occurs at 0.48; diiodotyrosine elutes too rapidly, 0.07, for accurate quantitation in this isothermal system, so that where this substance is important, temperature programming is necessary. The latter peak of T_3 predominates with longer reaction times and is the only peak after 5 hr. Slower methylation of the T_3 phenol compared to

T_4 is consistent with the lesser acidity, i.e., pK_a 8.4 compared to pK_a 6.6 [88]. Tetraiodothyroacetic acid gives a peak at relative retention time 1.02, but this offers no advantage as an internal standard, other than reaction control, over the steroid ester which is available in a controlled form.

Methylation of T_4 leads to a major peak, which is 93% of the total area, and one less mobile peak. The major peak exhibits no tailing and a symmetry of 0.93 due to the presence of another minor, but more mobile, methylated T_4 species. Initial NMR observations on the analogous diiodotyrosine suggest complete methylation of both phenolic and acid hydroxyls with possible methylation of the amine. Removal of excess diazomethane prior to injection is necessary to prevent side-product formation.

On the other hand, it was reported that alternative liquid phases were studied: OV-61 and OV-17, which consist of 2:1 and 1:1, respectively, methyl-phenyl radicals in the polysiloxane. These gave much greater resolution but required much greater temperatures and carrier flow, whereas a 1% OV-1 column showed distinct overload effects with samples in excess of 5 µg of thyroxine but allowed the detection of less than 50-ng samples using flame ionization.

2. Methyl Ester/Trifluoroacetyl Derivative

In 1966, Richards and Mason [67] developed a GC procedure for the separation of some iodinated-compounds present in serum; namely, 3-iodotyrosine (3-MITY), 3,5-diiodotyrosine (3,5-DITY), 3,5-diiodothyronine (3,5-T_2), 3,3',5-triiodothyronine (T_3), and 3,3',5,5'-tetraiodothyronine (T_4), which were converted to N,O-bistrifluoroacetyl methyl ester derivatives using a modified procedure employed for amino acids [89].

Sample preparation for subsequent GC analysis consisted of the following: Suspensions containing 10 µmoles of each of the compounds cited above in 10 ml of anhydrous methanol were treated with dry HCl gas for several minutes to ensure saturation. Each solution was then stirred for 30 min and taken to dryness under reduced pressure. After storing under vacuum with sodium hydroxide and phosphorus pentoxide for 2 hr, each residue was redissolved in 1 ml of trifluoroacetic anhydride, 0.9 ml of dichloromethane, and 0.1 ml of dimethylformamide. After stirring for 30 min, 1- to 3-µl aliquots were withdrawn and injected into a F&M model 402 gas chromatograph equipped with a flame ionization detector and a 4-ft glass column packed with 3.8% SE-30 coated on 80-100 mesh Diatoport S.

To obtain retention times for the methyl ester/trifluoroacetyl derivatives of 3-MITY, 3,5-DITY, $3,5-T_2$, T_3, and T_4 of 0.50, 1.23, 7.93, 18.52, and 42.00 min, respectively, the GC operating parameters were maintained as follows: injector temperature, 270°C; column temperature, 250°C; detector temperature, 250°C; helium carrier-gas flow rate, 75 ml/min.

Richards and Mason indicated that "further work is in progress to increase sensitivity by utilizing an electron-capture detection system and to apply this technique to the analysis of biologic materials. The potential sensitivity utilizing such a detector is appreciably greater than is achieved with the ceric-arsenite color reaction. Use of the electron-capture detector for determining thyroid hormones was first suggested by Lovelock [90]."

3. Methyl Ester/Heptafluorobutyryl Derivative

The analysis of thyroid hormones as their methyl ester/heptafluorobutyryl derivatives was reported by Petersen and his co-workers [68-70] using GC and GC-MS instrumentation.

In 1976, Petersen et al. [68] developed a methodology involving equilibrium dialysis and gas chromatography to measure concurrently the concentration of the dialyzable (i.e., free) fractions of thyroxine (T_4) and 3,3',5-triiodothyronine ($3,3',5-T_3$), which provide the most indicative index of thyroid function [91].

To circumvent problems and constraints imposed by the large molecular weights of these hormones (about 1000), the lability of their iodine atoms, their tendency to adsorb onto solid surfaces, and their presence and availability in only trace amounts in serum (in the free form), the isolation of free from protein-bound hormone was approached effectively by means of equilibrium dialysis [92,93] followed by a cation-exchange resin cleanup of the dialysate [Bio-Rad cation-exchange resin AG 50W-X2 (H^+), 100-200 mesh]. Derivatization of the free thyroid hormones was as described below:

The eluent from the cation-exchange column containing the thyroid hormones was dried under a stream of nitrogen at 40°C for 20 min. To the residue was added 0.5 ml of the 25% (w/w) HCl-methanol solution, the vial was sealed with a PTFE septum and heated at 60°C for 1 hr in order to esterify the acids. After this time, the reaction mixture was allowed to reach room temperature before removing the septum. The esterifying solution was evaporated to dryness at 40°C with a stream of nitrogen for 15 min. Acetylation was accomplished by adding separately 50 µl of heptafluorobutyric anhydride and 200 µl of acetonitrile to the residue, mixing on a vortex for 3 min, and heating to 60°C for 30 min. After removing the acetylating solution under a stream of nitrogen at 40°C, the reaction vial was sealed with a Minienert cap. This cap was used so that aliquots could be added or removed without exposure of the sample to the atmosphere.

The residue in the vial was taken up in 20 µl of acetonitrile and mixed on a vortex for 5 min. Injections into the chromatograph were made by removal of aliquots from the solution via the septum port valve on the Minienert cap. Injection volumes were 5 µl.

In this investigation, Petersen et al. separated these methyl ester/ heptafluorobuyryl derivatives with a Hewlett-Packard model 5730A gas chromatograph equipped with a 15-mCi ^{63}Ni-plated electron-capture detector and a 6-ft by 4-mm-i.d. glass column packed with 3% SE-30 on 80-100 mesh Suplecoport. Using injector and column temperatures of 250°C, a detector temperature of 300°C, and a carrier gas of 5% methane-95% argon maintained at 60 ml/min, the retention times of the N,O-diheptafluorobutyryl/methyl ester derivatives of T_3 (3,3',5-T_3), reverse T_3 (3,3',5'-T_3), and T_4 were approximately 16.95, 24.60, and 34.70 min, respectively. Having a lower detection limit of about 0.2 pg, they noted that the recovery of T_3 and T_4 from the cation-exchange column was essentially quantitative when the column was pretreated with 15 pg of T_2 (diiodothyronine); added on the assumption that losses were due in part to adsorption on the polyethylene column, based on observations made by Lee and Pileggi [94]. Adsorption problems on the glassware were eliminated by silanization, which was conducted using a 4% (v/v) solution of trimethylchlorosilane in dry toluene for 10 min at room temperature.

Molecular weights of the derivatives were verified using a Nuclide 12-90-G single-focusing magnetic-deflection mass spectrometer operated as follows: accelerating potential, 3 kV; electron energy, 70 eV; ion source temperature. 250°C. From the mass spectra of the thyroid hormone derivatives, they noted that molecular ion peaks (M^+) were of high intensity, each compound possessed a base peak at m/e values corresponding to $(M-213)^+$, and significant fragment peaks (relative intensities greater than 40%) were observed at m/e values of $(M-284)^+$, $(M-410)^+$, and $(M-538)^+$.

In a subsequent paper, Petersen et al. [70] described a simultaneous, absolute analysis for free (dialyzable) T_3 and T_4 in serum by the sequence: dialysis, internal standard addition to the dialysate, cation-exchange chromatography, derivatization, and gas chromatography with electron-capture detection. The procedure sequence was essentially the same as given previously [68], with the following exceptions: (1) the GC column was packed with 3% OV-17 on 80-100 mesh Suplecoport; (2) the injector, column, and detector were isothermally held at 300, 277, and 300°C, respectively; (3) an internal standard (3,5-diiodo-3',5'-dibromothyronine) was synthesized as described [95] and added as a solution (e.g., 60 pg in 50 μl of phosphate buffer) to the dialysate immediately after completion of the dialysis; and (4) the dialysis membrane was prepared by soaking in six changes of water during an hour, just before use.

Using the modified GC conditions and column, the retention times for the methyl ester/heptafluorobutyryl derivatives of T_3, internal standard, reverse T_3, and T_4 were 11.43, 14.10, 16.50, and 27.70 min, respectively.

They summarized some of their findings as follows:

The detection limit is 0.2 pg and the precision (repeatability) in the range of 4 to 20 ng/liter is 1.6%. Mean values for free T_3 and T_4 in 29 euthyroid sera were 4.2 and 18.9 ng/liter, respectively, in close agreement with accepted values [96]. Correlation coefficients for the two compounds were 0.99 and 0.97, respectively, when this procedure was compared with a method involving tracer dialysis and radioimmunoassay. A chromatographic peak was seen for free 3,3',5'-triiodothyronine (reverse T_3) in the analyses of two of eight hyperthyroid sera, and, with a larger sample volume, from a euthyroid serum.

The mean values for total, dialyzable fraction, and free thyroid hormones in euthyroid and pathological sera are listed in Table 2.17.

In 1977, Petersen and Vouros [69] examined the mass spectra of the methyl ester/heptafluorobutyryl derivatives of several thyroid hormones and their analogs. They noted that ions of significant relative intensity dominate the high mass (m/e > 700 amu) and, in view of the decreased interference of background peaks at this high mass region, this feature has been effectively utilized in the GC-MS analysis of thse compounds by selective-ion monitoring. Operated in this mode, detection limits of 0.5 pg were achieved.

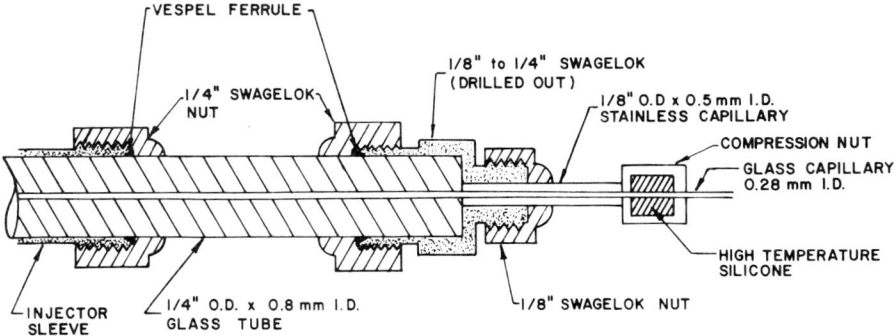

Figure 2.35. Schematic of capillary column connection to injection port of GC-MS system. From Petersen and Vouros [69], courtesy of Analytical Chemistry.

Whereas low-resolution mass spectra of the thyroid hormone derivatives were obtained with a Nuclide 12-90-G mass spectrometer by direct insertion probe (accelerating potential, 4 kV; electron energy, 70 eV; ionization current, 50 μA; ion source temperature, 300°C), integrated GC-MS analysis was performed with a Varian 2700 gas chromatograph interfaced to the mass spectrometer via a direct-transfer line which possessed high-capacity diffusion pumps and equipped with a 20-m by 0.15-mm-i.d. glass capillary coated with 1% OV-101. With regard to the GC-MS analysis, the authors noted that:

> The injector system of the GC was modified for direct capillary injection without splitting by inserting a glass sleeve (1/4 in. o.d. by 0.80 mm i.d.) into the injection port and maintained at 350°C. A 1/4-in. to 1/8-in. reducing union was drilled out so that the capillary column connector could be attached to the glass sleeve without excessive dead volume. The glass capillary was connected to the system with high-temperature silicone septums. A schematic diagram of this capillary column connection is shown in Figure [2.35]. The carrier gas was ultrahigh-purity helium (99.999%; Matheson) and the flow rate was 2 ml/min. The column was operated at 290°C to separate all the thyroid hormone derivatives and at 275°C during SIM of

TABLE 2.17

Values for Total, Dialyzable Fraction, and Free Thyroid Hormones in Euthyroid and Pathological Sera[a]

Sample	Total T_3 by RIA[b] (μg/liter)	Dialyzable fraction of T_3 (X 100) by tracer dialysis[c]	Free T_3 by tracer dialysis- RIA[d] (ng/liter)
Euthyroid			
X ± S.D.	1.48 ± 0.28	0.148 ± 0.021	2.2 ± 0.5
Hypothyroid			
X ± S.D.	0.62 ± 0.32	0.137 ± 0.021	0.9 ± 0.5
Hyperthyroid			
X ± S.D.	3.81 ± 1.74	0.180 ± 0.041	7.2 ± 5.1

[a] Adapted from Petersen et al. [70].
[b] Larsen procedure [97].
[c] Boston Medical Laboratory.
[d] Total value X dialyzable fraction.

the T_3 and reverse T_3 derivatives. The effluent from the GC was monitored using the total ion current detector while the output from the electron multiplier was monitored using a strip chart and the oscillographic recorder. The valve system, transfer line, and ion source were maintained at 300°C during GC-MS. Ionization conditions were identical to those cited above using the mass spectrometer with the direct-insertion probe.

By monitoring m/e 844 (M-213)⁺ which is common to the spectra of the ME-HFB derivatives of both T_3 and RT_3 (reverse T_3) comprising over 20% of the total ion current, it was possible to analyze both compounds in view of their significantly different retention times, as shown in Figure 2.36, which compares TIC and SID chromatograms.

With regard to the GC-MS studies, to assess the general applicability of their preliminary results, Petersen and Vouros further noted that:

Free T_3 by present method (ng/liter)	Total T_4 by RIA[b] (μg/liter)	Dialyzable fraction of T_4 (X 100) by tracer dialysis[c]	Free T_4 by tracer dialysis- RIA (ng/liter)	Free T_4 by present method (ng/liter)
4.2 ± 0.6	80 ± 14	0.024 ± 0.006	19.3 ± 9	18.9 ± 4.4
2.0 ± 0.8	22 ± 12	0.016 ± 0.003	3.7 ± 2.2	6.5 ± 0.6
14.9 ± 13.1	163 ± 62	0.028 ± 0.008	46.5 ± 27.3	48.6 ± 34.0

We examined a physiological sample of known concentrations of RT_3 (2 pg/ml). The ratio of free T_3 to free RT_3 in this sample had previously been established at 4:1 by dialysis-GC-ECD. After dialysis, ion exchange chromatography, derivatization, and concentration of a 20-ml euthyroid serum sample, an aliquot was analyzed by GC-MS and monitoring of the m/e 844 ion. The oscillographic recording of this analysis is shown in Figure [2.37]. Note that although the physiological concentrations of T_3 is four to five times higher than that of RT_3, no signal was detected at its expected retention time (i.e., about 11 min), whereas the response for the RT_3 derivative is clearly evident. Based on our calibration data, the signal obtained corresponds to approximately 1 pg injected, or a free concentration of 2 pg/ml of serum, i.e., well within the expected value. It should be noted that several blanks containing solvent and reagents exhibited no signal under the same conditions at m/e 844. In view of the

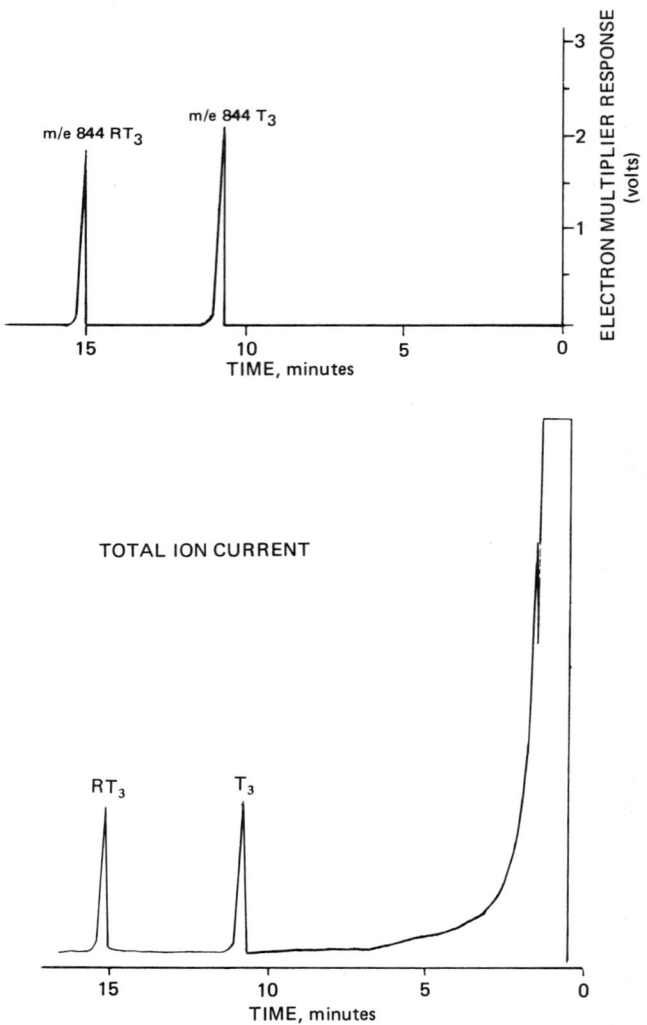

Figure 2.36. Gas chromatographic separation of 100 ng each of the HFB-ME derivatives of T_3 and RT_3. Simultaneous recording of the total ion current (bottom) and electron multiplier response (SIM of m/e 844; top). GC conditions: 20-m X 0.28-mm-i.d. glass capillary coated with 1% OV-101, gas flow 2 ml/min, temperature 275°C, isothermal. From Petersen and Vouros [69], courtesy of Analytical Chemistry.

THYROID HORMONES AND DRUGS 359

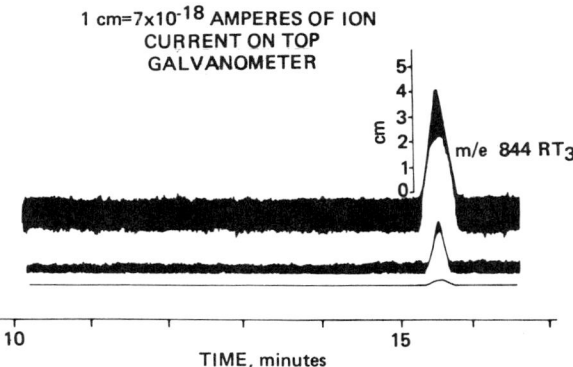

Figure 2.37. Oscillographic response to m/e 844 during GC-MS-SIM of a physiological sample containing RT_3 and T_3 as their HFB-ME derivatives. Galvanometer sensitivity 30 (top), 10 (middle), 1 (bottom). Electron multiplier gain, $G = 10^8$. Chromatographic conditions as in Figure 2.36. From Petersen and Vouros [69], courtesy of Analytical Chemistry.

extremely low concentrations involved, it is not entirely clear at this point whether the RT_3 detected represents the physiologically free forms or may result from mono deiodination of T_4 during dialysis. However, our data clearly indicate its presence.

As for the interpretation of the mass spectra of the thyroid hormone derivatives, the compounds examined were the derivatives of 3,5-diiodothyronine (T_2; 1), 3,3',5-triiodothyronine (T_3; 2), 3,3',5'-triiodothyronine (RT_3; 3), 3,3',5,5'-tetraiodothyronine (T_4; 4), 3',5'-dibromo-3,5-diiodothyronine (Br_2T_2; 5), 3',5'-dichloro-3,5-diiodothyronine (Cl_2T_2; 6), and 3,3',5,5'-tetrachlorothyronine (Cl_4T_0; 7). Their spectra are summarized in Table 2.18; their structures are illustrated on page 360.

4. Methyl Ester/Pivalyl Derivative

In 1966, Stouffer et al. [71] described the first successful GC separation of the thyroid hormones as methyl ester/pivalyl derivatives, of which the structure of thyroxine is shown on the following page.

After the conversion of thyroxine and the other iodinated amino acids to their respective methyl esters by esterification using methanol and thionyl chloride at room temperature, acylation was carried out with pivalic anhydride in the presence of triethylamine. To separate these derivatives,

ANTIHYPERTENSIVE, HYPOGLYCEMIC, AND THYROID DRUGS

$$C_3F_7-\overset{O}{\underset{\|}{C}}-O-\underset{X^4}{\overset{X^3}{\bigcirc}}-O-\underset{X^2}{\overset{X^1}{\bigcirc}}-CH_2-\underset{\underset{C_3F_7}{\overset{NH}{|}}}{\overset{}{CH}}-CO_2CH_3$$
$$\overset{}{\underset{}{}}\quad C=O$$

1 (T_2) : $X^1 = X^2 = I$; $X^3 = X^4 = H$

2 (T_3) : $X^1 = X^2 = X^3 = I$; $X^4 = H$

3 (RT_3) : $X^1 = X^3 = X^4 = I$; $X^2 = H$

4 (T_4) : $X^1 = X^2 = X^3 = X^4 = I$

5 (Br_2T_2) : $X^1 = X^2 = I$; $X^3 = X^4 = Br$

6 (Cl_2T_2) : $X^1 = X^2 = I$; $X^3 = X^4 = Cl$

7 (Cl_4T_0) : $X^1 = X^2 = X^3 = X^4 = Cl$

$$H_3C-\underset{\underset{CH_3}{|}}{\overset{\overset{CH_3}{|}}{C}}-\overset{O}{\underset{\|}{C}}-O-\underset{I}{\overset{I}{\bigcirc}}-O-\underset{I}{\overset{I}{\bigcirc}}-CH_2-\underset{\underset{\underset{\underset{CH_3}{|}}{H_3C-\overset{|}{C}-CH_3}}{\overset{|}{C=O}}}{\overset{\overset{H}{|}}{\underset{\underset{}{H-N}}{C}}}-\overset{O}{\underset{\|}{C}}-OCH_3$$

Methyl Ester/ N,O-Dipivalyl Derivative of Thyroxine (T_4)

Stouffer et al. used a Barber-Colman model 5000 gas chromatograph equipped with a flame ionization detector and a 6-ft U-shaped column packed with 0.5% SE-30 coated on 80-100 mesh Gas Chrom Q. With the column programmed from 130 to 305°C at a heating rate of 10°C/min (injector-detector temperatures and the carrier gas and its flow rate not specified), the retention times based on a published chromatogram of the methyl ester/pivalyl derivatives of tyrosine, monoiodotyrosine, diiodotyrosine, T_3, and T_4 were approximately 5.86, 8.12, 10.00, 15.50, and 17.00 min, respectively. On the other hand, if the gas chromatograph was temperature programmed from 175 to 305°C, the retention times indicated for the monoiodotyrosine, diiodotyrosine, T_3, and T_4 derivatives were considerably shortened, being 3.07, 5.08, 10.95, and 12.40 min, respectively.

In 1967, Jaakonmaki and Stouffer [72] described a GC system for the separation and detection of the thyroid hormones at the very low levels of substances found circulating in the blood.

Derivatization of the hormones was carried out as previously described [71] after their extraction from human blood samples which consisted of the following steps:

TABLE 2.18

Significant Ions and Relative Intensity of Methyl Ester/HFB Derivatives of Thyroid Hormones (Section I) and of Compounds Related to Thyroid Hormones (Section II)[a]

Section I

Major ions	Compound			
	1 (X = H)	2 (X = I)	3 (X = I)	4 (X = I)
$(M)^+$	931 (62)[b]	1057 (67)	1057 (63)	1183 (60)
$(M-213)^+$	718 (100)	844 (100)	844 (70)	970 (100)
$(M-284)^+$	647 (22)	773 (67)	773 (100)	899 (48)
$(M-410)^+$	521 (36)	647 (25)	647 (15)	773 (28)
$(M-213-I, X)^+$	590 (14)	590 (22)	590 (14)	716 (36)
$(M-284-I, X)^+$	519 (32)	519 (35)	519 (38)	645 (30)
$(M-410-I, X)^+$	393 (17)	393 (6)	393 (5)	519 (8)
$(M-284-I, X-197)^+$	322 (33)	322 (21)	322 (32)	448 (21)

Section II

Major ions	Compound		
	5 (X_1 = I, X_3 = Br)[c]	6 (X_1 = I, X_3 = Cl)[d]	7 (X_1 = Cl, X_3 = Cl)[d]
$(M)^+$	1087 (24)	999 (75)	815 (7)
$(M-213)^+$	874 (100)	786 (100)	602 (82)
$(M-284)^+$	803 (47)	715 (42)	531 (69)
$(M-410)^+$	677 (23)	589 (20)	405 (100)
$(M-213-X_1, X_3)^+$	668 (29)	624 (8)	532 (8)[e]
$(M-284-X_1, X_3)^+$	597 (26)	553 (9)	461 (6)
$(M-410-X_1, X_3)^+$	471 (6)	427 (5)	335 (7)
$(M-284-X_1, X_3-197)^+$	400 (12)	356 (7)	264 (9)

[a] Adapted from Petersen and Vouros [69], courtesy of Analytical Chemistry.
[b] Fragment m/e ion with relative intensity shown in parentheses.
[c] m/e values based on ^{79}Br in ion peak cluster.
[d] m/e values based on ^{35}Cl in ion peak cluster.
[e] Percent relative intensity corrected for isotopic composition from m/e 531; i.e., $(M-284)^+$.

Samples of human serum were extracted with n-butanol which had been previously saturated with 0.1 N H_2SO_4 in a manner similar to that described by Kono, van Middlesworth, and Astwood [98]. Three to five milliliters of serum was extracted three times with 2.5 volumes of acid-butanol and centrifuged to remove precipitated proteins and the aqueous serum layer. The combined extracts were neutralized with 2 N NH_4OH and evaporated to a small volume on a rotary evaporator. The concentrated butanol solution was then filtered to remove salts and the filter washed with 3 ml of n-butanol. An equal volume of chloroform was added to the combined filtrate and extracted once with an equal volume of 2 N NH_4OH and twice with one-half volumes of 2 N NH_4OH. The aqueous ammonia layer was evaporated to dryness and the derivatives prepared as previously described.

The GC separations of these derivatives were performed with a Barber-Colman model 5360 gas chromatograph equipped with a 0.056-mCi high-temperature radium detector at an applied voltage of 25 to 30 V and either a 3-ft by 1-mm column packed with 1% polysulfone on 80-100 mesh Gas Chrom Q or a 3-ft by 2-mm column filled with 3% OV-17 coated on 80-100 mesh Gas Chrom P. Maintaining a nitrogen carrier-gas flow rate of 60-80 ml/min for the column and 100 ml/min for the scavenger, an injector temperature of 320°C, and a detector temperature of 300°C, the derivatives were separated isothermally using column temperatures of 230 or 280°C. For example, with the 1% polysulfone column, the retention time of 3-monoiodotyrosine at 230°C relative to 3,5-diiodotyrosine (1.00) was 0.30. On the other hand, at 283°C, the retention time of T_3 relative to T_4 on the same column was 0.44.

Jaakonmaki and Stouffer also reported that, with the 3% OV-17 column, excellent separation of T_3 and T_4 was possible, as shown in Figure 2.38, whereas good linearity of response for T3 in the physiological range is evident, as indicated in Figures 2.39 and 2.40. When the method was applied to the determination of T_3 and T_4 in human serum, a typical chromatogram such as that shown in Figure 2.41 was obtained.

To improve the GC analysis of thyroid hormones, Stouffer [75] in 1969 developed a procedure for the extraction of these hormones which would permit the removal of proteins and other substances which might interfere with either derivative formation or with the subsequent GC column separation and detection. Based on a modified version of the extraction procedure described by Nauman, Nauman, and Werner [99] as outlined on page 363, the dried samples are converted to their methyl ester/pivalyl derivatives by means of the two-step procedure; the reactions of which are shown on page 365.

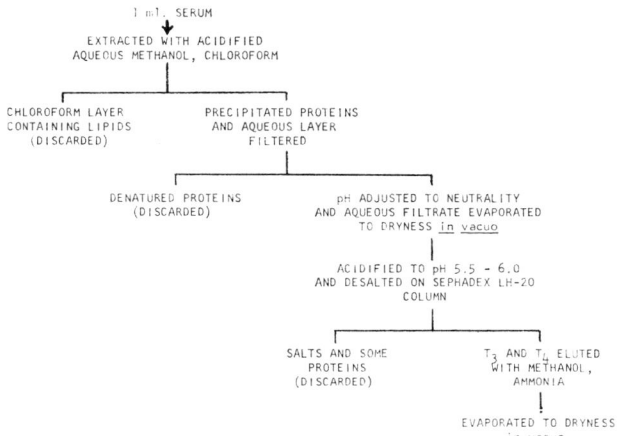

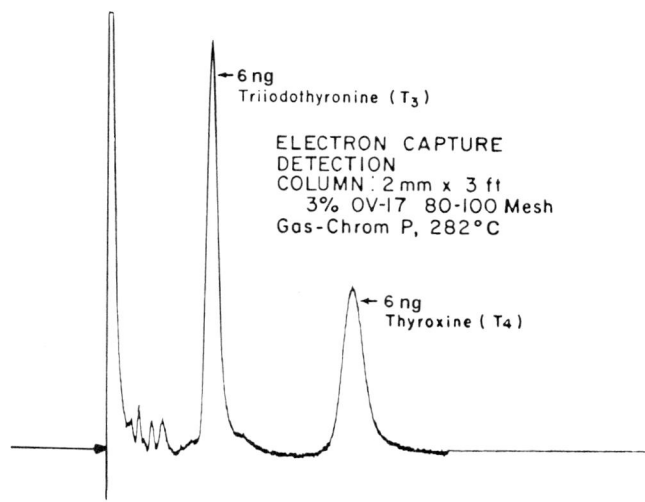

Figure 2.38. Separation of 3,3',5-triiodothyronine and thyroxine (T_4) on 3% OV-17. From Jaakonmaki and Stouffer [72], courtesy of the Journal of Chromatographic Science.

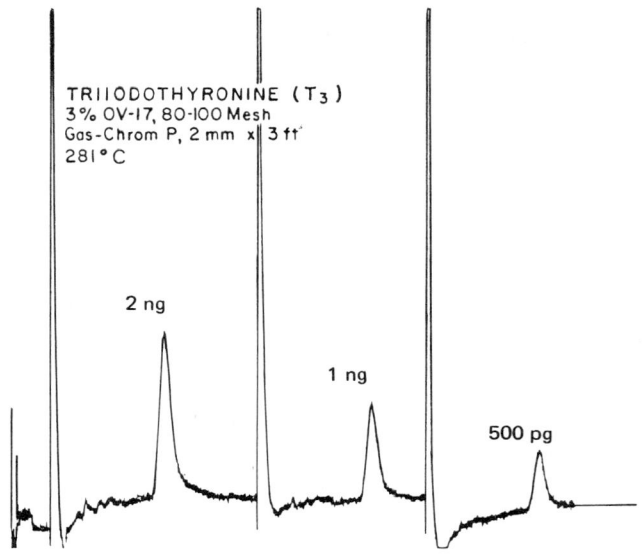

Figure 2.39. Chromatogram showing injection of 2 ng, 1 ng, and 500 pg of 3,3',5-triiodothyronine (T_3); 3% OV-17. From Jaakonmaki and Stouffer [72], courtesy of the Journal of Chromatographic Science.

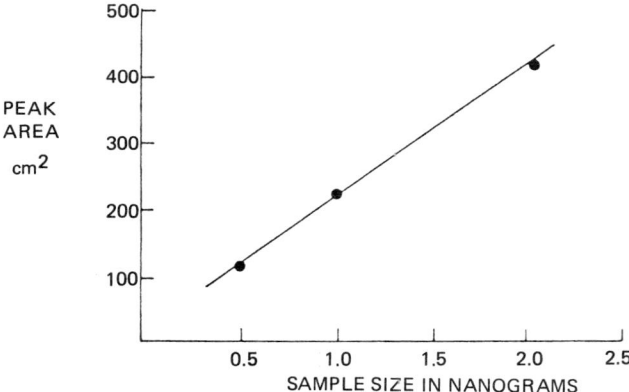

Figure 2.40. Linearity of detector response with respect to sample load for T_3. From Jaakonmaki and Stouffer [72], courtesy of the Journal of Chromatographic Science.

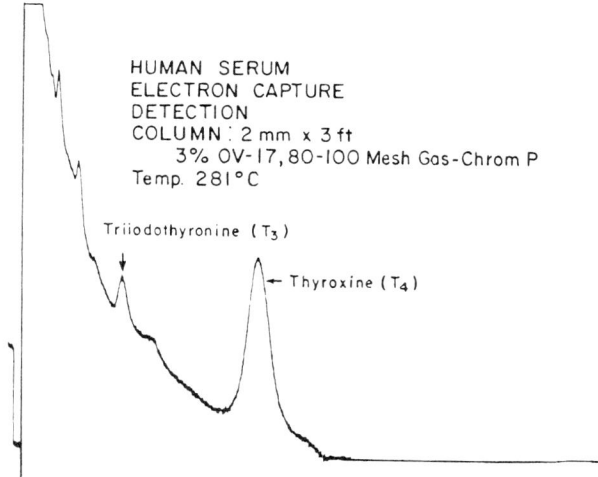

Figure 2.41. Chromatogram showing extract of human serum, 3% OV-17. From Jaakonmaki and Stouffer [72], courtesy of the Journal of Chromatographic Science.

Using a Barber-Colman GC instrument equipped with a flame ionization detector and a 4-ft by 2-mm column packed with 5% OV-17 on 80-100 mesh Gas Chrom Q and temperature programmed from 225 to 325°C at 5°C/min (no other parameters specified), a chromatogram was reproduced in which the retention times of the derivatives of tyrosine, 3-monoiodotyrosine, 3,5-diiodotyrosine, T_1 (thyronine), diiodothyronine (T_2), T_3, and T_4 were nearly 2.70, 6.04, 10.20, 11.85, 19.15, 23.70, and 32.50 min, respectively.

With a Barber-Colman model 5360 gas chromatograph equipped with a ^{226}Ra electron-capture detector and the following column/operating condi-conditions,

> Column: 5% OV-17, 80-100 mesh Gas Chrom Q, 1 mm X 3 ft
> Temperature: Column, 272°C; injector, 320°C; detector, 298°C
> Detector Voltage: 50 V, dc mode
> Electrometer: 2×10^{-10} A
> Flow Rates: Column, 22 ml/min; scavenger, 150 ml/min
> Carrier Gas: N_2

T_3 and T_4 were eluted in 13.55 and 32.30 min, respectively.

Stouffer also noted that with a ^{63}Ni electron-capture detector and a 1000-μsec pulse, T_3 could be readily detected at levels as low as 20×10^{-12} g, which, because of its high molecular weight, corresponds to only about 10^{-13} mole.

In 1971, Docter and Hennemann [76] prepared and compared the methyl ester/trifluoroacetyl and methyl ester/pivalyl derivatives of T_2, T_3, and T_4 using a Varian Aerograph model 2100 gas chromatograph equipped with a ^{63}Ni electron-capture detector and two column systems: system 1 for the separation of methyl ester/trifluoroacetyl derivatives, 3-ft by 2-mm U-shaped column packed with 2% SE-30 on 100-120 mesh Gas Chrom Q and programmed after an initial hold for 30 sec at 200°C to 260°C at 12°C/min (nitrogen carrier-gas flow rate, 30 ml/min); system 2 for the separation of methyl ester/pivalyl derivatives, 3-ft by 2-mm U-shaped column packed with 2.3% OV-1 on 100-120 mesh Gas Chrom Q and operated isothermally at 290°C with other GC conditions being injector temperature 320°C; detector temperature 320°C; nitrogen carrier-gas flow rate 62 ml/min.

Prior to GC analysis, derivatization of the thyroid hormones was carried out in the following manner:

1. Methyl ester/trifluoroacetyl derivatives: 100 to 200 μg of the iodo-aminoacids were heated with about 500 μl of methanol containing 25% anhydrous HCl for 1 hr at 80°C. After the solution was evaporated to dryness, the methyl ester derivatives were acylated with 100 μl of trifluoroacetic anhydride, 90 μl of dichloromethane, and 10 μl of dimethylformamide for 30 min at 80°C. After evaporation to dryness, the derivatives were dissolved in dichloromethane and appropriate aliquots were withdrawn and injected onto the 2% SE-30 column.

2. Methyl ester/pivalyl derivatives: The methyl esters prepared as described above were acylated by heating for 1 hr with 200 µl of pivalic acid anhydride and 50 µl of triethylamine. After evaporation, the residue was dissolved in dichloromethane from which aliquots were withdrawn and injected onto the 2.3% OV-1 column.

Using the 2% SE-30 column and the conditions previously specified, the retention times of the methyl ester/trifluoroacetyl derivatives of T_2, T_3, and T_4 were 5.45, 7.58, and 11.40 min, respectively. On the other hand, with the 2.3% OV-1 column operated isothermally at 290°C, the retention times of the methyl ester/pivalyl derivatives of T_2, T_3, and T_4 were approximately 2.22, 4.37, and 8.53 min, respectively. The minimum accurately measurable amount was found to be nearly 1.5 ng for T_3 and 2.5 ng for T_4 using the ^{63}Ni detector with a linear response obtained for these compounds from 1 to 16 ng.

Nihei and co-workers [77] also measured T_3 and T_4 in human serum by a gas chromatographic procedure that consisted of five fundamental steps: (1) extraction of T_3 and T_4 from serum by passage through a cation-exchange resin column (Bio-Rad resin AG 50W-X2, 100-200 mesh, in the hydrogen form), (2) preparation of stable, volatile methyl ester/pivalyl derivatives, (3) purification of the derivatives with an anion-exchange resin column (Amberlite IR 45 ion-exchange resin), (4) gas chromatographic separation and quantitation, and (5) correction for methodological conversion (deiodination) of T_4 to T_3.

The GC separations of these derivatives were performed with a Micro-Tek model MT 220 gas chromatograph equipped with a ^{63}Ni electron-capture detector and 2-ft by 4-mm-i.d. U-shaped glass columns packed with 5% OV-1 on Chromosorb W-HP. To obtain reported retention times of approximately 33 and 38 min, respectively, for the methyl ester/pivalyl derivatives of T_3 and T_4 as shown in Figure 2.42, the following GC conditions were maintained: injector temperature, 280°C; column temperature, held isothermally for 12 min at 220°C, then programmed at 3°C/min to 300°C with a final temperature hold for 5 min; detector temperature, 350°C; pulse rate, 1.1×10^4/sec; pulse width, 0.5 µsec.

With regard to the recovery of T_3 added in nanogram amounts to hypothyroid serum, the recoveries (based on four experiments) were 93.4, 99.2, 99.5, and 101.4% with the addition of 5, 11, 20, and 27 ng of T_3/ml of serum for which the mean value was 98.6%.

Studies performed to determine the conversion of T_4 to T_3 showed that, over a concentration range of 1.0 to 15.0 µg of added T_4/100 ml, the identical percentage of T_4 was converted to T_3, averaging 1.69 ± 0.05% through ten separate analyses.

Capable of detecting T_3 and T_4 at concentration levels of 50 and 100 pg, respectively, the procedure was applied to the determination of T_3 in man.

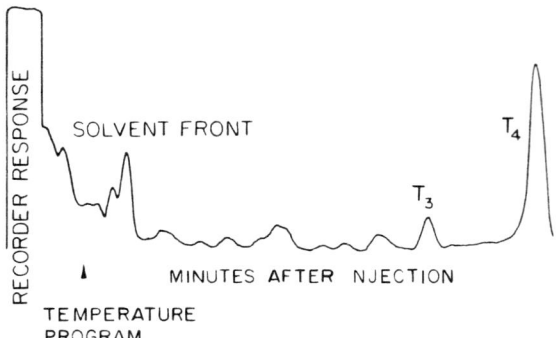

Figure 2.42. Gas chromatogram of serum sample: tracing of derivatized serum extract from a normal subject. The isothermal portion of the program, which ends at the arrowhead, is 12 min long and the T_3 and T_4 retention times were 33 and 38 min, respectively. Adapted from Nihei et al. [77].

Expressed as ng % (mean ± S.D.), T_3 values obtained for normal, hypothyroid, and hyperthyroid subjects were 137 ± 23, 68 ± 12, and 510 ± 131, respectively.

In 1973, Tajuddin and Elfbaum [78] evaluated the use of Dexsil 300, a polycarboranesiloxane, as the stationary phase for the GC analysis of the methyl ester/pivalyl derivatives of pure T_3 and T_4, and T_3 from human serum.

The GC characteristics of the derivatives were examined with a Perkin-Elmer model 900 gas chromatograph equipped with a ^{63}Ni electron-capture detector and a 81-cm by 6.4-mm-o.d. glass column packed with 3% Dexsil 300 on 80-100 mesh Chromosorb W-HP. Using the specified operating conditions [injector temperature, 320°C; column temperature, 305°C; detector temperature, 310°C; argon-methane (9:1 by volume) carrier-gas flow rate, 110 ml/min; pulse rate of 100 μsec of polarizing voltage (50 V) and 1 μsec duration], the retention times of T_3 and T_4 were 8 and 16 min, respectively.

When applied to clinical studies, a 162-cm by 6.4-mm-o.d. glass column packed with 3% Dexsil 300 on 80-100 mesh Chromosorb W-HP was used isothermally at 305°C with all other conditions maintained as previously noted above. With this column, the T_3 and T_4 derivatives were eluted in approximately 16 and 32 min, respectively, as shown in Figure 2.43.

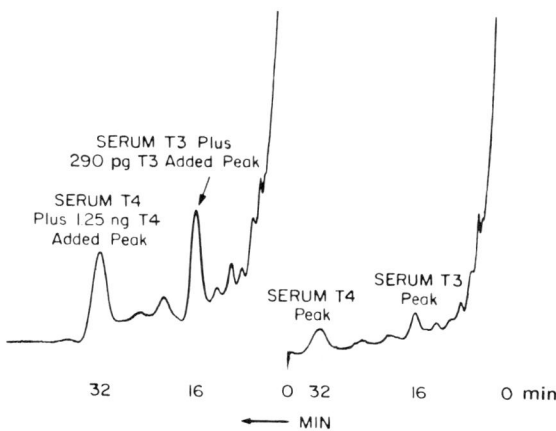

Figure 2.43. Chromatogram obtained from the "normal" pool, with and without added T_3. 3% Dexsil 300 GC on Chromosorb WHP 80-100 mesh; 162-cm by 6.4-mm-o.d. glass column; column temperature 305°C isothermal; range 10; attenuation 16. From Tajuddin and Elfbaum [78], courtesy of Clinical Chemistry.

5. Silyl Derivatives

In 1968, Hansen [79] undertook a study to develop a method for the quantitative determination of the physiologically active components of thyroid drug preparations by gas chromatography; the compounds of interest being tyrosine, 3,5-diiodotyrosine, 3,5-diiodothyronine (T_2), T_3, reverse T_3, and T_4.

The procedure adopted for sample preparation prior to GC analysis consisted of evaporating an appropriate aliquot of a mixed standard to dryness in a 2-dram vial, adding 100 μl of reagent mixture [5.00 ml of tetrahydrofuran, 2.00 ml of bis-(trimethylsilyl)acetamide (BSA), 5 drops of trimethylchlorosilane], sealing the vial with a foil-lined screw cap, and heating the mixture on the front edge of a water bath in a hood for 1 min. After the 1-min reaction period, the solution was cooled to room temperature; the sample then being suitable for GC analysis.

The GC separations were carried out with a Barber-Colman model 5000 gas chromatograph equipped with both flame ionization and electron-capture detectors, a 2-ft by 3-mm-i.d. glass column packed with 2% SE-33 on

100-120 mesh Chrom Q, and a splitting device for the simultaneous analysis of the separated sample with both detectors. With this splitting arrangement, 95% of the column effluent was diverted to the flame ionization detector and 5% to the electron-capture detector. The other GC conditions employed were injector temperature, 270°C; column temperature, programmed from 150 to 280°C at 10°C/min; nitrogen carrier-gas flow rate, 50 ml/min. Under these conditions the internal standard (squalene) and the silyl derivatives of tyrosine, 3,5-diiodotyrosine, T_2, T_3, reverse T_3, and T_4 were 8.38, 2.12, 6.62, 10.90, 12.70, 13.55, and 14.80 min, respectively.

Alexander and Scheig [80] also described the GC separation of the trimethylsilyl derivatives of tyrosine, 3-monoiodotyrosine, 3,5-diiodotyrosine, thyronine, 3,3',5-triiodothyronine (T_3), and thyroxine (T_4).

With the silylation reaction carried out as described by Klebe, Finkbeiner, and White [100], the rate of silylation of the amino acids was measured by comparing their peak areas to that of added trimethylsilyldocosanoic acid. The reaction kinetics were based on peak area measurements of com-components separated with a Barber-Colman model 5000 gas chromatograph equipped with a flame ionization detector and 4-ft and 6-ft by 3-mm U-shaped glass columns packed with 3% OV-1 on 60-80 mesh Gas Chrom Q. Using the 6-ft column and the specified GC operating conditions (injector temperature, 270°C; column temperature, programmed at 7.5°C/min from 150 to 225°C after a 3-min isothermal period; detector temperature, 275°C; nitrogen carrier-gas flow rate, 200 ml/min at 150°C), the retention times, in minutes, of the silylated derivatives of tyrosine, 3-monoiodotyrosine, docosanoic acid, 3,5-diiodotyrosine, and thyronine were 5.7, 9.7, 13.0, 13.6, and 15.0, respectively. With the 4-ft by 3-mm column programmed at 15°C/min from 190 to 250°C after a 3-min isothermal period, injector and detector temperatures set at 295°C, and the carrier-gas flow rate maintained at 200 ml/min (measured at 190°C), the retention times of the silyl derivatives of docosanoic acid, T_3, and T_4 were 6.0, 15.0, and 2 23.0 min, respectively. Figure 2.44 shows that the trimethylsilyl derivatives of tyrosine (Tyr), 3-monoiodotyrosine (MIT), 3,5-diiodotyrosine (DIT), thyronine (T), T_3, and T_4 are readily separated as sharp, symmetrical peaks within 30 min when the column temperature was programmed from 165 to 265°C.

Backer and Pileggi [81] described in 1968 the gas chromatographic behavior of the four principal iodoamino acids as their trimethylsilyl derivatives as well as a number of iodinated radiographic contrast media known to interfere with the chemical determination of these compounds.

Preparation of the TMSi derivatives consisted of evaporating 100 μl of a solution of the samples in methanol, singly or as a mixture (prepared at a concentration of 1 mg/ml methanol), to dryness, treating the residue with 100 μl of bis-(trimethylsilyl)acetamide containing 5% trimethylchlorosilane,

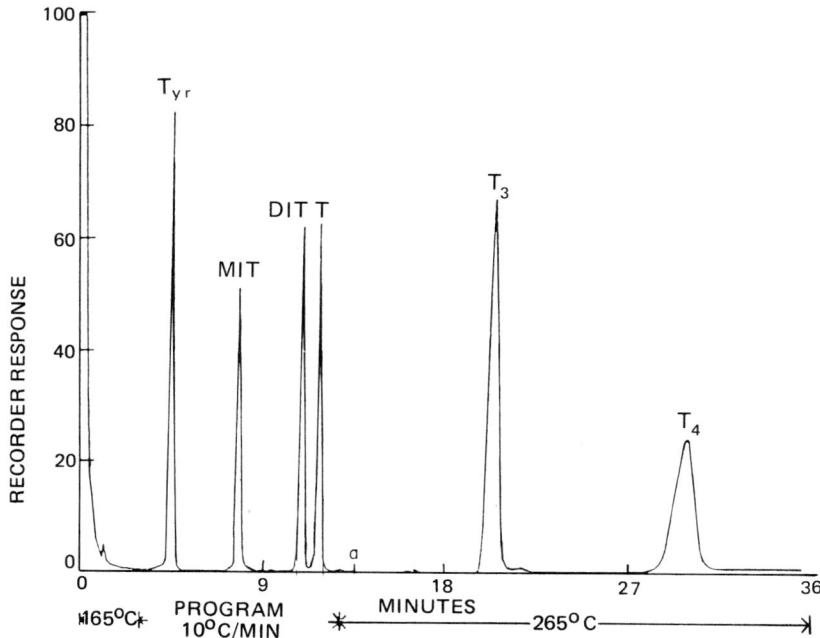

Figure 2.44. Gas chromatogram of the trimethylsilyl derivatives of tyrosine, thyronine, iodotyrosines, and iodothyronines. The separation was carried out on a 4-ft by 3-mm glass U column containing OV-1. An isothermal temperature of 165°C was maintained for 3 min and then programmed at 10°C/min as indicated. Nitrogen was the carrier gas at 30 psig (60 ml/min at 165°C). Injector temperature was 280°C, and detector 285°C. Maximum recorder response was 3×10^{-9} A up to point a, when it was changed to 9×10^{-10} A. The amount of each compound injected, in micrograms, was Tyr 3.8, MIT 4.5, DIT 13.2 T 4.5, T_3 13.2, and T_4 14.6. From Alexander and Scheig [80], courtesy of <u>Analytical Biochemistry.</u>

and heating this reaction mixture for 20 min at 50°C in a closed vial. After the reaction vial had been cooled to room temperature, 1- to 3-μl aliquots were withdrawn for GC analysis and injected into a Beckman GC-4 gas chromatograph equipped with flame ionization and electron-capture detection and a 5-ft by 2-mm glass column packed with 3% OV-1 on 100-120 mesh Gas Chrom Q. With the helium carrier-gas flow rate maintained at 70 ml/min, the column was run isothermally or with temperature programming from 210 to 220°C at 2°C/5 min.

When operated isothermally at 285°C (injector and detector temperature not specified), the retention times of the TMSi derivatives of T_3 and T_4 were 3.34 and 6.80 min, respectively, whereas those for derivatized 3-monoiodotyrosine and 3,5-diiodotyrosine at a column temperature of 210°C were 3.00 and 8.62 min, respectively. Using the flame ionization detector, the limits of detection were in the submicrogram range; for example, diiodotyrosine, 100 ng; T_3, 300 ng. However, with respect to the electron-capture detector, the limits of detection for 3-monoiodotyrosine, 3,5-diiodotyrosine, T_3, and T_4 were 0.3, 1.0, 5.0, and 30.0 ng, respectively.

On the other hand, when performing the separation of 3-monoiodotyrosine, 3,5-diiodotyrosine, Urokon, Telepaque, Teridax, Bilopaque, Orabilix, Hypaque, Miokon, and Conray as their TMSi derivatives (these trade-name materials being contrast media) by temperature programming from 210 to 220°C at 4°C/5 min, their respective retention times in minutes were 1.59, 5.18, 7.30, 7.91, 9.17, 16.90, 17.83, 19.30, 22.60, and 23.30. Backer and Pileggi noted that the contrast media, eluted from the column at much lower temperatures than the thyroid hormones, did not interfere with the separation of the hormones carried out at 285°C.

Shahrokhi and Gehrke [82] reported their results obtained for two methods investigated for the preparation of TMSi derivatives of iodine-containing amino acids: (1) trimethylsilylation with a hexamethyldisilazane-trimethylchlorosilane reagent mixture and (2) trimethylsilylation with bis-(trimethylsilyl)acetamide.

Reaction kinetics were monitored and the separations of the TMSi derivatives were performed with a F&M model 300 gas chromatograph equipped with a flame ionization detector and a 1.0-m by 3.5-mm-i.d. borosilicate glass column packed with 0.5% SE-30 coated on acid-washed, dimethylchlorosilane-treated, 60-80 mesh Chromosorb G. For this study, the other GC conditions were injector and detector temperatures, not specified; column temperature, programmed from 75 to 250°C at 4.6°C/min; nitrogen carrier-gas flow rate, 40 ml/min; hydrogen flow rate, 36 ml/min; air flow rate, 450 ml/min.

Using the above conditions, Table 2.19 includes the average relative molar response for various iodoamino acids prepared by the two silylating methods, as well as the elution temperatures and retention times of the derivatives.

Shahrokhi and Gehrke summarized their study and findings in the following manner:

Two procedures were developed and compared to prepare the volatile TMSi derivatives of iodinated amino acids. The volatile derivatives of 3-monoiodotyrosine, 3,5-diiodotyrosine, 3,5-diiodothyronine, 3,3',5-triiodothyronine (T_3), and thyroxine (T_4) were synthesized

TABLE 2.19

Relative Molar Responses (RMR), Elution Temperatures,
and Retention Times of TMSi Derivatives
of Iodoamino Acids[a]

Compound	RMR[b]		Elution temp. (°C)	Retention time (min)
	BSA[c]	HMDS-TMCS[d]		
Tyrosine	1.00	1.00	127	12.4
3-Monoiodotyrosine	1.11	0.94	150	17.1
3,5-Diiodotyrosine	1.30	1.04	175	21.9
3,5-Diiodothyronine	1.36	1.29	212	29.5
3,3',5-Triiodothyronine	1.47	1.02	225	32.6
Thyroxine	1.31	1.07	245	35.8

[a] Adapted from Shahrokhi and Gehrke [82].
[b] Relative molar response = (amino acid response/mole)/(tyrosine response/mole).
[c] 0.25 ml of BSA and 0.75 ml of acetonitrile in a screw-cap vial at 150°C for 30 min.
[d] 0.2 ml of HMDS plus 0.1 ml of TMCS, and 0.7 ml of pyridine refluxed at ca. 125°C for 90 min.

using HMDS-TMCS and bis-(trimethylsilyl)acetamide (BSA). The reaction conditions to obtain maximum yield with BSA were 150°C for 30 min in a closed tube. Reference derivatives were prepared on a macro scale and empirical formulas were established by elemental analyses and infrared spectra. Yields greater than 97% were obtained with BSA as the silylation reagent compared to values as low as 66% with HMDS-TMCS. The TMSi derivatives were chromatographed on a 1.0-m by 3.5-mm-i.d. borosilicate-glass column packed with Chromosorb G, 60-80 mesh, acid-washed, DMCS-treated, and coated with 0.5% SE-30. Complete chromatographic separation of the five iodoamino acids was achieved in 37 min. The minimum detectable response was found to be about 20 ng using the flame ionization detector (signal/noise = 2).

Funakoshi and Cahnmann [83] presented in detail in 1969 their procedure for the determination of a large variety of iodinated compounds and discussed various characteristics of the TMSi derivatives of the iodoamino acids. The compounds consisted not only of the known iodinated tyrosines (tyrosine, 3-monoiodotyrosine, 3,5-diiodotyrosine) and thyronines (thyronine, 3-iodothyronine, 3,5-diiodothyronine, 3,3'-diiodothyronine, 3,5',5-triiodothyronine, 3,3',5'-triiodothyronine, thyroxine), but also their deamino, position, and side-chain analogs as well as various intermediates in the synthesis of the thyroid hormones. The structures of the various iodinated compounds containing either one or two benzene rings are shown in Table 2.20. All compounds in Table 2.20 were silylated with 50 or 100 µl of BSA (for quantitative determinations and for the detection of picogram and nanogram amounts) or BSA containing 10% acetonitrile (for qualitative purposes), either at room temperature or at 80°C. With the mixed BSA/acetonitrile reagent solution, heating at 80°C for 5 to 7 min was sufficient to convert the iodoamino acids and related compounds to their TMSi derivatives.

For the GC separation of these silyl derivatives, a Chromalab (flame ionization detector) or a Micro-Tek MT-220 (^{63}Ni electron-capture detector) was used in conjunction with glass columns packed with either 1% OV-1 or 1% OV-17 on 80-100 mesh Chromosorb W-HP. The length of the columns ranged from 2 to 6 ft and their internal diameters from 1.7 to 3.3 mm. As noted by the authors, column temperatures ranged from about 130 to 285°C. Carrier-gas (nitrogen or argon with the flame ionization detector; argon-10% methane when a pulsed power supply was used with the electron-capture detector) flow rates usually ranged from 40 to 60 ml/min, even when narrow-bore columns were used in conjunction with EC detection.

In Table 2.21 are listed the retention times for the various silyl derivatives of iodinated compounds containing one or two benzene rings as well as the carrier-gas flow rate and column temperature used to obtain the RT values noted.

Using the flame ionization detector and the 6-ft by 1.7-mm column of 1% OV-1 which was temperature programmed from 135 to 225°C at 5°C/minute (injector temperature, 280°C; detector temperature, 295°C), the retention times for the completely resolved TMSi derivatives of tyrosine, 3-monoiodotyrosine, 3,5-diiodotyrosine, thyronine, 3-iodothyronine, 3,5-diiodothyronine, 3,3'-diiodothyronine, 3,3',5-triiodothyronine (T_3), 3,3',5'-triiodothyronine (reverse T_3), and thyroxine (T_4) were approximately 2.70, 5.65, 9.55, 11.30, 14.45, 16.42, 17.65, 20.10, 21.60, and 23.60 min.

Heinl et al. [85] described a quick and exact routine GC method suited for purity control of thyroid hormone preparations as well as for trace analysis of iodoamino acids in drugs containing thyroid hormones. In their investigation, silyl derivatives were made using BSA as silylating reagent and analyzed with a Philips-Pye-Unicam gas chromatograph equipped with flame ionization and electron-capture detectors and 50-cm by 3-mm glass columns packed with 3% OV-17 coated on 80-100 mesh Diatomite CQ.

TABLE 2.20

Structures of Various Iodinated Compounds Containing Either One (1-22) or Two (23-48) Benzene Rings

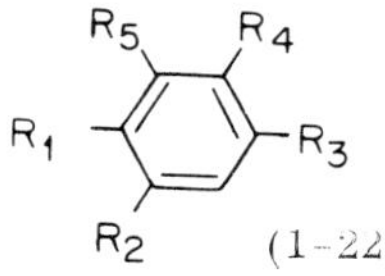

Compound Number	R_1	R_2	R_3	R_4	R_5
1	O	I	O	H	I
2	OH	I	OH	H	I
3	OH	H	CHO	H	I
4	OH	I	CHO	H	I
5	OH	I	CH_2COOH	H	I
6	OH	I	$(CH_2)_2COOH$	H	I
7	OH	I	$(CH_2)_3COOH$	H	I
8	OH	I	$CH_2CH(CH_3)COOH$	H	I
9	OH	I	$CH(OH)COOH$	H	I
10	OH	I	$CH_2CH(OH)COOH$	H	I
11	OH	I	$CH(OH)CH(OH)COOH)$	H	I
12	OH	H	$CH_2CH(NH_2)COOH$	H	I
13	OH	I	$CH_2CH(NH_2)COOH$	H	I
14	I	OH	$CH_2CH(NH_2)COOH$	I	H
15	OH	I	CH=CHCOOH	H	I
16	OH	I	$CH_2CH(COOH)_2$	H	I
17	AcO	H	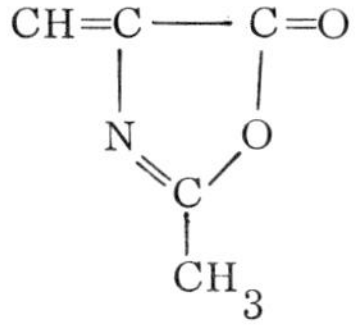 (see structure below)	H	I

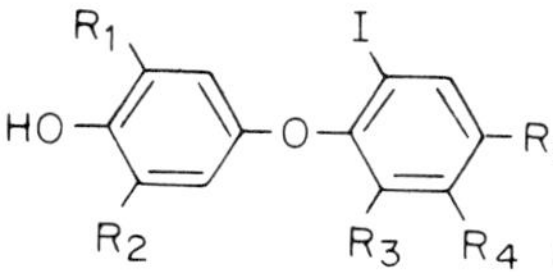

Compound 17, R_3:

$$\text{CH}=\text{C}-\text{C}=\text{O}$$
with N and O forming a ring closed by $C-CH_3$

TABLE 2.20 (continued)

Compound Number	R_1	R_2	R_3	R_4	R_5
18	AcO	I	See Compound 17	H	I
19	OH	I	COCOOH	H	I
20	OH	H	$CH_2COCOOH$	H	I
21	OH	I	$CH_2COCOOH$	H	I
22	OH	I	$CH(OH)CH_2NH_2 \cdot HCl$	H	I

Compound Number	R_1	R_2	R_3	R_4	R_5
23	I	I	I	H	COOH
24	H	H	H	H	CH_2COOH
25	H	H	I	H	CH_2COOH
26	I	H	H	H	CH_2COOH
27	I	H	I	H	CH_2COOH
28	I	I	I	H	CH_2COOH
29	H	H	H	H	$(CH_2)_2COOH$
30	H	H	I	H	$(CH_2)_2COOH$
31	I	H	H	H	$(CH_2)_2COOH$
32	I	H	I	H	$(CH_2)_2COOH$
33	I	I	H	H	$(CH_2)_2COOH$
34	I	I	I	H	$(CH_2)_2COOH$
35	H	H	I	H	$(CH_2)_3COOH$
36	I	H	I	H	$(CH_2)_3COOH$
37	I	I	I	H	$(CH_2)_3COOH$
38	I	I	I	H	$CH_2CH(OH)COOH$
39	H	H	H	H	$CH_2CH(NH_2)COOH$
40	H	H	I	H	$CH_2CH(NH_2)COOH$

TABLE 2.20 (continued)

Compound Number	R_1	R_2	R_3	R_4	R_5
41	I	H	H	H	$CH_2CH(NH_2)COOH$
42	I	H	I	H	$CH_2CH(NH_2)COOH$
43	I	I	H	H	$CH_2CH(NH_2)COOH$
44	I	I	I	H	$CH_2CH(NH_2)COOH$
45	I	I	I	H	$CH_2COCOOH$
46	H	H	H	$CH_2CH(NH_2)COOH$	I
47	I	H	I	$CH_2CH(NH_2)COOH$	I
48	I	I	I	$CH_2CH(NH_2)COOH$	I

[a] Adapted from Funakoshi and Cahnmann [83].

Using the specified GC conditions (column temperature, 285°C; FID detector temperature, 300°C; nitrogen carrier-gas flow rate, 40 ml/min; hydrogen flow rate, 40 ml/min; air flow rate, 600 ml/min), the retention times reported for the silyl derivatives of 3-monoiodotyrosine, 3,5-diiodothyronine, 3,3'-diiodothyronine, 3',5'-diiodothyronine, 3,3',5-triiodothyronine, 3,3',5'-triiodothyronine, and thyroxine were about 1.25, 2.08, 2.71, 3.54, 4.80, 6.88, and 12.92 min, respectively, whereas their respective retention index values calculated from GC data obtained with the OV-17 column operated isothermally at 285°C were 3310 ± 14, 3550 ± 6, 3660 ± 5, 3760 ± 5, 3930 ± 5, 4097 ± 5, and 4350 ± 5. Using the same GC conditions the retention index of silylated thyronine was 2900 ± 15.

Heinl et al. summarized their investigations and findings as follows:

The derivatization of iodoamino acids for gas chromatography by silylation with N,O-bis(trimrthylsilyl)acetamide proved to be advantageous. Isothermal gas chromatography was found best suited for qualitative and quantitative work. Quantitative evaluation was achieved by use of 3,5-diiodothyronine as internal standard. All iodothyronines and their isomers can be separated and determined quantitatively. Results on analysis of several commercially available iodoamino acids of 0.01-0.05% can be identified using sample sizes of 2 mg. When using a flame ionization detector the detection limit for

TABLE 2.21

Retention Times of Iodinated Compounds Containing One (1–22) or Two (23–48) Benzene Rings[a]

Compound no.	Col. temp. (°C)	CG flow (ml/min)	RT (min)	Compound no.	Col. temp (°C)	CG flow (ml/min)	RT (min)
1	132	50	2.53	23	275	56	2.43
2	160	50	4.18	24	227	53	1.95
3	132	50	1.88	25	227	53	3.83
4	160	50	2.77	26	227	53	4.65
5	197	50	1.95	27	275	56	1.42
6	197	50	2.77	28	275	56	2.73
7	197	50	3.73	29	237	53	1.82
8	197	50	2.73	30	228	50	4.75
9	202	54	1.97	31	237	53	3.87
10	202	54	3.37	32	275	56	1.95
11	202	54	4.23	33	275	56	2.40
12	208	50	1.38	34	275	56	3.62

13	208	50	3.17	35	237	50	4.10
14	204	53	2.92	36	275	56	2.27
15	204	54	4.25	37	275	56	4.42
16	212	50	3.90	38	274	56	4.95
17	213	50	1.42	39	250	50	1.82
18	213	50	3.08	40	250	50	2.92
19	199	53	1.70	41	250	50	3.60
20	199	53	2.48	42	276	56	2.23
21	199	53	6.52	43	276	56	2.95
22	200	50	2.11	44	276	56	4.50
				45	285	55	2.05
				46	275	55	0.87
				47	275	55	2.55
				48	282	55	3.53

[a] Adapted from Funakoshi and Cahmmann [83].

Column: 6 ft by 3.3 mm, 1% OV-1; inlet and detector temperatures were 10–20°C above column temperature.

Note: See Table 2.20 for identification of components.

thyronine and 3,5-diiodothyronine amounts to 5 ng, for thyroxine to 20 ng. Iodoamino acids with retention times between thyronine and thyroxine exhibit detection limits from 5 to 20 ng, accordingly.

In 1973, Bilous and Windheuser [86] reported a GC method for the quantitative analysis of liothyronine (3,3',5-triiodothyronine) and thyroxine in dried thyroid. In their procedure, three basic steps were employed: (1) barium hydroxide hydrolysis of the dried thyroid to release the iodoamino acids from their protein linkage, (2) separation of liothyronine and thyroxine from the interfering substances by extraction (n-butanol saturated with 0.1 N sodium thiosulfate) and column chromatography (a Sephadex G-10, 27- by 2.1-cm column using an aqueous ammonia-methanol solution to elute the T_3/T_4 components), and (3) detection and quantitation by gas chromatography.

The T_3/T_4 components eluted from the Sephadex column were subsequently converted to silyl derivatives with N,O-bis(trimethylsilyl)acetamide. The GC analysis of these derivatives was performed with a Nuclear-Chicago series 5000 gas chromatograph equipped with a flame ionization detector and a 6-ft by 3-mm-i.d. U-shaped borosilicate glass column packed with 1% OV-1 on 60-80 mesh Gas Chrom Q. To determine the T_3 and T_4 compounds, the following GC conditions were maintained: injector temperature, 240°C; column temperature, programmed from 165 to 285°C at 5°C/min; detector temperature, 330°C; nitrogen carrier-gas flow rate, 50 ml/min. Using these GC conditions, the retention times of the silyl derivatives of liothyronine (T_3), 3,3',5'-triiodothyronine (reverse T_3), and thyroxine were 14.39, 15.33, and 16.85 min, respectively.

In addition to the determination of liothyronine (T_3), 3,3',5'-triiodothyronine (reverse T_3 or T_3'), and thyroxine in dried thyroid (a typical chromatogram of the dried thyroid hydrolysate is shown in Fig. 2.45), the GC method was used to monitor the recovery of T_3 and T_4 (1) after hydrolysis and (2) from Sephadex G-10 columns. The mean recovery (n = 4) of T_3 and T_4 after hydrolysis was 100.6 ± 1.2% and 98.92 ± 2.22%, respectively, whereas their respective values from Sephadex G-10 columns were 101.9 ± 1.1% and 103.5 ± 1.3%.

B. Antithyroid Drugs

Although the introduction of thiouracils by Astwood [101] in 1943 was followed by extensive investigation of many chemical analogs to determine relative antithyroid activities and toxicities, few have achieved therapeutic stature. In the United States the most frequently used are propylthiouracil (PTU) and methimazole, whereas methylthiouracil and carbimazole are preferred in Europe [102]; the structures of these drugs are shown in Figure 2.46.

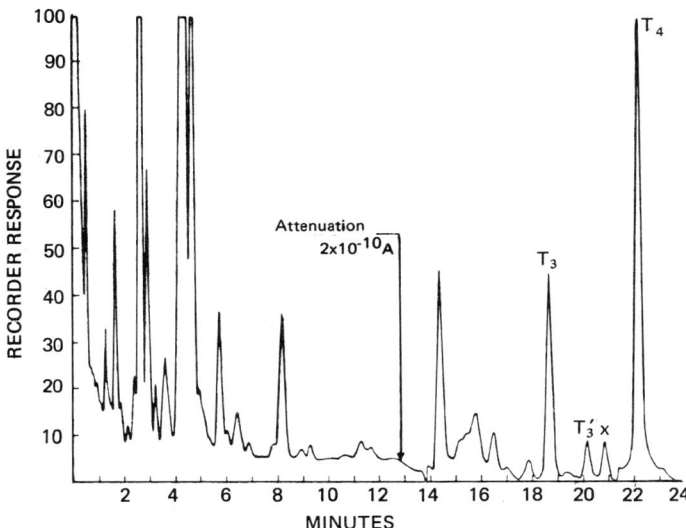

Figure 2.45. Chromatograms of dried thyroid hydrolysate. The thyroid hormones were liothyronine (T_3), 3,3',5'-triiodothyronine (T'_3), thyroxine (T_4), and an unknown, X. From Bilous and Windheuser [86], courtesy of the Journal of Pharmaceutical Sciences.

With regard to the gas chromatographic separation of these compounds, very little has been reported in the literature. Of a more qualitative nature, Moffat [13] reported retention indices of 1670 and 1550 for carbimazole and methimazole, respectively. On the other hand, Schuppan et al. [102] in 1973 developed a GC method to investigate the pharmacokinetics of propylthiouracil in humans.

In the method of Schuppan et al., sample preparation for subsequent analysis by GC consisted of adding 1 ml of plasma to 1 ml of $(NH_4)_2SO_4$ solution which was then acidified with dilute sulfuric acid to a pH of 4. This mixture was extracted with 5 ml of diethyl ether by shaking in a cradle for 1 hr. As noted, the addition of 1 ml of saturated ammonium sulfate solution to the plasma adjusted to pH 4 resulted in a 95 ± 1% recovery of PTU during extraction with 5 ml of ether. To this ether extract, 1 ml of an ether solution containing 5 μg of pentobarbital as internal standard was added. Following the centrifugation of this mixture, a 5-ml aliquot of the ether layer was withdrawn and transferred to a screw-cap conical test tube. The ether phase was then reextracted using 50 μl of a

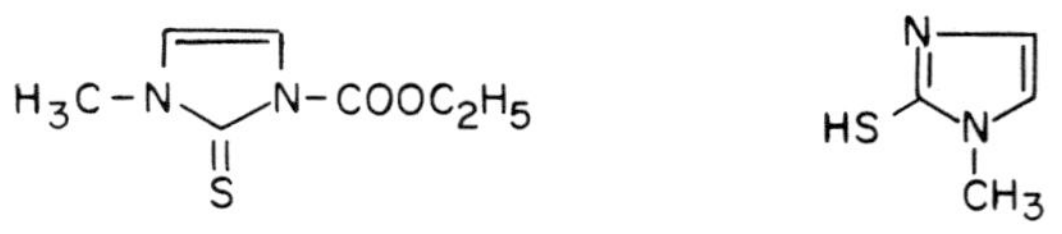

Carbimazole
(1-Ethoxycarbonyl-3-methyl-2-thio-4-imidazoline)

Methimazole
(1-Methylimidazole-2-thiol)

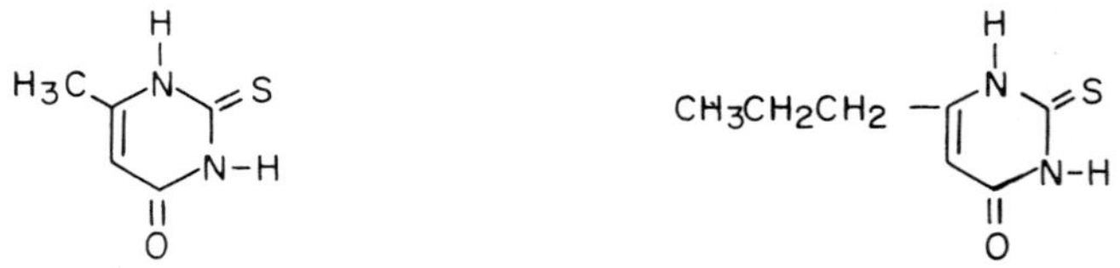

Methylthiouracil
(6-Methyl-2-thiouracil)

Propylthiouracil
(6-n-Propyl-2-thiouracil)

Figure 2.46. Structures of several antithyroid drugs.

5% solution of tetrapropylammonium hydroxide in order to convert the PTU and the internal standard into their salt forms, which completely transferred into the aqueous phase. The ether extract/TPAH system was shaken for 1 min on a Vortex mixer and then centrifuged for 5 min. After the removal of the ether phase, a 3-μl aliquot of the aqueous base solution was injected for analysis into a Varian Aerograph model 1200 gas chromatograph equipped with a flame ionization detector and a 11-ft by 0.125-in.-i.d. stainless steel column packed with 3% OV-1 on Gas Chrom Q. To obtain retention times of approximately 2.9 and 3.8 min for the propyl derivatives of PTU and pentobarbital, respectively, the following GC conditions were maintained: injector temperature, 325°C; column temperature, 185°C; detector temperature, 330°C; nitrogen carrier-gas flow rate, 27 ml/min; hydrogen flow rate, 27 ml/min; air flow rate, 270 ml/min. As noted by these investigators, it was necessary, between every two or three injections, to heat the oven to about 220°C in order to flush out extraneous, slowly eluting compounds and, at the end of each day, 30 μl of Silyl 8 was injected as a conditioning agent for the column.

Using calibration curves prepared by plotting peak height ratios versus PTU concentrations, the curve was linear over the concentration range studied, namely, between 0.4 and 30.0 μg/ml of PTU.

Using the GC procedure described above, Table 2.22 is a summary of physical, chemical and pharmacokinetic data on euthyroid and hyperthyroid subjects.

TABLE 2.22

Physical, Chemical, and Pharmacokinetic Data on Euthyroid and Hyperthyroid Subjects[a]

Subject	Sex	Age (yrs)	Weight (kg)	Clinical state	Dose/weight (mg/kg)	Half-life, $t_{1/2}$ (min)	t_{max}	Plasma clearance (ml/min)
A	M	32	63	EU[b]	3.2	63	90	324
B	M	31	68	EU	2.9	67	45	336
C	F	24	50	EU	3.0	57	120	304
D	M	50	80	EU	2.9	61	60	426
E	M	29	70	EU	2.5	58	15	444
F	F	17	51	HT[c]	18.0	44	120	338
G	F	42	51	HT[c]	17.6	62	60–120	243
H	M	60	54	HT[d]	8.4	105	90	700
I	F	27	50	HT[c]	8.9	47	60	257

[a] Adapted from Schuppan et al. [102].
[b] Euthyroid.
[c] Hyperthyroid, but under clinical control at the time.
[d] Hyperthyroid, but not under clinical control.

REFERENCES

1. Proelss, H. F. and Lohmann, H. J., Clin. Chem., 17, 222 (1971).
2. Finkle, B. S., Cherry, E. J., and Taylor, D. M., J. Chromatog. Sci., 9, 393 (1971).
3. Finkle, B. S., Foltz, R. L., and Taylor, D. M., J. Chromatog. Sci., 12, 304 (1974).
4. Foltz, R. L., Clark, P. A., Knowlton, D. A., and Hoyland, J. R., The Rapid Identification of Drugs from Mass Spectra, Final Report, R01-DA-00108, Batelle, Columbus, Ohio, Jan. 17, 1974.
5. Douglas, J. F., Smith, N. B., and Stockage, J. A., J. Pharm. Sci., 58, 145 (1969).
6. Rabinowitz, M. P., Reisberg, P., and Bodin, J. I., J. Pharm. Sci., 61, 1974 (1972).
7. Douglas, J. F., Kelley, T. F., Smith, N. B., and Stockage, J. A., Anal. Chem., 39, 956 (1967).
8. Beckett, A. H., Tucker, G. T., and Moffat, A. C., J. Pharm. Pharmacol., 19, 273 (1967).
9. Lebish, P., Finkle, B. S., and Brackett, J. W., Jr., Clin. Chem., 16, 195 (1970).
10. Finkle, B. S., Taylor, D. M., and Bonelli, E. J., J. Chromatog. Sci., 10, 312 (1972).
11. Caddy, B., Fish, F., and Scott, D., Chromatographia, 6, 251 (1973).
12. Caddy, B., Fish, F., and Scott, D., Chromatographia, 6, 293 (1973).
13. Moffat, A. C., J. Chromatog., 113, 69 (1975).
14. Berry, D. J. and Grove, J., J. Chromatog., 61, 111 (1971).
15. Caddy, B., Fish, F., and Scott, D., Chromatographia, 6, 335 (1973).
16. Boon, P. F. G. and Sudds, W., J. Pharm. Pharmacol., 19, 88S (1967).
17. Jack, D. B., Brechbuhler, A., Degen, P. H., Zbinden, P., and Reiss, W., J. Chromatog., 115, 87 (1975).
18. Melander, A., Danielson, K., Hanson, A., Rudell, B., Schersten, B., Thulin, T., and Wahlin, E., Clin. Pharmacol. Ther., 22, 104 (1977).
19. Haegele, K. D., Skrdlant, H. B., Robie, N. W., Lalka, D., and McNay, J. L., Jr., J. Chromatog., 126, 517 (1976).
20. Smith, K. M., Johnson, R. N., and Kho, B. T., J. Chromatog., 137, 431 (1977).
21. Talseth, T., Clin. Pharmacol. Ther., 21, 715 (1977).

REFERENCES

22. The United States Pharmacopeia, 19th rev., Mack Printing, Easton, Pa., 1974, p. 234.
23. Zak, S. B., Bartlett, M. F., Wagner, W. E., Gilleran, T. G., and Lukas, G., J. Pharm. Sci., 63, 225 (1974).
24. Hengstmann, J. H., Falkner, F. C., Watson, J. T., and Oates, J., Anal. Chem., 46, 34 (1974).
25. Erdtmansky, P. and Goehl, T. J., Anal. Chem., 47, 750 (1975).
26. Malcolm, S. L. and Marten, T. R., Anal. Chem., 48, 807 (1976).
27. Lennard, M. S., Silas, J. H., Smith, A. J., and Tucker, G. T., J. Chromatog., 133, 161 (1977).
28. Draffan, G. H., Clare, R. A., Murray, S., Bellward, G. D., Davies, D. S., and Dollery, C. T., in Proceedings of the Third International Symposium on Mass Spectrometry in Biochemistry and Medicine, Sardinia, Italy, June 1975.
29. Dollery, C. T., Davies, D. S., Draffan, G. H., Dargie, H. J., Dean, C. R., Reid, J. L., Clare, R. A., and Murray, S., J. Clin. Pharmacol. Ther., 19, 11 (1976).
30. Davies, D. S., Wing, L. M. H., Reid, J. L., Neill, E., Tippett, P., and Dollery, C. T., Clin. Pharmacol. Ther., 21, 593 (1977).
31. Reid, J. L., Wing, L. M. H., Mathias, C. J., Frankel, H. L., and Neill, E., Clin. Pharmacol. Ther., 21, 375 (1977).
32. Hodges, P., J. Pharm. Pharmacol., 28, 61 (1976).
33. Sadee, W., Finn, C., Castagnoli, N., and Garland, W., in P. D. Klein and S. V. Peterson (Eds.), Proceedings of the First International Conference on Stable Isotopes in Chemistry, Biology, and Medicine, Argonne National Laboratory, Argonne, Ill., 1973, pp. 346-352.
34. Sadee, W., Segal, J., and Finn, C., J. Pharmacokin. Biopharmaceut., 1, 295 (1973).
35. Settimj, G., Di Simone, L., and Del Giudice, M. R., J. Chromatog., 116, 263 (1976).
36. Zacchei, A. G. and Wishousky, T., J. Pharm. Sci., 65, 1770 (1976).
37. Sabih, K. and Sabih, K., J. Pharm. Sci., 59, 782 (1970).
38. Wickramasinghe, J. A. F. and Shaw, S. R., J. Pharm. Sci., 60, 1669 (1971).
39. Prescott, L. F. and Redman, D. R., J. Pharm. Pharmacol., 24, 713 (1972).
40. Simmons, D. L., Ranz, R. J., and Picotte, P., J. Chromatog., 71, 421 (1972).
41. Taylor, J. A., Clin. Pharmacol. Ther., 13, 710 (1972).
42. Matin, S. B. and Rowland, M., J. Pharm. Pharmacol., 25, 186, (1973).
43. Matin, S. B. and Rowland, M., Anal. Lett., 6, 865 (1973).

44. Aggarwal, V. and Sunshine, I., Clin. Chem., 20, 200 (1974).
45. Knight, J. B. and Matin, S. B., Anal. Lett., 7, 529 (1974).
46. Matin, S. B., Wan, S. H., and Karam, J. H., Clin. Pharmacol. Ther., 16, 1052 (1974).
47. Braselton, W. E., Jr., Ashline, H. C., and Bransome, E. D., Jr., Anal. Lett., 8, 301 (1975).
48. Braselton, W. E., Jr., Bransome, E. D., Jr., Ashline, H. C., Stewart, J. T., and Honigberg, I. L., Anal. Chem., 48, 1386 (1976).
49. Midha, K. K., McGilveray, I. J., and Charette, C., J. Pharm. Sci., 65, 576 (1976).
50. Williams, R. L., Blaschke, T. F., Meffin, P. J., Melmon, K. L., and Rowland, M., Clin. Pharmacol. Ther., 21, 301 (1977).
51. Belvedere, G., Fanelli, R., Frigerio, A., Malen, E., and Hugon, P., J. Chromatog. Sci., 13, 54 (1975).
52. Kleber, J. W., Galloway, J. A., and Rodda, B. E., J. Pharm. Sci., 66, 635 (1977).
53. Grostic, M. F., Wnuk, R. J., and MacKellar, F. A., J. Amer. Chem. Soc., 88, 4664 (1966).
54. Sabih, K., Mass Spectrom., 1, 163 (1974).
55. Kumar, D., Mehtalia, S. D., and Miller, L. V., J. Ass. Phys. India, 21, 275 (1973).
56. Knauff, R. E., Fajans, S. S., Ramirez, E., and Conn, J. W., Ann. N.Y. Acad. Sci., 74, 603 (1959).
57. Brook, R., Schrogie, J. J., and Solomon, H. M., Clin. Pharmacol. Ther., 9, 314 (1968).
58. Brotherton, P. M., Grieveson, P., and McMartin, C., Clin. Pharmacol. Ther., 10, 505 (1969).
59. Seiber, J. N., J. Agr. Food Chem., 20, 443 (1972).
60. McGilveray, I. J., Midha, K. K., and Sved, S., paper presented at the Pharmaceutical Analysis and Control Section, APhA Academy of Pharmaceutical Sciences, New Orleans, November 1974.
61. Wickramasinghe, J. A. F. and Shaw, S. R., J. Chromatog., 71, 265 (1972).
62. Matin, S. B., Karam, J. H., and Forsham, P. H., Anal. Chem., 47, 545 (1975).
63. Mottale, M. and Stewart, C. J., J. Chromatog., 106, 263 (1975).
64. Alkalay, D., Volk, J., and Bartlett, M. F., J. Pharm. Sci., 65, 525 (1976).
65. Alkalay, D., Khemani, L., Wagner, W. E., Jr., and Bartlett, M. F., J. Clin. Pharmacol., 15, 446 (1975).
66. Zimmerer, R. O., Jr. and Grady, L. T., J. Pharm. Sci., 60, 493 (1971).
67. Richards, A. H. and Mason, W. B., Anal. Chem., 38, 1751 (1966).

REFERENCES

68. Petersen, B. A., Hanson, R. N., Giese, R. W., and Karger, B. L., J. Chromatog., 126, 503 (1976).
69. Petersen, B. A. and Vouros, P., Anal. Chem., 49, 1304 (1977).
70. Petersen, B. A., Giese, R. W., Larsen, P. R., and Karger, B. L., Clin. Chem., 23, 1389 (1977).
71. Stouffer, J. E., Jaakonmaki, P. I., and Wenger, T. J., Biochem. Biophys. Acta, 127, 261 (1966).
72. Jaakonmaki, P. I. and Stouffer, J. E., J. Gas Chromatog., 5, 303 (1967).
73. Hollander, C. S., Trans. Ass. Amer. Physicians, 81, 96 (1968).
74. Jaakonmaki, P. I. and Stouffer, J. E., in A. Zlatkis (Ed.), Advances in Gas Chromatography, Preston Tech. Abstr. Co., Evanston, Ill., 1967, p. 149.
75. Stouffer, J. E., J. Chromatog. Sci., 7, 124 (1969).
76. Docter, R and Hennemann, C., Clin. Chim. Acta, 34, 297 (1971).
77. Nihei, N. N., Gershengorn, M. C., Mitsuma, T., Stringham, L. R., Cordy, A., Kuchmy, B., and Hollander, C. S., Anal. Biochem., 43, 433 (1971).
78. Tajuddin, M. and Elfbaum, S. G., Clin. Chem., 19, 109 (1973).
79. Hansen, L. B., Anal. Chem., 40, 1587 (1968).
80. Alexander, N. M. and Scheig, R., Anal. Biochem., 22, 187 (1968).
81. Backer, E. T. and Pileggi, V. J., J. Chromatog., 36, 351 (1968).
82. Shahrokhi, F. and Gehrke, C. W., Anal. Biochem., 24, 281 (1968).
83. Funakoshi, K. and Cahnmann, H. J., Anal. Biochem., 27, 150 (1969).
84. Funakoshi, K. and Cahnmann, H. J., in Proceedings of the Third International Congress on Endocrinolgy, Mexico City, 1968, Excerpta Medica Foundation, New York, p. 416.
85. Heinl, B. M. R., Ortner, H. M., and Spitzy, H., J. Chromatog., 60, 51 (1971).
86. Bilous, R. and Windheuser, J. J., J. Pharm. Sci., 62, 274 (1973).
87. Searcy, R. L., Diagnostic Biochemistry, McGraw-Hill, New York, 1969.
88. Tata, J. R., Biochem. J., 72, 214 (1959).
89. Zomzely, C., Marco, G., and Emery, E., Anal. Chem., 34, 1414 (1962).
90. Lovelock, J. E., Nature, 189, 729 (1961).
91. Larsen, P. R., Med. Clin. N. Amer., 59, 1063 (1975).
92. Sterling, K. A. and Hegedus, A., J. Clin. Invest., 41, 1031 (1962).
93. Levinson, S. S. and Rieder, S. V., Clin. Chem., 20, 1568 (1974).
94. Lee, N. D. and Pileggi, V. J., Clin. Chem., 17, 166 (1971).
95. Dibbo, A., Sly, J. C. P., and Stephensen, L., J. Chem. Soc., 2890 (1961).

96. Larsen, P. R., Metabolism, 21, 1073 (1972).
97. Larsen, P. R., in N. R. Rose and H. Friedman (Eds.), Manual of Clinical Immunology, American Society for Microbiology, Washington, D.C., 1976, pp. 222-230.
98. Kono, T., van Middlesworth, L., and Astwood, E. B., Endocrinology, 66, 845 (1960).
99. Nauman, J. A., Nauman, A., and Werner, S. C., J. Clin. Invest., 46, 1346 (1967).
100. Klebe, J. F., Finkbeiner, H., and White, D. M., J. Amer. Chem. Soc., 88, 3390 (1966).
101. Astwood, E. B., J. Amer. Med. Ass., 122, 78 (1943).
102. Schuppan, D., Riegelman, S., Lehmann, B., Pilbrant, A., and Becker, C., J. Pharmacokin. Biopharmaceut., 1, 307 (1973).

AUTHOR INDEX

Numbers in parentheses are reference numbers and indicate that an author's work is referred to although his name is not cited in the text. Underlined numbers give the page on which the complete reference is listed.

A

Aandahl, V., 95(236), 196(236), 247
Abraham, C. V., 80(206), 80(213), 97, 246
Abramson, F. P., 115, 116, 117, 118, 119, 120, 121, 249
Abuki, H., 164(313), 251
Adams, R. F., 80(163), 80(208), 105, 105(208), 244, 246
Adjepon-Yamoah, K. K., 79(125), 243
Affrime, M., 35(53), 240
Aggarwal, V., 288(44), 307, 386
Agurell, S., 80(193), 81(211), 109(193), 246, 247
Ahrens, E. H., Jr., 218(357), 223(357), 252
Albani, M., 80(188), 95(188), 245
Albert, K. S., 97(239), 248
Alexander, N. M., 344(80), 350(80), 370, 371, 387
Alkalay, D., 332(64), 332(65), 341, 341(64), 342, 346, 386

Alvarez-Ude, K., 233(376), 253
Anbar, M., 28, 30, 239
Ando, M., 164(313), 251
Anthony, G. M., 123(268), 123(269), 249
Araujo, O. E., 27, 28, 29, 239
Arnold, K., 34(37), 239
Ashline, H.C., 288(47), 288(48), 309(47), 311(47), 312(47), 314(47), 316(47), 316(48), 318(48), 319(48), 320(48), 322(48), 323(48), 386
Astwood, E. B., 362, 380, 388
d'Athis, P., 213(364), 253
Atkinson, A. J., Jr., 48, 48(70), 48(83), 48(84), 48(85), 48(88), 56, 58, 58(83), 58(84), 58(85), 58(88), 58(93), 64, 64(83), 65, 66, 70(93), 74(84), 76(83), 76(84), 76(85), 77(84), 78(84), 79(85), 79(117), 79(119), 79(120), 79(126), 79(128), 79(131), 241, 242, 243
Axenrod, T., 95(235), 196(340), 197(340), 247, 252

AUTHOR INDEX

Azarnoff, D. L., 218(360), 218(369), 224, 233(369), 233(370), 235(360), 235(369), 236(369), 236(370), 253

B

Bacallao, C. Z., 80(137), 243
Backer, E. T., 344(81), 350(81), 370, 372, 387
Baer, D. T., 58(92), 65, 67, 67(97), 68, 242
Baggett, B., 33, 37(56), 240
Bagnasco, G., 79(103), 242
Bailey, B. K., 165(319), 165(320), 170, 173, 251
Bailey, D. B., 80(196), 246
Baker, K. M., 111(253), 248
Ballard, B. E., 79(129), 243
Bareggi, S. R., 111(253), 248
Barkan, S., 40, 41(63), 42(63), 240
Barkus, J. C., Jr., 58(92), 65, 67, 68, 242
Barrett, A. M., 227, 253
Barrett, J., 80(146), 95(146), 244
Bartlett, M. F., 267(23), 332(64), 332(65), 341(64), 341(65), 342(65), 346(64), 385, 386
Battista, H., 80(139), 95(139), 243
Baylis, E. M., 80(149), 80(169), 244, 245
Becker, C., 380(102), 381(102), 383(102), 388
Beckett, A. H., 79(109), 79(112), 132(289), 135, 136, 139, 242, 250, 255(8), 384
Beermann, B., 196(346), 196(350), 206(346), 208, 212(350), 213, 252
Bellet, S., 35(50), 240
Bellward, G. D., 277(28), 278(28), 280(28), 385

Belvedere, G., 288(51), 327, 328, 386
Benet, L. Z., 48(86), 48(87), 58(86), 58(87), 61(86), 61(87), 63(87), 67(87), 72, 241, 242
Benowitz, N., 79(121), 243
Bergfors, P. G., 81(220), 247
Berlin, A., 80(193), 109, 218(363), 228(363), 230, 231, 246, 253
Berlin, I., 58(94), 65(94), 242
Berman, M., 78, 242
Berry, D. J., 80(162), 95(162), 244, 255(14), 384
Bianchetti, G., 165(328), 189, 251
Biemann, K., 79(135), 243
Bigger, J. T., 34(38), 239
Bilous, R., 344(86), 350(86), 380, 381, 387
Bine, R., Jr., 6(15), 238
Bishara, R. H., 129, 131, 132, 133, 249
Blair, D., 4(10), 238
Bland, C., 6(15), 238
Blankenhorn, D. H., 6, 19(16), 239
Blaschke, T. F., 80(186), 95(186), 245, 288(50), 325(50), 330(50), 331(50), 386
Blumer, J., 79(119), 243
Bodin, J. I., 255(6), 384
Bocrogi, L., 196(353), 215(353), 217(353), 252
Bogaert, M. G., 131(283), 131(284), 137(298), 137(299), 146, 148, 149, 249, 250
Bogan, J., 110, 248
Bonelli, E. J., 36(57), 79(57), 80(57), 80(159), 95(57), 240, 244, 255(10), 288(10), 384
Booker, H. E., 80(201), 105(201), 107, 108, 109, 110, 246
Boon, P. F. G., 255(16), 384
Boreus, L. O., 81(221), 247
Borga, O., 34(36), 80(193), 80(204), 81(218), 81(220),

[Borga] 105(204), 108(204), 109(193), 239, 246, 247
Boyes, R. N., 79(109), 79(118), 242, 243
Boza, O., 35(50), 240
Brachet-Liermann, A., 80(182), 245
Brackett, J. W., Jr., 123(270), 249, 255(9), 384
Bransome, E. D., Jr., 288(47), 288(48), 309(47), 311(47), 312(47), 314(47), 316(47), 316(48), 318(48), 319(48), 320(48), 322(48), 323(48), 386
Braselton, W. E., Jr., 288(47), 288(48), 309, 310, 311, 312, 314, 316, 318, 319, 320, 322, 323, 386
Brechbuhler, A., 256(17), 259(17), 264(17), 384
Breck, G. D., 79(115), 242
Bredesen, J. E., 48(77), 56(77), 57(77), 241
Bridgman, J. F., 233(374), 253
Briggs, W. A., 35(52), 45(52), 48(82), 58(82), 67(82), 69(82), 240, 241
Brochmann-Hanssen, E., 32, 240
Brodie, B. B., 45, 58(94), 65(94), 239, 240, 242
Brook, R., 315(57), 386
Brooks, C. J. W., 81(226), 123(268), 123(269), 247, 249
Brotherton, P. M., 315(58), 386
Brown, P., 29(31), 239
Brown, R. E., 79(114), 242
Brown, S. A., 165, 165(315), 165(316), 166, 169, 170, 171, 172, 251
Bruderlein, H., 218(361), 226, 227, 228, 229, 233, 253
Brunzell, J. D., 218(367), 233, 253
Bruschweiler, F., 29(31), 239
Buckmaster, H. S., 80(148), 244

Burnett, D., 80(170), 95(170), 245
Burris, B. C., 79(128), 243
Butler, C., 80(180), 80(198), 81(198), 82(198), 83(198), 84(198), 85(198), 88(198), 90(198), 91(198), 92(198), 93(198), 245, 246
Byars, B., 79(107), 242
Byers, S. O., 6(15), 238

C

Caddy, B., 255(11), 255(12), 255(15), 384
Cahnmann, H. J., 344(83), 344(84), 350(83), 373, 377, 379, 387
Camera, E., 137, 137(290), 141, 142, 250
Cameron, J. D., 79(127), 243
Canevari, R. J., 154(304), 250
Carroll, D. I., 81(227), 84(230), 86(232), 87(232), 247
Castagnoli, N., 281(33), 385
Catabeni, F., 115(263), 249
Cervoni, P., 152(339), 156, 158, 252
Chamberlain, J., 196(352), 215, 215(352), 252
Chang, T., 80(138), 80(172), 95(138), 97(237), 111(237), 243, 245, 248
Charette, C., 40, 42, 43, 44, 45, 240, 288(49), 319(49), 324(49), 325(49), 326(49), 386
Chasseaud, L. F., 236, 253
Cherry, E. J., 27, 36(28), 48(28), 79(28), 80(28), 123(28), 137(28), 152(28), 165(28), 180(28), 196(28), 204(28), 206(28), 218(28), 219(28), 239, 255(2), 256(2), 288(2), 384
Chidomere, E. C., 132(289), 135, 136, 139, 250
Chidsey, C. A., 111(253), 248

Chin, D. A., 80(157), 137(301), 151, 152, 153, 244, 250
Chow, M. S. S., 2, 4, 32, 34, 35(51), 238, 240
Christensen, H. D., 108, 248
Christensen, M., 4(10), 238
Christopher, G. T., 48(81), 58(81), 61(81), 62(81), 241
Chuang, C. M., 165(321), 170(321), 177(321), 178(321), 179(321), 251
Chucot, L., 97(237), 111(237), 248
Cimbura, G., 80(179), 245
Clare, R. A., 81(219), 247, 277(28), 277(29), 278(28), 280(28), 385
Clarke, P. A., 39(62), 79(62), 80(62), 95(62), 196(62), 197(62), 199(62), 215(62), 218(62), 219(62), 240, 255(4), 256(4), 384
Cohlmia, J. B., 218(360), 224, 235(360), 253
Collinsworth, K. A., 79(131), 243
Coltart, D. J., 35(48), 240
Cometti, A., 79(103), 242
Conn, H. L., 35(54), 240
Conn, J. W., 315(56), 386
Connor, J. N., 218(365), 231, 253
Conradi, E., 111(258), 248
Consolo, S., 154(308), 250
Cook, C. E., 80(204), 105(204), 108(204), 108, 246, 248
Cooper, J. K., 165(326), 165(330), 165(333), 185(326), 186(326), 187(326), 188(326), 190, 190(326), 190(330), 192(330), 193(330), 251
Cooper, J. R., 58(94), 65(94), 242
Cooper, J. W., Jr., 80(209), 99(209), 100(209), 101(209), 246
Cooper, R. G., 80(158), 244

Cordy, A., 344(77), 350(77), 367(77), 368(77), 387
Corrodi, H., 154(306), 154(307), 250
Costa, E., 115, 248, 249
Cox, S., 48(73), 51(73), 53(73), 54(73), 55(73), 241
Cremers, H. M. H. G., 80(173), 95(173), 245
Crombez, E., 164, 251
Curtius, H. C., 123(273), 249
Cutler, R. E., 48(81), 58(81), 61(81), 62(81), 241

D

Dalen, E., 196(350), 212(350), 213(350), 252
Danielson, K., 256(18), 259(18), 260(18), 384
Darcey, B., 80(147), 107(147), 244
Darcey, B. A., 80(201), 105(201), 107, 108, 109, 110, 246
Dargie, H. J., 277(29), 385
Davidow, B., 80(157), 244
Davidson, I. W. F., 137(297), 144, 145, 147, 250
Davies, D. L., 196(348), 209(348), 210, 252
Davies, D. S., 277(28), 277(29), 277(30), 278, 278(28), 280, 280(28), 282, 284, 385
Davis, D. L., 218(355), 218(356), 219(355), 222(355), 252
Davis, H. L., 80(196), 246
Dean, C. R., 277(29), 385
Dean, R. R., 124(275), 249
De Boer, T. J., 229, 253
Deckert, F. W., 165(322), 165(323), 165(327), 181, 183, 184, 251
Degen, P. H., 256(17), 259(17), 264(17), 384

AUTHOR INDEX

Del Giudice, M. R., 284(35), 385
De Marchi, F., 158, 160, 251
De Moerloose, P., 164, 251
Desager, J. P., 111(260), 196(351), 213, 213(351), 215, 248, 252
Dessouky, Y. M., 80(141), 244
De Villiers, L. S., 80(210), 100, 246
Diamond, I., 80(174), 245
Dibbo, A., 354(95), 387
Dicarlo, F. J., 137(297), 144(297), 145(297), 147(297), 250
Di Fazio, C. A., 79(114), 242
Dill, W. A., 99(237), 111, 248
Di Salle, E., 111(253), 248
Di Simone, L., 284(35), 385
Dobson, V. F., 246, 249
Docter, R., 344(76), 350(76), 366, 387
Doherty, J. E., 4(11), 238
Dollery, C. T., 81(219), 247, 277, 277(28), 277(29), 277(30), 278(28), 278(30), 280(28), 282(30), 284(30), 385
Donike, M., 123(272), 249
Dosa, S., 233(375), 253
Douglas, J. F., 255(5), 255(7), 384
Draffan, G. H., 81(219), 247, 277(28), 277(29), 278, 280, 385
Drayer, D. E., 48(75), 48(89), 58, 58(89), 65(95), 70, 241, 242
Driessen, O., 80(183), 245
Driscoll, P., 43, 240
Dubois, M., 80(182), 245
Duchateau, A. M. J. A., 125, 249
Dufresne, L., 65, 242
Duhme, D. W., 4(9), 238
Dujovne, C. A., 218(369), 233(369), 233(370), 235, 236, 236(370), 253
Dumont, P. A., 80(195), 246
Dutcher, J. S., 48(84), 48(85), 58(84), 58(85), 74(84),
[Dutcher] 76(84), 76(85), 77(84), 78(84), 79(85), 241
Dutta, J., 165(324), 170, 180, 182, 251
Dvornik, D., 218(361), 226, 228(361), 229(361), 233(361), 253
Dzidic, I., 81(227), 84(230), 86(232), 87(232), 247

E

Eisen, A. A., 111(247), 248
Elander, M., 80(202), 94(202), 105(202), 246
Elfbaum, S. G., 344(78), 350(78), 368, 369, 387
Elsom, L. F., 236, 253
Elson, J., 48(83), 58, 58(83), 58(93), 64, 70, 76(83), 241, 242
Emery, E., 351(89), 387
Emonds, A., 80(183), 245
Erdey, L., 80(141), 244
Erdtmansky, P., 268(25), 270, 272, 385
Eriksson, E., 34(42), 240
Ervik, M., 111(259), 196(343), 204, 206, 207(343), 212(343), 248, 252
Estas, A., 80(195), 246
Evans, G. H., 35(46), 35(47), 240
Evenson, M. A., 80(147), 107, 244

F

Fajans, S. S., 315(56), 386
Fales, H. M., 95(235), 95(236), 196(236), 196(340), 197(340), 247, 252
Falk, K. J., 80(196), 246

Falkner, F. C., 268(24), 270(24), 271(24), 385
Fanelli, R., 152, 154(308), 250, 288(51), 327(51), 386
Farnebo, L. O., 154(307), 250
Fastlich, E., 80(157), 244
Feher, T., 196(353), 215(353), 217, 252
Feit, P. W., 196(347), 206(347), 209, 209(347), 210, 211, 252
Field, F. H., 39(60), 39(61), 240
Finkbeiner, H., 370, 388
Finkle, B. S., 27, 36, 38, 48(28), 79(28), 79(57), 79(58), 80(28), 80(57), 80(58), 95(57), 95(58), 123(23), 123(270), 137(28), 152(28), 152(58), 165(28), 180(28), 196, 196(28), 196(58), 197, 198(58), 199(58), 204(28), 206(28), 218(28), 218(58), 219, 219(28), 219(58), 239, 240, 249, 255, 255(2), 255(3), 255(9), 255(10), 256(2), 288(2), 288(3), 288(10), 384
Fischer, E. P., 218(355), 218(356), 219(355), 222(355), 252
Fish, F., 255(11), 255(12), 255(15), 384
Florey, K., 241
Foltz, R. L., 36(58), 38(58), 39, 79(58), 79(62), 80(58), 80(62), 95(58), 95(62), 152(58), 196, 196(58), 196(62), 197, 197(58), 198, 198(58), 199(58), 199(62), 215(62), 218(58), 218(62), 219, 219(58), 240, 255, 255(3), 255(4), 256(4), 288(3), 384
Fontan, C. R., 32, 123(267), 240, 249
Forsham, P. H., 332(62), 336(62), 338(62), 339(62), 386
Fossel, E. T., 137(291), 140, 250
Frankel, H. L., 277(31), 280(31), 385

Friedman, H., 388
Friedman, M., 6(15), 238
Friel, P., 80(175), 80(184), 80(192), 95(184), 245, 246
Frigerio, A., 111(253), 152, 248, 250, 288(51), 327(51), 386
Frislid, K., 48(77), 56, 57, 58, 241
Funakoshi, K., 344(83), 344(84), 350(83), 373, 377, 379, 387
Furuya, T., 165(318), 170, 171, 177, 251
Fuxe, K., 154(306), 154(307), 250
Fry, D. E., 80(149), 80(169), 244, 245

G

Gaffney, T. E., 111(249), 111(250), 111(251), 111(252), 111(254), 111(255), 117(251), 248
Galeazzi, R. L., 48(86), 48(87), 58(86), 58(87), 61, 61(86), 62, 63, 67(87), 241
Gallaher, E. G., 80(159), 80(177), 244, 245
Galli, C., 247
Galloway, J. A., 288(52), 328(52), 333(52), 386
Gardner-Thorpe, C., 80(165), 80(167), 95(165), 95(167), 196(167), 199(167), 244
Garland, W. A., 190(336), 190(337), 252, 281(33), 385
Garle, M., 80(202), 80(216), 81(218), 94(202), 105(202), 105(216), 246, 247
Garattini, S., 154(308), 250
Garrett, E. R., 126, 127, 249
Garrettson, L. K., 80(187), 95(187), 245
Gartiez, D. A., 111(250), 120(265), 248, 249

AUTHOR INDEX

Gauchell, F. D., 80(188), 95(188), 245
Gehrke, C. W., 344(82), 350(82), 372, 373, 387
Gerber, N., 34(37), 239
Gershengorn, M. C., 344(77), 350(77), 367(77), 368(77), 387
Giannelly, R. J., 34(43), 240
Gibb, B. H., 137(292), 141(292), 250
Gibson, D. G., 35(48), 240
Gibson, T., 35(52), 45(52), 240
Gibson, T. P., 48(82), 58(82), 67, 67(82), 69, 70, 241
Giese, R. W., 344(68), 344(70), 350(68), 350(70), 352(68), 352(70), 354(68), 354(70), 356(70), 387
Gillen, H. W., 80(142), 80(144), 95(144), 95(233), 244, 247
Gilleran, T. G., 267(23), 385
Giovanniello, T. J., 80(185), 95(185), 245
Gjerdum, K., 4(4), 4(7), 238
Glazko, A. J., 34(35), 80(138), 80(172), 95(138), 97(237), 111(237), 239, 243, 245, 248
Glogner, P., 165(331), 251
Gobbeler, K. H., 137(296), 250
Goehl, T. J., 268(25), 270, 272, 385
Goldbaum, L. R., 110, 248
Goldberg, A. P., 218(367), 233, 253
Gordos, J., 80(215), 103, 104, 246
Goth, A., 1, 80(1), 123(1), 137(1), 152(1), 165, 194, 195(1), 238
Goudie, J. H., 80(170), 95(170), 245
Grady, L. T., 233(368), 253, 344(66), 345, 350, 350(66), 386
Graffner, C., 48(79), 48(80), 58, 58(79), 58(80), 60, 67(79), 71, [Graffner] 71(79), 72, 73, 74, 75, 241
Graham, D. N., 65, 242
Greaves, M. S., 80(158), 244
del Greco, F., 48(88), 58(88), 64(88), 66(88), 241
Greeley, R. H., 105, 248
Green, J. B., 80(191), 245
Green, J. R., 80(175), 80(192), 245, 246
Greenblatt, D. J., 4(9), 238
Greenwood, N. D., 79(124), 243
Grego, J., 79(111), 242
Gregory, P., 80(180), 245
Gresham, D., 80(213), 97, 246
Grieveson, P., 315(58), 386
Griffiths, W. C., 80(174), 245
Grimmer, G., 80(142), 80(190), 244, 245
Groschinsky, M., 196(345), 206(345), 207(345), 252
Groschinsky-Grind, M., 196(346), 206(346), 208(346), 252
Grostic, M. F., 313(53), 386
Grove, J., 80(162), 95(162), 244, 255(14), 384
Gruber, V. F., 196(344), 206(344), 207(344), 252
Guichard, A., 34(40), 79(116), 239, 242
Gugler, R., 218(360), 218(366), 224, 225, 226, 232, 235, 253
Gustavii, K., 196(343), 204, 206, 207(343), 212(343), 252

H

Haas, L. B., 218(367), 233, 253
Haber, E., 4(3), 238
Haddock, R. E., 190(337), 190(338), 252
Haegele, K. D., 256(19), 260, 261, 262, 264, 265, 384
Halkin, H., 79(130), 243

Hallmark, M., 97(239), 248
Hamberger, B., 154(307), 250
Hamburg, E. L., 43, 240
Hammar, C. G., 81(225), 247
Hammer, R. H., 80(152), 80(194), 95(152), 111(194), 244, 246
Haney, W. G., 48(73), 51(73), 53(73), 54(73), 55(73), 241
Hansen, L. B., 344(79), 350(79), 369, 387
Hanson, A., 256(18), 259(18), 260(18), 384
Hanson, R. N., 344(68), 350(68), 352(68), 354(68), 387
Harasymiv, I., 80(153), 244
Harrison, D. C., 79(131), 243
Hartel, G., 45, 241
Harvengt, C., 111(260), 248
Hashimoto, H., 19(23), 239
Haut, H., 218(359), 224, 225, 253
Hawkins, D. F., 81(219), 247
Hawkins, D. R., 236, 253
Haythorn, P., 80(212), 246
Hebert, R. M., 218(355), 218(356), 219(355), 222(355), 252
Hefferen, J. J., 79(105), 242
Hegedus, A., 352(92), 387
Heinl, B. M. R., 344(85), 350(85), 374, 377, 387
Heller, W. M., 239
Henderson, W. M., 79(132), 243
Hengstmann, J. H., 268, 268(24), 270, 271, 385
Heni, N., 165(331), 251
Hennemann, C., 344(76), 350(76), 366, 387
Hensley, W. J., 80(153), 244
Hickert, P., 82(228), 247
Hignite, C. E., 45, 46, 240
Higuchi, S., 154, 251
Hill, J. G., 80(207), 105(207), 111, 113, 246
Hill, R. E., 80(211), 102, 103, 246

Hill, R. M., 80(176), 80(180), 80(181), 80(198), 80(217), 81(198), 81(217), 81(224), 82(198), 82(228), 82(229), 83(198), 84(176), 84(198), 85(198), 88(198), 90(198), 91(198), 92(198), 93(198), 245, 246, 247
Hinderling, P. H., 126, 127, 249
Hodges, P., 277(32), 281, 385
Hollander, C. S., 344(73), 344(77), 350(77), 367(77), 368(77), 387
Holmstedt, B., 81(225), 247, 248
Honigberg, I. L., 288(48), 316(48), 318(48), 319(48), 320(48), 322(48), 323(48), 386
Hoppel, C., 80(202), 80(216), 94, 105, 246, 247
Hoque, M., 165(324), 170, 180, 182, 251
Horning, E. C., 4, 5, 11, 12(20), 13(20), 14(20), 15(20), 16(20), 17(20), 80(217), 81(217), 81(227), 84(230), 86(232), 87(232), 218(355), 218(356), 219(355), 222(355), 238, 239, 247, 252
Horning, M. G., 80, 80(176), 80(180), 80(181), 80(198), 80(217), 81(217), 81(227), 82, 82(228), 82(229), 83, 84, 84(176), 84(230), 84(231), 85, 86(232), 87(232), 88, 90, 91, 92, 93, 218(355), 218(356), 219, 220, 221, 222, 245, 246, 247, 252
Houin, G., 218(364), 253
Houston, A. B., 35(49), 240
Hoyland, J. R., 39(62), 79(62), 80(62), 95(62), 196(62), 197(62), 199(62), 215(62), 218(62), 219(62), 240, 255(4), 256(4), 384

Huang, C. M., 48(88), 58(88), 64(88), 66(88), 241
Hubbard, J. W., 165(330), 190(330), 192(330), 193(330), 251
Hucker, H. B., 79(134), 159, 161, 233, 233(368), 235, 243, 251, 253
Huffman, D. H., 45, 46, 218(360), 218(369), 224, 233(369), 233(370), 235(360), 235(369), 236, 236(369), 240, 253
Hugon, P., 288(51), 327(51), 386
Hung, A., 84(231), 247
Hurwitz, A., 218(369), 233(369), 235(369), 236(369), 253
Hutsell, T. C., 124, 125, 126, 249
Hvidberg, E., 80(164), 244
Hwang, B., 196(351), 213(351), 252

I

Idzu, G., 162(312), 164(313), 251
Inman, J. K., 108, 248
Irgens, T. R., 79(132), 243
Ishibashi, M., 162(312), 164(313), 251
Ishizaki, T., 111(250), 111(252), 248
Izawa, T., 162(312), 251

J

Jaakonmaki, P. I., 344(71), 344(72), 344(74), 350(71), 350(72), 359(71), 360, 360(71), 362, 363, 364, 365, 387
Jack, D. B., 255, 255(17), 256, 256(17), 259, 264, 384
Jacine, G., 247
Jacob, J., 80(190), 245
Jacobsson, S. E., 79(108), 242
Jahnchen, E., 165(332), 192, 193, 251

Jalling, B., 81(221), 247
Jelliffe, R. W., 4(13), 6, 19(16), 24, 238, 239
Jensen, C., 218(366), 232, 253
Jervell, J., 4(7), 238
Jessen, B., 80(205), 105(205), 110(205), 112(205), 246
Johnson, G. F., 80(200), 93(200), 218(365), 231, 246, 253
Johnson, R. N., 256(20), 265(20), 384
Johnson, S. A., 6, 8(17), 9(17), 10(17), 19(17), 239
Johnsson, G., 48(79), 58(79), 60(79), 67(79), 71(79), 241
Jones, P., 80(147), 107(147), 244
Jordan, D. B., 80(205), 105(205), 110(205), 112(205), 246
Jordan, G. L., Jr., 218(355), 218(356), 219(355), 222(355), 252
Jori, A., 154(308), 250
Joslin, H. D., 80(206), 97, 246
Julian, D. B., 239
Jusko, W. J., 80(187), 95(187), 245

K

Kaiser, D. G., 165(325), 183, 184, 185, 251
Kallberg, N., 81(221), 247
Kalman, S. M., 24, 26, 27(26), 239
Kananen, G., 80(168), 94(168), 101, 245
Kaplar, L., 80(141), 244
Karam, J. H., 288(46), 306(46), 308(46), 332(62), 336(62), 338(62), 339(62), 386
Karger, B. L., 344(68), 344(70), 350(68), 350(70), 352(68), 352(70), 354(68), 354(70), 356(70), 387

Karim, A., 124(275), <u>249</u>
Karlsen, J., 165(317), <u>251</u>
Karlsson, E., 48(72), 48(74), 58, 71(72), <u>241</u>
Karmen, A., 218(359), 224, 225, <u>253</u>
Katz, J., 79(110), <u>242</u>
Kaydan, H. J., 58(94), 65(94), <u>242</u>
Kaye, C. M., 132(287), <u>250</u>
Kazyak, L., 79(102), 80(102), 165(102), 169, <u>242</u>
Keenaghan, J. B., 49(90), 79(90), 79(118), <u>241</u>, <u>243</u>
Kellaway, P., 80(181), <u>245</u>
Kelley, T. F., 255(7), <u>384</u>
Kelley, J. G., 132, 132(285), 134, <u>250</u>
Kepler, J. A., 108, <u>248</u>
Kern, H., 48, 48(69), 79(69), <u>241</u>
Kerr, D. N. S., 233(376), <u>253</u>
Kessler, K. M., 35(52), 45, <u>240</u>
Khanna, U., 186(335), <u>251</u>
Khemani, L., 332(65), 341(65), 342(65), <u>386</u>
Kho, B. T., 137(301), 151(301), 153(301), <u>250</u>, 256(20), 265(20), <u>384</u>
Kibbe, A. H., 27, 28, 29, <u>239</u>
Kiddie, M. A., 132(286), 132(287), <u>250</u>
Kirk, P. L., 123(267), <u>249</u>
Klebe, J. F., 370, <u>388</u>
Kleber, J. W., 288(52), 328, 332, 333, <u>386</u>
Klein, M. W., 80(205), 105(205), 110(205), 112(205), <u>246</u>
Klein, P. D., <u>385</u>
Klein, S. W., 35(44), 56, 56(44), 58(44), 76, 77, <u>240</u>
Kleinberg, S. I., 137(293), 137(295), 142(293), 144(293), 144(295), <u>250</u>
Knapp, D. R., 111(254), 111(255), <u>248</u>

Knauff, R. E., 315(56), <u>386</u>
Knight, J. B., 80(159), <u>244</u>, 288(45), 301, 304, 305, 306, 315, <u>386</u>
Knight, J. C., 29, 30, 31, <u>239</u>
Knoblock, E. C., 79(102), 80(102), 165(102), 169, <u>242</u>
Knowlton, D. A., 39(62), 79(62), 80(62), 95(62), 196(62), 197(62), 198(62), 215(62), 218(62), 219(62), <u>240</u>, 255(4), 256(4), <u>384</u>
Knuchel, V. F., 218(358), <u>252</u>
Koch-Weser, J., 4(9), 35(44), 35(45), 56, 56(44), 58(44), 65(45), 67(45), 76, 77, <u>238</u>, <u>240</u>
Koehler, H. M., 79(105), <u>242</u>
Kofoed, J., 80(179), <u>245</u>
Kojima, H., 165(318), 170, 171, 177, <u>251</u>
Konig, R., 165(327), <u>251</u>
Kono, T., 362, <u>388</u>
Korhonen, A., 45, <u>241</u>
Koslow, S. H., 115(263), <u>249</u>
Kraml, M., 218(361), 226, 228(361), 229(361), 233(361), <u>253</u>
Krauer, B., 81(219), <u>247</u>
Krumlovsky, F. A., 48(88), 58(88), 64(88), 66(88), <u>241</u>
Kubo, K., 19(23), <u>239</u>
Kuc, J., 165(321), 170(321), 177(321), 178(321), 179(321), <u>251</u>
Kuchmy, B., 344(77), 350(77), 367(77), 368(77), <u>387</u>
Kumar, D., 315(55), <u>386</u>
Kupferberg, H. J., 80(150), 80(166), 80(192), 108, <u>244</u>, <u>246</u>, <u>248</u>
Kutt, H., 34(38), <u>239</u>

L

Ladinsky, H., 154(308), 250
Lalka, D., 67(97), 242, 256(19), 260(19), 262(19), 264(19), 265(19), 384
Lant, A. F., 196(348), 209(348), 210(348), 252
Larsen, N. E., 80(164), 95(234), 244, 247
Larsen, P. R., 344(70), 350(70), 352(70), 352(91), 354(70), 354(96), 356(70), 356(97), 387, 388
Latham, A. N., 80(211), 102, 103, 246
Latini, R., 165(328), 189(328), 251
Lau, H. L., 10, 239
Laubie, M. J., 154(304), 154(305), 350
Laurie, W. A., 39(60), 240
Law, M. R., 80(160), 244
Law, N. C., 95(236), 196, 196(236), 197, 247
Lawrence, R. C., 123, 249
Least, C. J., Jr., 80(200), 93, 246
Lebish, P., 123(270), 249, 255(9), 384
Le Douarec, J. C., 154(304), 154(305), 350
Lee, K. P., 186(335), 251
Lee, N. D., 353, 387
Lee, W. K., 48(83), 48(84), 48(85), 58(83), 58(84), 58(85), 64(83), 74(84), 76(83), 76(84), 76(85), 77(84), 78(84), 79(85), 241
Lehmann, B., 380(102), 381(102), 383(102), 388
Lennard, M. S., 268(27), 274, 385
Lertratanangkoon, K., 80(176), 80(180), 80(181), 81(227), 82(229), 84(176), 245, 247

Levandoski, P., 196(351), 213(351), 252
Levine, J., 40, 41(63), 42(63), 240
Levinson, S. S., 352(93), 387
Levy, G., 81(222), 165(329), 186(329), 247, 251
Levy, M., 65(95), 242
Levy, R. H., 48(76), 48(81), 52, 54, 58(81), 61(76), 61(81), 62(81), 79(122), 79(123), 241, 243
Lewis, R. J., 190(336), 252
Lhuguenot, J. C., 123(271), 249
Li, H., 152(339), 156, 158, 252
Lin, Y. J., 111(261), 249
Lind, M., 81(220), 247
Linde, H. H. A., 18(22), 239
Lindner, A., 48(81), 58(81), 61(81), 62(81), 241
Lindstrom, B., 196(345), 196(349), 196(350), 206(345), 207, 207(349), 208, 212, 212(349), 212(350), 213(350), 252
Lockwood, T., 48(86), 58(86), 61(86), 241
Lohmann, H. J., 80(155), 244, 255(1), 384
Lovelock, J. E., 352, 387
Lowden, J. A., 111(248), 248
Lowenthal, D. T., 35(52), 45(52), 240
Luchi, R. J., 35(54), 240
Lukas, D. S., 4(5), 4(8), 238
Lukas, G., 267(23), 385
Lund, L., 80(193), 109(193), 246
Lunde, P. K. M., 48(77), 56(77), 57(77), 241

M

MacGee, J., 80(145), 95(145), 101, 105, 109, 111(240), 244, 248
Machata, G., 80(139), 95(139), 243

AUTHOR INDEX

MacKellar, F. A., 313(53), 386
Maclean, I., 123(268), 249
Maggi, N., 79(103), 242
Maha, G. E., 233(368), 253
Maienthal, M., 40, 41(63), 42(63), 240
Malbica, J. O., 137(300), 150, 250
Malcolm, S. L., 268(26), 272, 274, 275, 276, 385
Malen, E., 288(51), 327(51), 386
Mallick, N. P., 233(375), 253
Manion, C. V., 67(97), 242
Marco, G., 351(89), 387
Marcus, M., 137(293), 137(295), 142(293), 144(293), 144(295), 250
Mardente, S., 158, 160, 251
Mark, L. C., 58(94), 65, 242
Marks, V., 80(149), 80(169), 244, 245
Marten, T. R., 268(26), 272, 274, 275, 276, 385
Martin, B., 33, 37(56), 240
Martin, R. S., 165(325), 183, 184, 185, 251
Martino, A. G., 4(8), 238
Mason, W. B., 344(67), 350(67), 351, 352, 386
Mather, L. E., 55, 242
Mathias, C. J., 277(31), 380(31), 385
Matin, S. B., 288(42), 288(43), 288(45), 288(46), 295, 295(42), 295(43), 296, 297(42), 298, 299, 300, 301, 302, 303, 304, 305, 306, 306(42), 307, 308, 315, 315(43), 325, 332(62), 336, 337, 338, 339, 385, 386
Matusik, E., 48(82), 58(82), 67(82), 69(82), 241
Matusik, J., 48(82), 58(82), 67(82), 69(82), 241
Maume, B., 11, 12, 13, 14, 15, 16, 17, 239

Maume, B. F., 123(271), 249
Mayersdorf, A., 80(152), 95(152), 244
Mayfield, D. E., 79(128), 243
McGilveray, I. J., 80(203), 95(203), 98(203), 165(326), 165(330), 185(326), 186(326), 187(326), 188(326), 190(326), 190(330), 192(330), 193(330), 246, 251, 288(49), 319(49), 324(49), 325(49), 325(60), 326(49), 386
McKenna, M. J., 80(160), 244
McMahon, F. G., 233(368), 253
McMartin, C., 315(58), 386
McNay, J. L., Jr., 256(19), 260(19), 262(19), 264(19), 265(19), 384
Meffin, P. J., 79(130), 243, 288(50), 325(50), 330(50), 331(50), 386
Mehtalia, S. D., 315(55), 386
Meijer, J. W. A., 80(189), 245
Melander, A., 256(18), 259, 260, 384
Melmon, K. L., 34(40), 79(116), 79(130), 80(186), 95(186), 239, 242, 243, 245, 288(50), 325(50), 330(50), 331(50), 386
Melville, R. S., 246, 249
Meola, J., 48(71), 49, 51, 79(71), 241
Merkus, F. W. H. M., 125(277), 249
Metaxas, J. M., 80(178), 95(178), 245
Meyer, K., 18(22), 239
Meyer, M. B., 67(97), 242
Michelucci, J., 137(301), 151(301), 153(301), 250
Michniewicz, B. M., 233(368), 253
Middleditch, B. S., 81(226), 123(269), 247, 249

Midha, K. K., 40, 42, 43, 44, 45, 80(203), 95, 95(203), 96, 98, 165(326), 165(330), 165(333), 185, 186, 187, 188, 190, 190(326), 190(330), 192, 193, 240, 246, 251, 288(49), 319, 323, 324, 325, 325(60), 326, 386
Millard, N. R., 196(348), 209(348), 210(348), 252
Miller, L. V., 315(55), 386
Milne, G. W. A., 95(235), 95(236), 196, 196(236), 196(340), 197, 247, 252
Mirkin, B. L., 81(223), 247
Mitsuma, T., 344(77), 350(77), 367(77), 368(77), 387
Miyada, D. S., 80(205), 105(205), 110(205), 112(205), 246
Miyazaki, H., 162, 164(313), 251
Moffat, A. C., 36, 39, 48(59), 79(59), 123(59), 152(59), 165, 180, 196, 196(59), 199, 218(59), 219, 240, 255, 255(8), 255(13), 256(13), 288(13), 381, 384
Molander, M., 196(345), 196(349), 206(345), 207(345), 207(349), 208(349), 212, 212(349), 252
Molin, L., 48(74), 241
Monson, K., 137(300), 150(300), 250
Morishita, N., 164(313), 251
Morrison, J. I., 111(256), 111(258), 248
Morselli, P. L., 111(253), 165(328), 189(328), 248, 251
Moss, A. J., 32(34), 239
Mottale, M., 332(63), 339, 341, 386
Mule, S. J., 80(156), 244
Muller, S. H., 48(69), 79(69), 241
Murray, M. H., 80(160), 244
Murray, S., 277(28), 277(29), 278(28), 280(28), 385

Murray, W. J., 137(292), 141(292), 250

N

Naestoft, J., 80(164), 95(234), 244, 247
Nakagawa, F., 97(238), 248
Nakamura, H., 218(357), 223(357), 252
Narasimhachari, N., 115, 249
Nau, H., 79(135), 243
Nauman, A., 362(99), 388
Nauman, J. A., 362(99), 388
Neflin, P. J., 80(186), 95(186), 245
Neill, E., 277(30), 277(31), 278(30), 280(31), 282(30), 284(30), 385
Neilson, K., 137(300), 150(300), 250
Nelson, H. A., 48(82), 58(82), 67(82), 69(82), 241
Nelson, M. B., 79(133), 243
Nelson, S. D., 79(133), 243
Nies, A. S., 35(47), 240
Nihei, N. N., 344(77), 350(77), 367, 368, 387
Nimmo, J., 132(285), 250
Nishihara, K., 97(238), 248
Norlander, B., 48(74), 241
Notari, R. E., 4(12), 238
Nowlin, J., 80(176), 80(180), 80(198), 80(217), 81(198), 81(217), 81(227), 82(198), 82(228), 82(229), 83(198), 84(176), 84(198), 85(198), 88(198), 90(198), 91(198), 92(198), 93(198), 245, 246, 247
Nursten, H. E., 79(124), 243

O

Oates, J., 268(24), 270(24), 271(24), 385
Ochs, H., 218(358), 252
Oder-Cederlof, A., 34(36), 239
Ogilvie, R. I., 65, 242
Oleksyk, S. K., 80(174), 245
Orme, M., 80(204), 105(204), 108, 109, 246
Ortengren, B., 79(108), 242
Ortner, H. M., 344(85), 350(85), 374(85), 387
Osiewicz, R., 80(168), 94(168), 101(168), 245
Ottestad, E., 171, 251
Owen, G., 80(158), 244

P

Palmer, K. H., 33, 37, 240
Papadopoulos, A. S., 80(169), 245
Parker, K. D., 123(267), 249
Parker, J. B. R., 79(109), 242
Parker, M., 48(70), 56(70), 58(70), 65(70), 79(120), 241, 243
Parsonage, M. J., 80(165), 80(167), 95(165), 95(167), 196(167), 199(167), 244
Pate, D., 34(40), 239
Patel, I. H., 79(123), 243
Patel, J. A., 79(136), 243
Patterson, D. A., 80(171), 245
Patton, R. D., 32(34), 239
Peat, M. A., 80(214), 105(214), 106, 246
Pecci, J., 80(185), 95(185), 245
Pecile, A., 247
Pellizzari, E. D., 165(321), 170, 177, 178, 179, 251
Pentikainen, P., 218(369), 233(369), 235(369), 236(369), 253
Perchalski, R. J., 80(194), 111, 246

Periroth, F., 79(131), 243
Perkins, W., 4(11), 238
Perkins, W. H., 6, 8(17), 9(17), 10(17), 19(17), 239
Perry, W. F., 35(49), 240
Petersen, B. A., 344(68), 344(69), 344(70), 350(68), 350(69), 350(70), 352, 353, 354, 354(68), 355, 356, 358, 359, 361, 387
Peterson, S. V., 385
Pettit, G. R., 29(31), 239
Picotte, P., 288(40), 293(40), 385
Pierides, A. M., 233(376), 253
Pilbrant, A., 380(102), 381(102), 383(102), 388
Pileggi, V. J., 344(81), 350(81), 353, 370, 372, 387
Pippenger, C. E., 80(144), 95(144), 95(233), 244, 247
Poet, R. B., 48(78), 241
Pohl, L. R., 190(337), 190(338), 252
Pratt, E. L., 79(111), 242
Pravisani, D., 137, 137(290), 141, 142, 250
Predmore, D. B., 80(177), 245
Prescott, L. F., 79(125), 132(285), 243, 250, 288(39), 292, 315(39), 316, 385
Privitera, P. J., 111(250), 111(254), 111(255), 121, 248, 249
Prcelss, H. F., 80(155), 244, 255(1), 384
Prue, D. G., 137(301), 151(301), 153(301), 250
Purnell, H., 245

R

Rabinowitz, M. P., 255(6), 384
Radin, H., 48(78), 241
Radzialowski, F. M., 124(275), 249

Rae, R., 132(285), 250
Ramirez, E., 315(56), 386
Rane, A., 80(216), 81(218), 105(216), 247
Rango, R. E., 65, 242
Ranney, R. E., 124(275), 249
Ranz, R. J., 288(40), 293(40), 385
Rapport, R. L., 108, 248
Rasmussen, K., 4(7), 238
Raymon, F., 79(128), 243
Redman, D. R., 288(39), 292, 315(39), 316, 385
Redweik, U., 123(273), 249
Regnier, G., 154(304), 250
Reichstein, T., 29(31), 239
Reid, J. L., 277(29), 277(30), 277(31), 278(30), 280, 282(30), 284(30), 385
Reidenberg, M. M., 35(52), 35(53), 45(52), 48(75), 48(89), 58(75), 58(89), 65(95), 240, 241, 242
Reisberg, P., 255(6), 384
Reiss, W., 256(17), 259(17), 264(17), 384
Resnick, G. L., 80(137), 243
Reuning, R. H., 4(12), 238
Reynolds, F., 79(112), 242
Rhodes, C. T., 80(209), 99(209), 100(209), 101(209), 246
Richards, A. H., 344(67), 350(67), 351, 352, 386
Richey, H. G., Jr., 10(18), 239
Richey, J. M., 10(18), 239
Rieder, S. V., 352(93), 387
Riedmann, M., 80(161), 244
Riegelman, S., 196(341), 196(342), 199(341), 199(342), 201, 201(341), 202(341), 203(341), 252, 380(102), 381(102), 383(102), 388
Ripley, J. E., 6, 8(17), 9(17), 10(17), 19, 19(17), 21, 22, 23, 24, 25, 239
Ritz, D. P., 80(197), 246

Robie, N. W., 256(19), 260(19), 262(19), 264(19), 265(19), 384
Robinson, W. T., 218(361), 226, 228(361), 229(361), 233(361), 253
Rodda, B. E., 288(52), 328(52), 333(52), 386
Roholt, K., 196(347), 206(347), 209(347), 210(347), 211(347), 252
Roman, L. R., 35(50), 240
Ronfeld, R. A., 2, 4, 32, 34, 35(51), 238, 240
Rose, N. R., 388
Rosen, A., 196(346), 206(346), 208(346), 252
Rosen, S. M., 233(374), 253
Ross, B., 40, 41(63), 42(63), 240
Rosseel, M. T., 131(283), 131(284), 137(298), 137(299), 146, 148, 149, 249, 250
Roth, R. J., 218(355), 218(356), 219(355), 222(355), 252
Rovenstine, E. A., 58(94), 65(94), 242
Rowland, M., 34(40), 79(116), 79(121), 79(122), 79(130), 80(186), 95(186), 239, 242, 243, 245, 288(42), 288(43), 288(50), 295, 295(42), 295(43), 296, 297(42), 298, 299, 300, 302, 303, 306(42), 315(43), 325, 330(50), 331(50), 385, 386
Royds, R. B., 132(286), 250
Rozanski, A., 31(33), 239
Rudell, B., 256(18), 259(18), 260(18), 384
Ruelius, H. W., 152(302), 250
Rutherford, B. S., 129, 131, 132, 133, 249
Ryhage, R., 81(225), 247

S

Sabih, K., 80(140), 80(151), 243, 244, 288, 288(37), 290, 293(37), 294, 313(54), 315(37), 317, 320, 385, 386
Sadee, W., 281, 281(33), 281(34), 283, 385
Sado, T., 154(309), 251
Saelens, D. A., 111(250), 111(254), 111(255), 121, 248, 249
Saitoh, Y., 97(238), 248
Sakimar, E., 97(239), 248
Sakmar, E., 4(10), 238
Sakurai, K., 19(23), 239
Samanin, R., 154(308), 250
Sampson, D., 80(153), 244
Sams, R. A., 4(12), 238
Sandberg, D. H., 80(137), 243
Sangster, I., 123(268), 249
Sarandis, S. G., 80(205), 105(205), 110(205), 112(205), 246
Sasaki, H., 154(309), 251
Sawlewicz, L., 18(22), 239
Schafer, H., 80(190), 245
Schaublin, J., 80(215), 103(215), 104(215), 246
Scheig, R., 344(80), 350(80), 370, 371, 387
Schersten, B., 256(18), 259(18), 260(18), 384
Schill, G., 79(104), 242
Schilling, P., 48(69), 79(69), 241
Schmidt, D. H., 34(38), 239
Schmitt, H., 154(305), 250
Schmitt, K. F., 165(332), 192, 193, 251
Schobben, F., 125(277), 249
Schraer, R., 10(18), 239
Schrogie, J. J., 315(57), 386
Schuppan, D., 380(102), 381, 383, 388
Schuppel, R. V., 165(327), 251

Schwartz, P. A., 80(209), 99, 100, 101, 246
Scott, D., 255(11), 255(12), 255(15), 384
Scott, D. B., 34(39), 239
Scott, E. M., 67, 67(98), 242
Scott, J. E., 80(144), 95(144), 244
Scott, K. N., 80(194), 111(194), 246
Searcy, R. L., 344, 344(87), 387
Sedaghat, A., 218(357), 223, 252
Sedman, A. J., 4(10), 238
Segal, J., 281(34), 385
Seiber, J. N., 319(59), 386
Sengupta, A., 80(214), 105(214), 106, 246
Serfontein, W. J., 80(210), 100, 246
Settimj, G., 284, 284(35), 385
Sevy, R. W., 48(75), 58(75), 241
Shah, V. P., 196(342), 199(342), 252
Shahrokhi, F., 344(82), 350(82), 372, 373, 387
Shand, D. G., 35(46), 35(47), 35(48), 240
Shanks, R. G., 132(285), 250
Shaw, S. R., 288(38), 290, 291, 332, 332(61), 385, 386
Shaw, T. R. D., 132(286), 250
Sheehan, M., 80(212), 246
Sheiner, L. B., 48(86), 48(87), 58(86), 58(87), 61(86), 61(87), 63(87), 67(87), 241
Shelley, L. L., 80(148), 244
Shelver, W. H., 79(132), 243
Sherber, P. A., 137(293), 137(295), 142, 144, 144(293), 250
Sherrard, D. J., 218(367), 233, 253
Sherwin, A. L., 111(247), 248
Shoeman, D. W., 218(360), 218(369), 224, 233(369),

[Shoeman] 233(370), 235(360), 235(369), 236(369), 236(370), 253
Shyluk, J. P., 165, 165(315), 166, 169, 170, 171, 172, 251
Siegfried, J., 123(273), 249
Silas, J. H., 268(27), 274(27), 385
Silvestri, S., 218, 218(354), 252
Simmons, D. L., 288(40), 293, 385
Simons, K. J., 48(76), 48(81), 52, 54, 58(81), 61, 61(76), 61(81), 62(81), 241
Sine, H. E., 80(160), 244
Singh, B. N., 132(288), 134, 250
Sisenwine, S. F., 152(302), 250
Sitar, D. S., 65, 242
Sjogren, J., 48(79), 58(79), 60(79), 67(79), 71(79), 241
Sjoqvist, F., 48(74), 80(193), 80(204), 80(216), 81(218), 81(220), 105(204), 105(216), 108(204), 109(193), 241, 246, 247
Skillen, A. W., 233(376), 253
Skinner, R. F., 80(159), 80(177), 244, 245
Skrdlant, H. B., 256(19), 260(19), 262(19), 264(19), 265(19), 384
Slotki, I. N., 233(375), 253
Sly, J. C. P., 354(95), 387
Smethurst, P. F., 80(165), 95(165), 244
Smith, A. J., 196(348), 209(348), 210(348), 252, 268(27), 274(27), 385
Smith, E., 40, 41, 42, 240
Smith, H., 110, 248
Smith, K. M., 256(20), 265, 267, 384
Smith, N. B., 255(5), 255(7), 384
Smith, T. W., 4(3), 4(9), 238
Sokolowski, C. D., 111(247), 248

Soldin, S. J., 80(207), 105(207), 111, 113, 246
Solomon, H. M., 80(200), 93(200), 218(365), 231, 246, 253, 315(57), 386
Solow, E. B., 80(178), 80(191), 95(178), 245
Sorensen, H., 196(347), 206(347), 209(347), 210(347), 211(347), 252
Spiehler, V., 80(205), 105(205), 110, 111, 112, 246
Spitzy, H., 344(85), 350(85), 374(85), 387
Spring, P., 80(215), 103(215), 104(215), 246
Sprissler, R., 137(300), 150(300), 250
Stachelski, S. J., 124, 125, 126, 249
Stafford, M., 80(180), 84(231), 247
Stauffer, S. C., 79(134), 159, 161, 233(368), 243, 251, 253
Steck, W., 165(319), 165(320), 170, 173, 251
Steele, J. M., 58(94), 65(94), 242
Steinhilber, E., 165(327), 251
Steinmann, B., 123(273), 249
Stephensen, L., 354(95), 387
Sterling, J., 48(73), 51, 53, 54, 55, 241
Sterling, K. A., 352(92), 387
Stewart, C. J., 332(63), 339, 341, 386
Stewart, J. T., 288(48), 316(48), 318(48), 319(48), 320(48), 322(48), 323(48), 386
Stillwell, R. N., 80(176), 80(181), 80(198), 81(198), 81(227), 82(198), 82(229), 83(198), 84(176), 84(198), 84(230), 85(198), 86(232), 87(232), 88(198), 90(198), 91(198),

[Stillwell] 92(198), 93(198), 245, 246, 247
Stillwell, W. G., 80(176), 80(180), 80(181), 80(198), 81(198), 81(227), 82(198), 82(228), 82(229), 83(198), 84(176), 84(198), 84(231), 85(198), 88(198), 90(198), 91(198), 92(198), 93(198), 245, 246, 247
St. John, G. A., 28, 30, 239
Stockage, J. A., 255(5), 255(7), 384
Stoll, R. G., 4(10), 238
Storstein, L., 4(6), 4(7), 238
Stouffer, J. E., 344(71), 344(72), 344(74), 344(75), 350(71), 350(72), 350(75), 359, 360, 360(71), 362, 363, 364, 365, 387
Stratton, C., 80(217), 81(217), 247
Street, H. V., 80(143), 244
Streiff, R. R., 80(152), 95(152), 244
Stringham, L. R., 344(77), 350(77), 367(77), 368(77), 387
Strong, J., 48(70), 56(70), 58(70), 65(70), 241
Strong, J. M., 48(83), 48(84), 48(85), 48(89), 58(83), 58(84), 58(85), 58(89), 58(93), 64(83), 70(93), 74, 76, 76(83), 76(84), 76(85), 77, 78(84), 79, 79(117), 79(119), 79(120), 79(126), 79(128), 79(131), 241, 242, 243
Sudds, W., 255(16), 384
Summers, T. R., 80(178), 95(178), 245
Sun, L., 80(205), 105(205), 110(205), 112(205), 246
Sung, C. Y., 34(41), 239
Sunshine, I., 80(168), 94(168), 101(168), 245, 288(44), 307, 386

Suzuki, T., 97(238), 248
Sved, S., 325(60), 386
Svendsen, A. B., 165(317), 171, 251
Svinhufvud, G., 79(108), 242
Szabo, E. I., 137(297), 144(297), 145(297), 147(297), 250

T

Tajuddin, M., 344(78), 350(78), 368, 369, 387
Takacs, J., 80(141), 244
Takayama, H., 162(312), 164(313), 251
Talseth, T., 256(21), 264, 266, 384
Tan, L., 17, 18, 20, 239
Tata, J. R., 351(88), 387
Taylor, D. M., 27, 36(28), 36(57), 36(58), 38(58), 48(28), 79(28), 79(57), 79(58), 80(57), 80(58), 95(57), 95(58), 123(28), 137(28), 152(28), 152(58), 165(28), 180(28), 196(28), 196(58), 197(58), 198(58), 199(58), 204(28), 206(28), 218(28), 218(58), 219(28), 219(58), 239, 240, 255(2), 255(3), 255(10), 256(2), 288(2), 288(3), 288(10), 384
Taylor, J. A., 288(41), 294, 295, 385
Teorell, T., 77(100), 242
Thebault, J. J., 218(364), 253
Thompson, E. D., 43, 240
Thomson, P. D., 34(40), 79(116), 239, 242
Thorp, J. M., 227(372), 233(374), 253
Thulin, T., 256(18), 259(18), 260(18), 384
Tigelaar, R. E., 108, 248

AUTHOR INDEX

Tindell, G. L., 111(249), 111(256), 248
Tippett, P., 277(30), 278(30), 282(30), 284(30), 385
Tompsett, S. L., 79(113), 242
Toothill, C., 80(165), 80(167), 95(165), 95(167), 196(167), 199(167), 244
Toseland, P. A., 80(162), 80(188), 95(162), 95(188), 244, 245
Trager, W. F., 79(115), 79(133), 190(336), 190(337), 190(338), 242, 243, 252
Tramell, P., 26, 239
Trezeguet, C., 80(182), 245
Troupin, A. S., 80(184), 95(184), 245
Trowell, J. M., 137(294), 143, 250
Truant, A. P., 34(41), 239
Tucker, G. T., 55, 242, 255(8), 268(27), 274(27), 384, 385
Tuong, A., 218(362), 228, 228(362), 253
Tuong, T. C., 218(362), 228, 228(362), 253

U

Udall, J. A., 165(329), 186(329), 251
Udenfriend, S., 45, 240
Ungerstedt, U., 154(306), 154(307), 250

V

Valentine, J. L., 43, 45, 240
Vandemark, F. L., 80(208), 105, 105(208), 246
Van Den Bossche, W., 164, 251
Vanden Heuvel, W. J. A., 4, 5, 196(344), 206, 206(344), 207, 238, 252
Vanderbist, M., 196(351), 213(351), 252
Van Durme, J. P., 131(283), 131(284), 249, 250
Van Meter, J. C., 80(148), 80(154), 95(154), 244
Van Middlesworth, L., 362, 388
Varadi, A., 196(353), 215(353), 217(353), 252
Verheesen, P. E., 80(173), 95(173), 245
Versille, C., 80(182), 245
Vessman, J., 79(104), 79(106), 242
Volk, J., 332(64), 341(64), 346(64), 386
Von Hagen, P., 165(317), 251
Vouros, P., 115, 249, 344(69), 350(69), 352(69), 354, 355, 356, 358, 359, 361, 387

W

Wagner, J. G., 4(10), 97(239), 111(261), 186(335), 238, 248, 249, 251
Wagner, W. E., Jr., 267(23), 332(65), 341(65), 342(65), 385, 386
Wahlin, E., 256(18), 259(18), 260(18), 384
Walker, R. W., 196(344), 206(344), 207(344), 252
Wall, M. E., 33, 37(56), 240
Wallace, E., 110, 248
Wallace, S. M., 196(341), 196(342), 199, 199(341), 199(342), 201, 201(341), 202, 203, 252
Walle, K., 111(258), 248
Walle, T., 80(199), 87, 111(249), 111(250), 111(251), 111(252), 111(254), 111(255), 111(256), 111(257), 111(258), 117(251), 120(265), 121, 246, 248, 249

Walwick, E. R., 80(205), 105(205), 110(205), 112(205), 246
Wan, S. H., 288(46), 306(46), 308(46), 386
Ward, J. W., 196(348), 209(348), 210(348), 252
Warner, C. R., 137(301), 151(301), 153(301), 250
Warner, H., 35(52), 45(52), 65(95), 240, 242
Warren, C. G., 80(197), 246
Warrington, H. P., 79(111), 242
Watkins, W. D., 111(253), 248
Watson, E., 24, 26, 27(26), 239
Watson, J. R., 123, 249
Watson, J. T., 268(24), 270(24), 271(24), 385
Webster, L. T., Jr., 79(128), 243
Weidler, D., 97(239), 111(261), 248, 249
Weidner, L., 128, 130, 249
Weiss, M. F., 78, 242
Welling, P. G., 186, 251
Wenger, T. J., 344(71), 350(71), 359(71), 360(71), 387
Werner, S. C., 362(99), 388
White, D. M., 370, 388
White, S. E., 233(368), 253
Wickramasinghe, J. A. F., 288(38), 290, 291, 332, 332(61), 385, 386
Wilder, B. J., 80(152), 80(194), 95(152), 111(194), 244, 246
Wilensky, A. J., 111(248), 248
Wilkinson, J., 48(82), 58(82), 67(82), 69(82), 241
Williams, A. F., 137(292), 141, 250
Williams, E. B., 165(321), 170(321), 177(321), 178(321), 179(321), 251
Williams, F. M., 81(219), 247
Williams, R. L., 288(50), 325, 330, 331, 386
Willis, P. W., 4(10), 238
Willox, S., 132(288), 134, 250

Wilson, A., 80(217), 81(217), 247
Wilson, D. L., 80(203), 95(203), 98(203), 246
Wilson, G. M., 196(348), 209(348), 210(348), 252
Wilson, W. E., 6, 8, 9, 10, 11, 12(20), 13(20), 14(20), 15(20), 16(20), 17(20), 19, 19(17), 21, 22, 23, 24, 25, 239
Windheuser, J. J., 344(86), 350(86), 380, 381, 387
Wing, L. M. H., 277(30), 277(31), 278(30), 280(31), 282(30), 284(30), 385
Winkle, R. A., 79(131), 243
Wishousky, T., 285, 285(36), 286, 287, 385
Wnuk, R. J., 313(53), 386
Wolf, F. J., 196(344), 206(344), 207(344), 252
Wolfensberger, M., 123(273), 249
Wright, R. C., 67, 67(98), 242

Y

Yacobi, A., 165(329), 186, 251
Yates, J. D., 4(10), 238
Ygge, H., 81(220), 247
Yoshii, E., 19(23), 239

Z

Zacchei, A. G., 128, 130, 249, 285, 285(36), 286, 287, 385
Zak, S. B., 267(23), 385
Zbinden, P., 256(17), 259(17), 264(17), 384
Zimmerer, R. O., Jr., 344(66), 345, 350, 350(66), 386
Zion, T. E., 80(181), 245
Zlatkis, A., 387
Zomzely, C., 351(89), 387

SUBJECT INDEX

A

Acenocoumarin, 180, 182, 183, 189, 190, 192
   detection limits of, 189, 192
   methyl derivative of, 190
   pentafluorobenzyl derivative of, 189
   recovery of, 189, 192
   silyl derivative of, 182
   structure of, 183
p-(Acetamido-d_3)-N-(2-diethylaminoethyl-1,1-d_2)-benzamide, see N-Acetylprocainamide, deuterated
Acetazolamide, 194, 195, 197, 198, 199-204
   binding of, to erythrocytes, 201, 204
     equation for, 201
   concentration in erythrocytes of, 201
     equation for, 201
   concentration in plasma of, 200, 201, 202, 203
     equation for, 201
   concentration in red blood fraction of, 200, 202, 203
     equation for, 200
   detection limits of, 200
   dissociation constant for, 201, 204

[Acetazolamide]
   maximum binding capacity of, 201, 204
   methyl derivative of, 200
   recovery of, 200
   structure of, 195
Acetic acid, 157, 219, 220, 221, 339
Acetic anhydride, 17, 21, 125
Acetohexamide, 289, 328, 332, 333
   metabolism of, 328
   methyl derivative of, 328
   pyrolysis of, 328
   pharmacokinetic data for, 333
   recovery of, 332
   structure of, 289
Acetone, 24, 26, 103, 171, 192, 200, 221, 224, 268, 327, 340
Acetonitrile, 111, 121, 122, 123, 263, 353, 373, 374
3-(α-Acetonylbenzyl)-4-hydroxycoumarin, see Warfarin
3-(α-Acetonyl-p-chlorobenzyl)-4-hydroxycoumarin, 184
   pentafluorobenzyl derivative of, 184
   recovery of, 184
3-(α-Acetonyl-p-nitrobenzyl)-4-methoxycoumarin, 190
Acetylacetone, 274

N-Acetylprocainamide, 47, 49, 52, 53, 54, 55, 56, 57, 58, 59, 61, 62, 63, 64, 65, 66, 67, 68, 69, 70, 71, 72, 73, 74, 75, 76, 77, 78, 79
  acid hydrolysis of, 55
  alkaline hydrolysis of, 55
  ^{13}C-labeled, 77, 78
  detection limits of, 65
  deuterated, 76, 77, 78
  dialysance, 65, 66
    equation for, 65
  dialytic clearance of, 65, 66
    equation for, 65
  half-life of, 64, 67, 68, 74, 77, 78
  one-compartment model for, 71
  pharmacokinetics of, 58, 65, 67, 68, 71, 72, 73, 74, 75, 76, 77, 78, 79
  plasma clearance of, 77, 78
  protein binding of, 65
  rate of change of, 72, 73, 74
    equations for, 72, 73, 74
  recovery of, 56, 65, 67
  renal clearance of, 68, 74, 77, 78
  structure of, 47, 50
  total body clearance of, 68
  three-compartment model for, 74, 76, 78
  volume of distribution of, 64, 68, 74, 77, 78
Aesculetin, 169, 171, 172, 176, 179
  acetate derivative of, 169, 172
  silyl derivative of, 171, 176, 179
  structure of, 169
Aesculetin dimethyl ether, 167, 169, 171, 180, 181
  structure of, 167
Aesculin, 179
  silyl derivative of, 179
Aglycone(s), 3, 4, 6, 14, 17, 21, 22, 23, 27
β-Alanine, 115, 118
  silyl derivative of, 115, 118

Aldactone, see Spironolactone
Aldadiene, 215, 216, 217
  detection limits of, 217
  recovery of, 217
  structure of, 216
Albumin, 331
Alkali ionization detector (GC), see Nitrogen detector
Alkaline phosphatase, 331
3-Allyl-5-isobutyl-2-thiohydantoin, 95
5-Allyl-5-phenylbarbituric acid, 105
  methyl derivative of, 105
Alprenolol, 120, 121, 134, 135
  heptafluorobutyryl derivative of, 135
  structure of, 121
Alseroxylon, 255
Amformin, 343
Amino acids, 115, 117, 118, 119, 374, 375, 376, 377, 378, 379
  iodinated, 374, 375, 376, 377, 378, 379
    silyl derivatives of, 374, 375, 376, 377, 378, 379
    structures of, 375, 376, 377
  silyl derivatives of, 115, 118, 119
p-Aminobenzoic acid, 47, 76
  acetyl derivative of, 76
  acetyl/methyl derivative of, 76
  methyl derivative of, 76
  structure of, 47
2-Amino-4-butylamino-6-chlorodifluoromethyl-s-triazine, 346
2-Amino-4-butylamino-6-heptafluoropropyl-s-triazine, 346
2-Amino-4-butylamino-6-pentafluoroethyl-s-triazine, 346
2-Amino-4-butylamino-6-trifluoromethyl-s-triazine, 346
2-Amino-4-chlorodifluoromethyl-6-(N-ethyl-N-phenethyl)amino-s-triazine, 346

SUBJECT INDEX

2-Amino-4-chlorodifluoromethyl-
6-(α-methylphenethyl)amino-
s-triazine, 346
2-Amino-4-chlorodifluoromethyl-
6-(p-methylphenethyl)amino-
s-triazine, 346
2-Amino-4-chlordifluoromethyl-
6-pentylamino-s-triazine,
346
2-Amino-4-chlorodifluoromethyl-
6-phenethylamino-s-triazine,
346
2-Amino-4-dichlorofluoromethyl-
6-phenethylamino-s-triazine,
346
p-Amino-N-(2-diethylaminoethyl)
benzamide, see Procainamide
2-Amino-4-dimethylamino-
6-trifluoromethyl-s-triazine,
346
p-Amino-N-(2-dipropylaminoethyl)
benzamide, 48, 49, 50, 52,
53, 56, 62, 64, 70, 74
  acetyl derivative of, 70, 74
  detection limits of, 52
  mass spectrum of, 50
  structure of, 50, 53
N-(2-Aminoethyl)octahydroazocine,
268, 269, 270, 271
  structure of, 268
  trifluoroacetyl derivative of, 269,
  270, 271
  structure of, 271
2-Amino-4-(N-ethyl-N-phenethyl)
amino-6-heptafluoropropyl-
s-triazine, 346
2-Amino-4-(N-ethyl-N-phenethyl)
amino-6-pentafluoroethyl-
s-triazine, 346
2-Amino-4-(N-ethyl-N-phenethyl)
amino-6-trifluoromethyl-
s-triazine, 346
2-Amino-4-heptafluoropropyl-6-
(α-methylphenethyl)amino-
s-triazine, 346

2-Amino-4-heptafluoropropyl-6-
(p-methylphenethyl)amino-s-
triazine, 346
2-Amino-4-heptafluoropropyl-6-
pentylamino-s-triazine, 346
2-Amino-4-heptafluoropropyl-6-
phenethylamino-s-triazine,
346
2-Amino-4-(p-methoxyphenethyl)
amino-6-trifluoromethyl-s-
triazine, 346
2-(Aminomethyl)benzo-1,4-dioxane,
270, 271
  trifluoroacetyl derivative of, 270,
  271
  structure of, 271
2-Amino-4-(α-methylphenethyl)
amino-6-pentafluoroethyl-s-
triazine, 346
2-Amino-4-(p-methylphenethyl)
amino-6-pentafluoroethyl-s-
triazine, 346
2-Amino-4-(α-methylphenethyl)
amino-6-trifluoromethyl-s-
triazine, 346
2-Amino-4-(p-methylphenethyl)
amino-6-trifluoromethyl-s-
triazine, 346
2-Amino-4-pentafluoroethyl-6-
pentylamino-s-triazine, 346
2-Amino-4-pentafluoroethyl-6-
phenethylamino-s-triazine,
346
2-Amino-4-pentylamino-6-tri-
fluoromethyl-s-triazine, 346
2-Amino-4-phenethylamino-6-
trifluoromethyl-s-triazine,
346
Aminopyrine, 164, 165
2-Amino-4-trifluoromethyl-6-
(2-phenethyl)amino-1,3,5-
triazine, 340
  structure of, 340
Amisometradine, 196, 199
  structure of, 199

Ammonium carbonate, 91, 92
Ammonium chloride, 62
Ammonium hydroxide, 206, 227, 281, 282, 362, 363, 380, 382
Ammonium sulfate, 381
Amobarbital, 309
Androst-4-ene-3,6,17-trione, 215, 217
Angelicin, 166, 167, 169, 170, 174, 177, 180, 181
  structure of, 167
β-Anhydrodigitoxigenin, 2
  structure of, 2
β-Anhydrodigoxigenin, 2
  structure of, 2
β-Anhydrogitoxigenin, 3
  structure of, 3
Anisindione, 180, 181
  structure of, 181
Antazoline, 277
Antiarrhythmic agents, 32-137
Antihyperlipidemia drugs, see Antisclerosis drugs
Antihypertensive drugs, 255-287
Antipyrine, 224
Antisclerosis drugs, 218-238
Antithyroid drugs, 380-383
Aprindine, 32, 129-131, 132, 133
  degradation products of, 132
  degradation study of, 131, 133
  recovery of, 131, 133
  structure of, 129
Aprobarbital, 307
Arachidic acid, 223
  methyl ester of, 223
Arbutin, 179
  silyl derivative of, 179
Argon (GC carrier gas), 4, 5, 6, 26, 135, 150, 156, 200, 206, 296, 337, 343, 353, 368, 374
Argon ionization detector (GC), 4, 5, 6, 169
Ascorbic acid, 124
Aspirin, 81

Atmospheric pressure ionization source, 84, 86, 87, 93
  detection limits of, 86, 87, 90
  negative ion spectra using, 93
Atropine, 32, 33, 36, 39, 40
Ayapin, 175, 180, 181
  structure of, 175

B

Barbital, 87, 91, 93
  pentafluorobenzyl derivative of, 87, 91, 93
  detection limits of, 91
Barium hydroxide, 380
Base peak, 38, 46, 47, 49, 75, 85, 93, 115, 192, 219, 263, 264, 353
Benzalkonium chloride, 124
Benzene, 18, 24, 26, 40, 41, 45, 56, 67, 74, 76, 122, 128, 135, 146, 150, 163, 206, 221, 228, 258, 271, 285
Benzoylglucosiduronic acid, 81
Benzylamine, 270, 271
  trifluoroacetyl derivative of, 270, 271
  structure of, 271
2-N-Benzylamino-5-chlorobenzophenone, 154, 155
  mass spectrum of, 155
  structure of, 155
Benzylbiguamide, 336, 337
  reaction with monochlorodifluoroacetic anhydride, 337
  structure of, 336
4-Benzyl-3-n-butylamino-5-sulfamylbenzoic acid, 209
  methyl derivative of, 209
Benzylmalonate methyl ester monoamide, 93, 94
  silyl derivative of, 94
Bergapten, 166, 168, 169, 170, 172, 177, 180, 181

SUBJECT INDEX

[Bergapten]
  structure of, 168
Bethanidine, 256, 269, 270, 271
  alkaline hydrolysis product(s) of, 269, 270, 271
    trifluoroacetyl derivative of, 269, 270, 271
    structure of, 271
  structure of, 256
Biguanides, 288, 289, 332-343, 346
  cyclization of, 336
  reaction with acid anhydrides, 336, 343
  structures of common, 289
Bile acids, 219, 220, 221
  methyl/silyl derivative of, 221
Bilirubin, 326, 330
Bishydroxycoumarin, 182, 183
  structure of, 183
Bis-(trimethylsilyl)acetamide, 11, 14, 17, 33, 123, 143, 286, 369, 370, 372, 373, 374, 377, 380
Bis-(trimethylsilyl)trifluoroacetamide, 31, 33, 40, 157, 220, 221
6-Bromo-3,4-dihydro-2H-1,2,4-benzothiadazine-7-sulfonamide-1,1-dioxide, 206, 207
  methyl derivative of, 206, 207
9-Bromophenanthrene, 87
Bufadienolides, 19
Buformin, 289, 332, 334, 335, 336, 337, 338, 341, 343
  detection limits of, 334, 337
  pyrolysis product(s) of, 334, 335
  reaction with monochlorodifluoroacetic anhydride, 337, 338
  structure of, 289, 336
Bumetanide, 194, 195, 209-212
  detection limits of, 210
  methylation sequence for, 209-210
  methyl derivative of, 209, 210
  recovery of, 210

[Bumetanide]
  structure of, 195, 210
Bunolol, 120, 121
  structure of, 121
n-Butanol, 164, 165, 362, 380
2-n-Butylamino-4,6-diamino-1,3,5-triazine, 334, 335
  structure of, 334
3-n-Butylamino-4-phenoxy-5-sulfamylbenzoic acid, see Bumetanide
Butylbiguanide, 233
1-Butyl-3-p-carboxyphenylsulfonylurea, 296, 297, 298, 299, 300, 301, 302, 303
  detection limits of, 298
  half-life of, 301
  pharmacokinetic data for, 301, 302, 303
  reaction product with 2,4-dinitrofluorobenzene, 297, 299
  recovery of, 298
  structure of, 296
1(n-Butyl)-3-p-chlorobenzenesulfonylurea, 291
  structure of, 291
  thermal degradation of, 291
Butyl-2,4-dinitroaniline, 296, 299, 300
1-Butyl-3-p-hydroxymethylphenylsulfonylurea, 297, 298, 299, 300, 301, 302, 303
  detection limits of, 298, 301
  half-life of, 301
  pharmacokinetic data for, 301, 302, 303
  reaction product with 2,4-dinitrofluorobenzene, 297, 299
  recovery of, 298
  structure of, 297
Butyric anhydride, 134
Byakangelicin, 175, 180, 182
  structure of, 175

C

Caffeic acid, 178
  silyl derivative of, 178
Caffeine, 55, 83, 134, 195, 197
Calibration factor, 140, 142
Camylofine, 164, 165
  alkaline hydrolysis of, 164
  recovery of, 165
  structure of, 164
Canrenone, see Aldadiene
Carbamazepine, 93, 94, 97, 99, 106, 107, 111, 113
  detection limits of, 93, 97
  methyl derivative of, 97, 99, 106, 107
  recovery of, 94, 97
  silyl derivative of, 94
Carbimazole, 380, 381, 382
  structure of, 382
Carbon disulfide, 52, 107, 115, 185, 186, 190
Carboxytolbutamide, 293, 309, 310, 315, 316, 317, 318, 319, 320, 321, 323, 325
  methyl derivative of, 293, 309, 310, 315, 316, 317, 318, 319, 320, 321, 323, 325
    deuterated, 317
  methyl/heptafluoropropionyl derivative of, 316, 317, 318, 319, 320, 321, 323
  methyl/pentafluoropropionyl derivative of, 316, 317, 318, 319, 320, 321, 323
  methyl/trifluoroacetyl derivative of, 309, 310, 315, 316, 317, 318, 319, 320, 321, 323
  trifluoroacetyl derivative of, 309, 310, 315, 316, 317, 318, 319, 320, 321, 323
3-Carboxytriazolophthalazine, 262, 263, 265
  structure of, 262

Cardadienolides, 17, 18, 19, 20
  acetyl derivative of, 17, 20
  mechanism of formation of, 19
  silyl derivative of, 17, 18, 20
  structure of, 18
Cardenolides, 12, 17, 18, 19, 20
  acetyl derivative of, 17, 20
  β-anhydro derivative of, 17
  silyl derivative of, 12, 17, 18, 20
  structure of, 18
Carotene, 344
Catechin, 179
  silyl derivative of, 179
Chalcone, 179
  silyl derivative of, 179
Charcoal, 49, 51
Chlordiazepoxide, 49, 51, 55
p-Chlorobenzenesulfonamide, 291, 292, 293, 295, 309
  structure of, 291
p-Chlorobenzenesulfonylurea, 294, 295, 309
  degradation of, 295
  half-life of, 295
  structure of, 294
Chlorobutanol, 124
Chlorodifluoroacetic anhydride, 343
2-Chloro-10-(3'-dimethylaminopropyl)phenothiazine-S-oxide, 214
p-Chlorodisopyramide, 125, 126
Chloroform, 31, 51, 52, 70, 76, 99, 102, 103, 107, 125, 126, 129, 157, 158, 186, 196, 220, 223, 225, 226, 227, 235, 261, 263, 268, 281, 288, 290, 291, 362, 363
Chlorogenic acid, 178
  silyl derivative of, 178
Chlorogenin, 5
Chloroglycerol dinitrate, 140

SUBJECT INDEX 415

7-Chloro-3-methyl-2H-1,2,4-
benzothiadiazine-1,1-
diazoxide, see Diazoxide
2-(4-Chloro-3-methylphenoxy)-
2-methylpropionic acid, 231,
methyl ester of, 231
Chlorophenoxyacetic acid, 224, 225,
231
butyl ester of, 231
methyl ester of, 224
recovery of, 231
p-Chlorophenoxyisobutyric acid,
219, 220, 221, 222, 223, 224,
225, 226, 227, 228, 229, 230,
231, 232
bound fraction in serum of, 232
butyl ester of, 231
detection limits of, 226, 227, 230,
231, 232
glucuronide of, 222, 225, 226
half-life of, 226
methyl ester of, 223, 224, 225,
226, 227, 228, 229, 230, 231,
232
protein binding of, 226
recovery of, 224, 226, 227, 231,
232
silyl derivative of, 219, 220, 222
structure of, 219, 230
unbound fraction in plasma of,
226, 232
equation for, 232
3-(p-Chlorophenoxy)propionic acid,
223, 224, 225, 231
butyl ester of, 231
methyl ester of, 223, 224
recovery of, 231
p-Chlorophenprocoumon, 192, 193,
194
recovery of, 194
(p-Chlorophenyl)(m-trifluoromethyl-
phenoxy)acetic acid, 233, 234,
235
glucuronide of, 235

[p-Chlorophenyl)(m-trifluoromethylphenoxy)acetic acid]
half-life of, 235
methyl ester of, 234, 235
structure of, 234
Chlorothiazide, 55, 194, 195, 196,
197, 198, 199, 255
structure of, 196
Chlorpropamide, 288, 289, 290,
292, 293, 294, 295, 296, 297,
299, 300, 309, 310, 311, 312,
313, 314, 315, 316, 317, 318,
319, 320, 321, 322, 323, 324,
325
detection limits of, 290, 315
half-life of, 295
metabolism of, 293, 294, 295
methyl derivative of, 288, 290,
292, 293, 294, 309, 310, 311,
312, 313, 314, 315, 316, 317,
318, 319, 320, 321, 322, 323
deuterated, 317
methyl enol ether of, 322
methyl/heptafluorobutyryl derivative of, 316, 317, 318, 319,
320, 321, 323
methyl/pentafluoropropionyl
derivative of, 316, 317, 318,
319, 320, 321, 323
methyl/trifluoroacetyl derivative
of, 310, 311, 312, 313, 314,
315, 316, 317, 318, 319, 320,
321, 323
structure of, 312
pharmacokinetic data for, 294,
295, 325
reaction product with 2,4-dinitro-
fluorobenzene, 296, 299
recovery of, 290, 293, 309, 324
structure of, 289, 294
trifluoroacetyl derivative of,
310, 311, 312, 313, 314, 315,
316, 317, 318, 319, 320, 321,
323

Chlorthalidone, 194, 195, 196,
    204-206, 207, 208, 212, 255
  detection limits of, 206
  ethyl derivative of, 206
  methyl derivative of, 204, 206,
    208
  recovery of, 208
  structure of, 195
Chlorzoxazone, 152
Cholestane, 5, 6, 129, 131
Cholesterol, 27, 28, 29, 214, 215,
    219, 221, 222, 236, 344
  silyl derivative of, 27, 28, 29,
    222
Cholic acid, 221
  ^{14}C-labeled, 221
Cholylglycine hydrolase, 221
Cinchona alkaloids, 42
  silyl derivative of, 42
Cinchonidine, 32, 40, 41, 42, 43,
    44, 45, 46, 47
  methyl derivative of, 41, 42, 43,
    44, 45, 46, 47
    fragmentation pattern of, 44
  recovery of, 41
  silyl derivative of, 40, 42
Cinchonine, 32, 40, 41, 42, 44
  methyl derivative of, 45
  silyl derivative of, 40, 41, 42
Cinnamic acid, 178
  silyl derivative of, 178
Citric acid, 124
Citropten, see 5,7-Dimethoxy-
    coumarin
Clofibrate, 218-233, 235, 236
  detection limits of, 224
  half-life of, 233
  metabolism of, 219, 225
  pharmacokinetics of, 224, 225,
    226, 228, 229, 230, 233
  recovery of, 224
  structure of, 218
Clonazepam, 189
Clonidine, 256, 277-281, 307

[Clonidine]
  amounts of drug absorbed, 279
    equation for, 279
  area under plasma concentration-
    time curve, 279, 280
    equation for, 280
  bioavailability of, 279, 280, 282
    equation for, 279
  detection limits of, 278
  deuterated, 277, 278
    methyl derivative of, 278
  half-life of, 277, 280, 282
  metabolism of, 281
  methyl derivative of, 278
  non-renal clearance of, 284
    definition of, 284
  pharmacokinetics of, 277-278
  plasma clearance of, 282, 283
  recovery of, 277
  renal clearance of, 279, 280, 284
    equation for, 279
  structure of, 256
  two-compartment model for,
    278-279, 280, 282-283
    equation for, 278-279
  volume of distribution of, 282,
    283
Cocaine, 32
Codeine, 32, 33, 55, 164, 165
Columbianetin, 174, 177
  structure of, 174
Column packing (solid substrate)
  adsorptivity of, 10, 151
  types of
    Anakrom-series, 140, 169
    Celite-type, 137
    Chromosorb-series, 21, 28, 31,
      36, 41, 45, 48, 49, 70, 75,
      76, 87, 92, 96, 99, 104, 105,
      107, 123, 125, 128, 129, 131,
      135, 136, 144, 156, 162, 165,
      170, 174, 177, 182, 183, 185,
      189, 190, 192, 193, 214, 215,
      224, 230, 259, 263, 284, 291,

SUBJECT INDEX 417

[Column packing (solid substrate)]
  [types of]
    [Chromosorb-series], 293, 296,
      308, 322, 337, 340, 343, 367,
      368, 369, 370, 372, 373, 374
    Diatomite-series, 52, 209, 215,
      217
    Diatoport S, 292, 352
    Embacel, 142
    Gas Chrom-series, 4, 5, 7, 11,
      17, 19, 21, 26, 27, 40, 45,
      52, 56, 58, 62, 67, 94, 95,
      102, 106, 111, 126, 134, 135,
      143, 146, 148, 150, 151, 154,
      159, 161, 165, 170, 184, 198,
      200, 206, 208, 212, 220, 223,
      225, 227, 230, 231, 232, 234,
      235, 237, 267, 269, 272, 275,
      276, 278, 283, 286, 289, 291,
      292, 309, 317, 327, 332, 345,
      360, 362, 363, 364, 365, 366,
      370, 371, 380, 382
    Glass beads, 49, 51, 58, 158,
      334
    Porapak-series, 165
    Supelcoport, 97, 129, 224, 310,
      317, 353, 354
Coronary vasodilators, 137-165
  non-organonitro compounds,
    137-152
  organonitro compounds, 152-165
m-Coumaric acid, 178
  silyl derivative of, 178
o-Coumaric acid, 178
  silyl derivative of, 178
p-Coumaric acid, 178
  silyl derivative of, 178
Coumarin, 165, 166, 167, 169, 174,
  176, 177, 178, 181, 182, 183
  structure of, 167
Coumarin-type anticoagulants,
  165-194
Coumurrayin, 174, 177
  structure of, 174

Creatine phosphokinase, 233, 236
Creatinine, 62, 65, 66, 69, 127,
  209, 213, 232, 284
  clearance of, 62, 65, 69, 127,
    213, 232
  dialytic clearance of, 65
Cyclandelate, 152
Cyclobenzaprine, 159, 161, 162
  ^{14}C-labeled, 162
  detection limits of, 161
  structure of, 159
Cyclohexane, 268, 310, 317
Cyclohexanecarboxylic acid, 106,
  107
  methyl derivative of, 106, 107
Cyclopentanone oxime, 163
Cyheptamide, 111

D

Dalbergin, 175, 180, 182
  structure of, 175
Daphnetin, 168, 169, 171, 172, 176
  acetate derivative of, 168, 172
  silyl derivative of, 172, 176
  structure of, 168
Debrisoquin, 256, 268, 269, 270,
  271, 272, 273, 274, 275, 276,
  277
  acetylacetone derivative of, 274,
    277
  alkaline hydrolysis product of,
    269, 270, 271
  trifluoroacetyl derivative of,
    269, 270, 271
    structure of, 271
  detection limits of, 274, 277
  deuterated, 272, 273, 274
    hexafluoroacetylacetone derivative of, 272, 273, 274
  hexafluoroacetylacetone derivative of, 272, 273, 274, 275
    mass spectrum of, 275
    structure of, 273

[Debrisoquin]
  pharmacokinetics of, 276
  structure of, 256, 273
d_{10}-Decadeuteriodebrisoquin, 272, 273, 274
  hexafluoroacetylacetone derivative of, 273, 274
Decadeuteropiperidine, 163
N-Deisopropylpropranolol, 117, 120, 121, 122, 123
  detection limits, 123
  heptafluorobutyryl derivative of, 117
  recovery of, 123
  structure of, 120
  trifluoroacetyl derivative of, 122, 123
    structure of, 122
    detection limits of, 123
Demerol, 83
Desdimethylcyclobenzaprine, 161, 162
  trifluoroacetyl derivative of, 162
Deserpidine, 255, 257, 258
  structure of, 257
Desmethylcyclobenzaprine, 161, 162
  trifluoroacetyl derivative of, 162
Diazepam, 55
Diazomethane, 76, 185, 186, 190, 214, 221, 224, 228, 229, 231, 234, 237, 283, 284, 286, 294, 301, 309, 310, 317, 319, 322, 345
Diazoxide, 256, 281-284
  deuterated, 281, 282, 283
    methyl derivative of, 283
    structure of, 282
    synethsis of, 282
  half-life of, 283
  methyl derivative of, 283
  pharmacokinetics of, 283, 284
  renal clearance of, 284
  structure of, 256
Dibenzylsuccinate, 123

Dibucaine, 52
2,4-Di-(n-butylamino)-6-amino-1,3,5-triazine, 334, 335
  structure of, 334
2-(2,6-Dichloroanilino)-2-imidazoline, see Clonidine
(6,7-Dichloro-2-cyclopentyl-2-methyl-1-oxo-5-indanyloxy) acetic acid, 285, 286
  methyl derivative of, 285, 286
Dichlorofluoroacetic anhydride, 343
[6,7-Dichloro-2-(4-hydroxyphenyl)-2-methyl-1-oxo-5-indanyloxy] acetic acid, 286, 287
  half-life of, 287
  methyl derivative of, 286
  methyl/silyl derivative of, 286
  pharmacokinetic data for, 287
  silyl derivative of, 286
  structure of, 286
Dichloromethane, see Methylene chloride
(6,7-Dichloro-2-methyl-1-oxo-2-phenyl-5-indanyloxy)acetic acid, 257, 285-287
  detection limits of, 287
  half-life of, 287
  metabolism of, 286
  methyl derivative of, 285, 286
  pharmacokinetic data for, 287
  recovery of, 287
  structure of, 257
2-(2,6-Dichlorophenylamino)-2-imidazoline-4,4,5,5-^{2}H, see Clonidine, deuterated
2,6-Dichlorophenylguanidine, 281
(2,4-Dichlorophenyl)(3-trifluoromethylphenoxy)acetic acid, 234, 235
  methyl derivative of, 234, 235
  structure of, 234
[2,3-Dichloro-4-(2-thienyl)phenoxy] acetic acid, see Tienilic acid
Dichlorphenamide, 196

SUBJECT INDEX

Dicumarol, 55
N-[2-(Diethylamino)ethyl]-2-
  phenylglycinate, see
  Camylofine
Diethylene glycol dinitrate, 137,
  140, 141, 142
Diethyl ether, 54, 76, 96, 106, 132,
  134, 135, 143, 151, 161, 199,
  209, 212, 214, 217, 218, 224,
  231, 234, 269, 277, 278, 283,
  297, 301, 310, 343, 381, 382
N,N-Diethyl-N'-(2-indanyl)-N'-
  phenyl-1,3-propanediamine,
  see Aprindine
N,N-Diethyl-N'-phenyl-1,3-
  propanediamine, 132
Diginatigenin, 23, 24
  17α epimer of, 23, 24
  CPK model of, 24
Digitalin, 27
Digitalis, 1, 6
  source of, 1
Digitalis-type glycosides, 1-32
Digitoxigenin, 2, 6, 7, 8, 9, 10,
  11, 12, 13, 14, 15, 16, 17,
  21, 22, 23, 25, 26, 27, 28,
  30
  acetyl derivative of, 21, 22, 23
  bisdigitoxoside, 25
    silyl derivative of, 25
  heptafluorobutyryl derivative of,
    26, 27
  monodigitoxoside, 25
    silyl derivative of, 25
  recovery of, 26
  silyl derivative of, 6, 7, 8, 9, 11,
    12, 13, 14, 15, 16, 17, 21,
    22, 23, 25
    mass spectrum of, 13, 15, 16
    structure of, 7
  structure of, 2, 30
Digitoxin, 2, 3, 4, 6, 9, 10, 19, 23,
  25, 26, 27, 32
  acetyl derivative of, 21

[Digitoxin]
  half-life of, 4
  heptafluorobutyryl derivative of,
    26, 27
  pharmacokinetics of, 4
  plasma protein-binding of, 4
  renal clearance of, 4
  silyl derivative of, 6, 19, 23, 25
  structure of, 2
  therapeutic concentration of, 4
  volume of distribution of, 4
Digoxigenin, 2, 6, 7, 8, 9, 10, 11,
  12, 14, 17, 19, 21, 22, 23,
  25, 26, 27, 28, 29
  acetyl derivative of, 21, 22, 23
  bisdigitoxoside of, 6, 7, 8, 25, 27
    heptafluorobutyryl derivative of,
      27
    silyl derivative of, 6, 7, 8, 25
  detection limits of, 26
  heptafluorobutyryl derivative of,
    26, 27
  monodigitoxoside of, 6, 7, 8, 25,
    27
    heptafluorobutyryl derivative of,
      27
    silyl derivative of, 6, 7, 8, 25
  recovery of, 26
  silyl derivative of, 6, 7, 8, 9, 10,
    11, 12, 14, 17, 19, 21, 22,
    23, 27, 28, 29
    structure of, 7
  structure of, 2
Digoxin, 2, 4, 6, 7, 8, 9, 10, 20,
  23, 24, 25, 26, 27, 32, 55,
  233
  bisdigitoxoside, 27
    heptafluorobutyryl derivative of,
      27
  half-life of, 4
  heptafluorobutyryl derivative of,
    24, 26, 27
  ^{3}H-labeled, 24
  monodigitoxoside, 27

[Digoxin]
  [monodigitoxoside]
    heptafluorobutyryl derivative of, 27
  pharmacokinetics of, 4
  plasma protein-binding of, 4
  renal clearance of, 4
  silyl derivative of, 6, 7, 8, 20, 23, 25, 27
  structure of, 2
  therapeutic concentration of, 4
  volume of distribution of, 4
Dihydrocinchonidine, 40, 41, 42
  silyl derivative of, 40, 41, 42
Dihydrocinchonine, 40, 42
  silyl derivative of, 40, 42
Dihydrodigoxigenin, 3, 11, 12, 22, 23, 25
  acetyl derivative of, 22, 23
  silyl derivative of, 11, 12, 22, 23, 25
  structure of, 3
3,4-Dihydro-1-methyl-2(1H)-isoquinoline carboxamidine, 270, 272, 274, 277
  acetylacetone derivative of, 274, 277
  detection limits of, 272
  structure of, 270
  trifluoroacetylacetone derivative of, 272
  structure of, 272
3,4-Dihydro-1-methyl-2(1H)-isoquinoline carboxamidoxime, 256, 270
  metabolism of, 270
  structure of, 256, 270
Dihydroquinidine, 40, 41, 42
  silyl derivative of, 40, 41, 42
Dihydroquinine, 40, 42
  silyl derivative of, 40, 42
4,7-Dihydroxycoumarin, 171, 173, 176
  silyl derivative of, 171, 176

[4,7-Dihydroxycoumarin]
  structure of, 173
6,7-Dihydroxycoumarin, see Aesculetin
7,8-Dihydroxycoumarin, see Daphnetin
5-(3,4-Dihydroxy-1,5-cyclohexadien-1-yl)-5-phenylhydantoin, 80, 83, 95, 105
2,4-Dihydroxydiphenylhydantoin, 95
  methyl derivative of, 95
3,4-Dihydroxydiphenylhydantoin, 95
  methyl derivative of, 95
4,4'-Dihydroxydiphenylhydantoin, 95
  methyl derivative of, 95
Dihydroxyphenobarbital, 83
3,4-Dihydroxyphenylacetic acid, 178
  silyl derivative of, 178
Dihydroxysecobarbital, 80, 81, 83
  silyl derivative of, 81
3,5-Diiodo-3',5'-dibromothyronine, 354, 359, 360, 361
  heptafluorobutyryl derivative of, 354, 359, 360, 361
  methyl derivative of, 354, 359, 360, 361
  methyl/heptafluorobutyryl derivative of, 354, 359, 360, 361
  structure of, 360
3,5-Diiodo-3',5'-dichlorothyronine, 359, 360, 361
  heptafluorobutyryl derivative of, 359, 360, 361
  methyl derivative of, 359, 360, 361
  methyl/heptafluorobutyryl derivative of, 359, 360, 361
  structure of, 360
3,3'-Diiodothyronine, 349, 350, 365, 366, 367, 374, 377
  methyl derivative of, 350, 365, 366, 367

[3,3'-Diiodothyronine]
  methyl/methoxy derivative of, 350
  methyl/pivalyl derivative of, 365, 366, 367
  methyl/trifluoroacetyl derivative of, 366, 367
  pivalyl derivative of, 365, 366, 367
  silyl derivative of, 374, 377
  structure of, 349
  trifluoroacetyl derivative of, 366, 367
3,5-Diiodothyronine, 349, 350, 351, 352, 353, 359, 360, 361, 365, 366, 367, 369, 370, 372, 373, 374, 377, 380
  detection limits of, 373, 380
  heptafluorobutyryl derivative of, 359, 360, 361
  methyl derivative of, 350, 351, 352, 359, 360, 361, 365, 366, 367
  methyl/heptafluorobutyryl derivative of, 359, 360, 361
  structure of, 360
  methyl/pivalyl derivative of, 365, 366, 367
  methyl/trifluoroacetyl derivative of, 351, 352, 366, 367
  pivalyl derivative of, 365, 366, 367
  silyl derivative of, 369, 370, 372, 373, 374, 377,
  structure of, 349
  trifluoroacetyl derivative of, 351, 352, 366, 367
3',5'-Diiodothyronine, 349, 350, 365, 366, 367, 377, 380
  detection limits of, 380
  methyl derivative of, 350, 365, 366, 367
  methyl/methoxy derivative of, 350
  methyl/pivalyl derivative of, 365, 366, 367
  methyl/trifluoroacetyl derivative of, 366, 367

[3',5'-Diiodothyronine]
  pivalyl derivative of, 365, 366, 367
  silyl derivative of, 377
  structure of, 349
  trifluoroacetyl derivative of, 366, 367
3,5-Diiodotyrosine, 348, 350, 351, 352, 360, 362, 365, 367, 369, 370, 371, 372, 373, 374
  detection limits of, 372, 373
  methyl derivative of, 350, 351, 352, 360, 362, 365, 367
  methyl/methoxy derivative of, 350
  methyl/pivalyl derivative of, 360, 362, 365, 367
  methyl/trifluoroacetyl derivative of, 351, 352, 367
  pivalyl derivative of, 360, 362, 365, 367
  silyl derivative of, 369, 370, 371, 372, 373
  structure of, 348
  trifluoroacetyl derivative of, 351, 352, 367
4-Diisopropyl-2-(p-chlorophenyl)-2-(2-pyridyl)butyramide, see p-Chlorodisopyramide
4-Diisopropylamino-2-phenyl-2-(2-pyridyl)butyramide, see Disopyramide
Dimethadione, 94
4,7-Dimethoxycoumarin, 173, 176
  structure of, 173
5,7-Dimethoxycoumarin, 173, 176
  structure of, 173
6,7-Dimethoxycoumarin, see Dimethylaesculetin
5,7-Dimethoxy-6-hydroxycoumarin, 173, 176
  silyl derivative of, 176
  structure of, 173
N,N-Dimethylacetamide, 231
Dimethylaesculetin, 171, 176, 177

N,N-Dimethyl-p-carboxytolbutamide, 309
N,N-Dimethyl-p-chlorobenzenesulfonamide, 309
Dimethylchlorosilane, 96, 158, 182, 183, 185, 190, 214, 215, 296, 322, 337, 372, 373
N,N-Dimethyl-5H-dibenzo-(a,d)-cycloheptene-Δ^5-α-ethylamine, 161
N,N-Dimethyl-5H-dibenzo-(a,d)-cycloheptene-Δ^5,α-propylamine, see Cyclobenzaprine
2,6-Dimethyl-4-dihydropyridine-3,5-dicarboxylic acid 3-[3-(N-benzyl-N-methylamino] propyl ester 5-isopropyl ester, 156, 157
  mass spectrum of, 157
  pyridine analog of, 156, 157
  mass spectrum of, 157
1,3-Dimethyl-5,5-diphenylhydantoin, 96, 103
Dimethylformamide, 351, 366
Dimethylmesuol, 180, 182
1,3-Dimethyl-5-(4-methoxyphenyl)-5-phenylhydantoin, 96
1,3-Dimethyl-5-(4-methylphenyl)-5-phenylhydantoin, 96, 103
α,α-Dimethyl-β-methylsuccinimide, 102, 103
2,6-Dimethyl-4-(3-nitrophenyl)-1,4-dihydropyridine-3,5-dicarboxylic acid 3-[2-(N-benzyl-N-methylamino)]ethyl ester 5-methyl ester, see YC-93
1-(2',6'-Dimethyl)phenoxy-2-aminopropane, see Mexiletine
1-(2',6'-Dimethyl)phenoxypropan-2-ol, 135, 136, 138
  detection limits of, 135
  recovery of, 138
  structure of, 136

[1-(2',6'-Dimethyl)phenoxypropan-2-ol]
  trifluoroacetyl derivative of, 138
1-(2',6'-Dimethyl)phenoxypropan-2-one, 135, 136, 138
  detection limits of, 135
  recovery of, 138
  structure of, 136
1-(2',6'-Dimethyl)phenoxypropan-2-one oxime, 135, 136, 138
  detection limits of, 135
  recovery of, 138
  silyl derivative of, 138
  structure of, 136
Dimethylphthalate, 143
1-(3,5-Dimethylpyrazole) phthalazine, 265, 267
  structure of, 267
Dimethylsebacate, 143
Dimethyl sulfate, 225, 235, 288, 292, 293, 316, 317, 328
  deuterated, 317
Dimethylsulfoxide, 102, 345
α,α-Dimethyl-4-(α,α,β,β-tetrafluorophenethyl)benzylamine, 32, 128-129
  recovery of, 129
  structure of, 128
  trifluoroacetyl derivative of, 128, 129
N,N-Dimethyl-p-toluenesulfonamide, 309
m-Dinitrobenzene, 143, 144
2,4-Dinitrofluorobenzene, 296, 297
1,2-Dinitroglycerol, 143, 148
  detection limits of, 148
  silyl derivative of, 143
1,3-Dinitroglycerol, 143, 148
  detection limits of, 148
  silyl derivative of, 143
1,5-Dinitropentanediol, 137, 140, 141, 142
1,2-Dinitropropanediol, 137, 141, 142

SUBJECT INDEX 423

Diosgenin, 5, 30, 31
  silyl derivative of, 31
  structure of, 30
  trifluoroacetyl derivative of, 31
Dioxane, 6
Diphenadione, 180, 181
  structure of, 181
1,1-Diphenyl-3-hexamethyleneimino-
    butyronitrile, 159
1,1-Diphenyl-3-hexamethylene-
    iminopropane, see
    Hexadiphane
Diphenylhydantoin, 32, 34, 36, 39,
    79-111, 112, 113, 192, 224,
    226
  apparent dissociation constant of,
    99, 100
  ^{13}C-labeled, 85, 86, 87, 88, 91
  methyl derivative of, 85, 86, 88,
    89
  mass spectrum of, 85, 89
  comparison of GC/HPLC methods
    for, 113
  comparison of GC/UV methods
    for, 97, 98
  comparison of RIA/EMIT/GC/
    SPECT methods for, 112
  detection limits of, 93, 95, 97,
    104, 106
  half-life of, 34
  ^{3}H-labeled, 110
  methyl derivative of, 36, 85, 86,
    88, 94, 95, 97, 99, 102, 103,
    104, 105, 106, 107, 109, 111,
    192
  mass spectrum of, 85, 88
  negative ions of, 93
  pentafluorobenzyl derivative of,
    87, 91, 93
  detection limits of, 91
  plasma protein-binding of,
    34
  pharmacokinetic data for, 34,
    98, 105

[Diphenylhydantoin]
  recovery of, 94, 95, 97, 103, 104,
    106, 107, 192
  renal clearance of, 34
  silyl derivative of, 94
  solubility of, 99, 100, 101
  equation for, 99
  structure of, 103
  therapeutic concentration of, 34
  volume of distribution of, 34
1,2-Diphenyl-3-methoxy-4-n-
    butyl-5-oxopyrazoline, 186
1,2-Diphenyl-4-methyl-4-(2-
    butanone)-3,5-dioxopyrazo-
    line, 191
Diphenylpyraline, 158, 159
Dipyridamole, 152
Dipyrone, 164, 165
Disopyramide, 32, 124-128
  acetyl derivative of, 125
  apparent volume of distribution of,
    127
  detection limits of, 126
  half-life of, 124, 127
  metabolic clearance of, 127
  metabolite of, 124, 125, 126, 127,
    128
  pharmacokinetics of, 124, 126,
    127
  recovery of, 126
  renal clearance of, 127
  structure of, 124
  two-compartment model for, 127
2,6-Disubstituted-4-monochloro-
    difluoromethyl-1,3,5-
    triazine(s), 336, 337
Diuretics, 194-217
Diuril, see Chlorothiazide
Docosane, 158
Docosanoic acid, 370
  silyl derivative of, 370
Dopamine, 115, 116, 117, 118
  heptafluorobutyryl derivative of,
    115, 116

[Dopamine]
[heptafluorobutyryl derivative of]
mass spectrum of, 116
isocyanate derivative of, 115
isocyanate/silyl derivative of, 115, 116
mass spectrum of, 116
silyl derivative of, 115, 117, 118
mass spectrum of, 117
structure of, 117

E

Electron affinity detector (GC), 24, 26, 87, 122, 123, 128, 134, 141, 142, 143, 144, 146, 147, 148, 150, 151, 154, 156, 184, 189, 200, 201, 206, 207, 212, 214, 215, 235, 259, 270, 272, 286, 287, 294, 296, 298, 306, 317, 319, 336, 343, 352, 353, 354, 357, 363, 365, 366, 367, 368, 369, 370, 371, 372, 374
Elution temperature, 145, 373
Epinephrine, 123, 124
silyl derivative of, 123, 124
Epiquinidine, 42
silyl derivative of, 42
Epiquinine, 42
silyl derivative of, 42
Erythritol tetranitrate, 140, 145
structure of, 140
Erythromycin, 55
Estradiol benzoate, 345, 351
Ethacrynic acid, 194, 196, 199, 213, 233
structure of, 196
Ethanol, 32, 126, 134, 140, 141, 152, 163, 215, 288, 339, 340
Ethchlorvynol, 196
Ethosuccinimide, see Ethosuximide
Ethosuximide, 94, 97, 99, 102, 103, 106, 107, 111, 113, 114

[Ethosuximide]
methyl derivative of, 99, 103, 106, 107
Ethotoin, see 3-Ethyl-5-phenylhydantoin
1-Ethoxycarbonyl-3-methyl-2-thio-4-imidazole, see Carbimazole
Ethoxzolamide, 194, 195, 196, 199
structure of, 195
Ethyl acetate, 26, 48, 56, 74, 91, 143, 146, 150, 151, 161, 206, 267, 268, 269, 277, 278, 281, 310, 317
Ethylbiscoumacetate, 180, 182, 183
structure of, 183
Ethylene chloride, see Ethylene dichloride
Ethyl-p-chlorophenoxyisobutyrate, see Clofibrate
Ethylene dichloride, 183, 185, 186, 190, 192
Ethylene glycol dinitrate, 137, 141, 142
detection limits of, 141
N-Ethyl-N'-(2-indanyl)-N'-phenyl-1,3-propanediamine, 132
5-Ethyl-3-methyl-5-phenyl-hydantoin, 95
1-Ethyl-1-phenethylbiguanide, 343
3-Ethyl-5-phenylhydantoin, 95, 106, 107
methyl derivative of, 106, 107
5-Ethyl-5-phenylhydantoin, 95

F

Factor VIII (proconvertin), 165
Factor IX (Christmas), 165
Factor X (Stewart-Power), 165
Ferulic acid, 178
silyl derivative of, 178
Flame ionization detector (GC), 7, 11, 19, 21, 28, 31, 33, 40,

SUBJECT INDEX 425

[Flame ionization detector (GC)],
   41, 45, 48, 49, 51, 52, 56,
   61, 67, 70, 87, 94, 97, 99,
   101, 102, 104, 105, 106, 107,
   123, 125, 129, 135, 142, 143,
   144, 146, 148, 154, 158, 159,
   161, 165, 170, 177, 180, 182,
   183, 185, 190, 192, 193, 208,
   209, 215, 217, 223, 225, 227,
   230, 231, 232, 234, 267, 269,
   274, 275, 277, 284, 286, 287,
   289, 291, 293, 308, 310, 311,
   314, 315, 322, 324, 327, 328,
   332, 340, 343, 345, 351, 352,
   360, 365, 369, 370, 371, 372,
   373, 374, 377, 380, 382
Florisil, 24
Fluoranthene, 200
Fluorene, 97, 99
Fluorescamine, 51
Formic acid, 268, 290
Fraxetin, see 6-Methoxy-7,8-
   dihydroxycoumarin
Fraxinol, see 5,7-Dimethoxy-6-
   hydroxycoumarin
Furosemide, 194, 195, 207, 210,
   212-213, 233, 255
   apparent volume of distribution of,
      213
      equation for, 213
   detection limits of, 212
   ethyl derivative of, 212
   half-life of, 213
   methyl derivative of, 212
   plasma clearance of, 213
      equation for, 213
   recovery of, 212
   renal clearance of, 213
   ^{35}S-labeled, 213
   structure of, 195

G

Genin, 3
Gitogenin, 5, 30, 31

[Gitogenin]
   silyl derivative of, 31
   structure of, 30
   trifluoroacetyl derivative of, 31
Gitoxigenin, 3, 6, 8, 11, 12, 14,
   17, 21, 22, 23, 25
   acetyl derivative of, 21, 22, 23
   silyl derivative of, 8, 11, 12, 14,
      17, 21, 22, 23, 25
   structure of, 3
Gitoxin, 3, 19, 23, 25
   acetyl derivative of, 21
   silyl derivative of, 19, 23, 25
   structure of, 3
Glibenclamide, 233
Glucose, 332, 333
Glucose-6-phosphate, 107, 265
   dehydrogenase, 107
β-Glucuronidase, 96, 157, 226
Glusulase, 263
Glutethimide, 55
Glycerine, 124, 143
Glycerol trinitrate, see
   Nitroglycerine
Glycine, 115, 118
   silyl derivative of, 115, 118
Guanethidine, 256, 268-277
   alkaline hydrolysis of, 268, 269,
      270, 271
   trifluoroacetyl derivative of,
      269, 270, 271
   detection limits of, 269
   structure of, 256
Guanido-containing drugs,
   268-277
Guanoxan, 256, 270, 274, 277
   acetylacetone derivative of, 274,
      277
   alkaline hydrolysis product of,
      270, 271
   trifluoroacetyl derivative of,
      270, 271
   structure of, 271
   structure of, 256

H

Halofenate, 218, 233-236
  ^{14}C-labeled, 235
  metabolism of, 233, 234, 235
  structure of, 218
Hecogenin, 5
Helium (GC carrier gas), 19, 27, 46, 51, 53, 75, 106, 125, 129, 131, 134, 135, 137, 140, 143, 154, 158, 161, 162, 166, 174, 177, 197, 198, 230, 235, 237, 263, 272, 276, 278, 283, 286, 289, 290, 291, 292, 308, 310, 317, 328, 332, 334, 341, 345, 352, 355, 371
Hematocrit, 200, 201
Heptabarbital, 106, 107
  methyl derivative of, 106, 107
Heptafluorobutyric anhydride, 24, 26, 27, 135, 317, 343, 353
n-Heptane, 161, 234, 236, 288
Herniarin, see 7-Methoxycoumarin
Hexadiphane, 158, 159, 160
  recovery of, 160
  structure of, 159
Hexafluoroacetylacetone, 271, 272, 273, 274, 275
  structure of, 273
Hexamethyldisilazane, 6, 11, 17, 21, 27, 33, 135, 171, 181, 372, 373
n-Hexane, 164, 206, 212, 230, 292, 296, 297, 298, 343
Hexatriacontane, 58
Hexobarbital, 87, 91, 102, 103
  methyl derivative of, 103
  pentafluorobenzyl derivative of, 87, 91
    detection limits of, 91
Homatropine, 32
D-Homo-172-oxandrostan-1,4-diene-3,17-dione, see Δ^1-Testololactone
Hydralazine, 255, 256, 258-268

[Hydralazine]
  bioavailability of, 259
  ^{14}C-labeled, 260, 263
  detection limits of, 259
  deuterated, 260
  effect of HCl/NaNO$_2$ on, 258
  half-life of, 261, 266
  hydroxylated phenyl ring derivative of, 262
    structure of, 262
  metabolic pathways of, 260, 262
  metabolic products of, 260, 262
  4-methyl analog of, 256, 258
  pharmacokinetics of, 259, 260-261, 264, 265, 266
  reaction with 2,4-pentanedione, 265, 267
  recovery of, 263
  structure of, 256, 258, 262, 267
Hydrastine, 32
1-Hydrazino-4-methylphthalazine, 258, 259
  effect of HCl/NaNO$_2$ on, 258
  structure of, 258
1-Hydrazinophthalazine, see Hydralazine
1-Hydrazinophthalazine acetone hydrazone, 260, 262, 263, 264, 265
  structure of, 262
1-Hydrazionophthalazine pyruvic acid hydrazone, 260, 262, 263, 264, 265
  recovery of, 263
  silyl derivative of, 263, 264
  structure of, 262
Hydrochloric acid, 6, 32, 55, 65, 76, 93, 95, 96, 102, 106, 107, 132, 133, 134, 156, 157, 161, 163, 192, 209, 212, 214, 218, 223, 225, 227, 234, 235, 258, 259, 263, 268, 270, 277, 278, 290, 296, 297, 301, 310, 336, 343, 345, 351, 352, 365, 366

Hydrochlorothiazide, 194, 195, 196, 206-209
  bromo analog of, 206, 207
  methyl derivative of, 206, 207
  ^{14}C-labeled, 208
  detection limits of, 206, 208
  half-life of, 208
  methyl derivative of, 206, 207, 208
  pharmacokinetics of, 207
  recovery of, 208
  structure of, 195
  two-compartment model for, 208
p-Hydroxybenzoic acid, 178
  silyl derivative of, 178
2-Hydroxychalcone, 179
  silyl derivative of, 179
2-Hydroxychlorpropamide, 294, 295, 309, 325
  half-life of, 295
  methyl derivative of, 309, 325
  degradation of, 325
  structure of, 294
3-Hydroxychlorpropamide, 294, 295, 325
  methyl derivative of, 325
  degradation product of, 325
  structure of, 294
3-Hydroxycoumarin, 173, 176
  silyl derivative of, 176
  structure of, 173
4-Hydroxycoumarin, 173, 176, 181, 182, 183, 184
  acetyl derivative of, 183, 184
  silyl derivative of, 176, 181, 182, 183, 184
  structure of, 173
  trichloroacetyl derivative of, 183, 184
  trifluoroacetyl derivative of, 183, 184
7-Hydroxycoumarin, see Umbelliferone

4-Hydroxydebrisoquin, 272, 273, 274, 275, 276, 277
  acetylacetone derivative of, 274, 277
  detection limits of, 274
  hexafluoroacetylacetone derivative of, 272, 273, 274, 275
  mass spectrum of, 275
  structure of, 273
  pharmacokinetics of, 276
  structure of, 273
5-(4-Hydroxy-3,5-dideuterophenyl)-5-phenylhydantoin, see p-Hydroxydiphenylhydantoin, deuterated
1-(4'-Hydroxy-2',6'-dimethyl) phenoxy-2-aminopropane, 135, 136, 138
  detection limits of, 135
  recovery of, 138
  silyl derivative of, 138
  structure of, 136
  trifluoroacetyl derivative of, 138
1-(4'-Hydroxy-2',6'-dimethyl) phenoxypropan-2-ol, 135, 136, 139
  detection limits, 135
  silyl derivative of, 139
  structure of, 136
  trifluoroacetyl derivative of, 139
3-Hydroxydiphenylhydantoin, see 5-(3-Hydroxyphenyl)-5-phenylhydantoin
p-Hydroxydiphenylhydantoin, 80, 81, 94, 95, 96, 97, 98, 105, 106, 108, 109, 111
  detection limits of, 97
  deuterated, 95
  glucuronide of, 80
  methyl derivative of, 94, 95, 96, 106, 109, 111
  pharmacokinetic data for, 98, 105
  recovery of, 95, 97
  silyl derivative of, 81

6-Hydroxydopamine, 115, 118
  silyl derivative of, 115, 118
p-(1-Hydroxyethyl)-N-methyl-
    benzenesulfonamide, 332
Hydroxyhexamide, 328, 332, 333
  methyl derivative of, 328
  pyrolysis of, 328
  pharmacokinetic data for, 333
  recovery of, 332
  structure of, 328
Hydroxylamine, 163
4-Hydroxy-7-methoxycoumarin,
    173, 176
  silyl derivative of, 176
  structure of, 173
6-Hydroxy-7-methoxycoumarin,
    171, 173, 176
  silyl derivative of, 171, 176
  structure of, 173
7-Hydroxy-8-methoxycoumarin,
    168, 172
  acetate derivative of, 168, 172
  structure of, 168
4-Hydroxy-4'-methylphenylhy-
    dantoin, 95
  methyl derivative of, 95
1-(2'-Hydroxymethyl, 6'-methyl)
    phenoxy-2-aminopropane,
    135, 136, 139
  detection limits of, 135
  recovery of, 139
  silyl derivative of, 139
  structure of, 136
  trifluoroacetyl derivative of, 139
1-(2'-Hydroxymethyl, 6'-methyl)
    phenoxypropan-2-ol, 135,
    136, 139
  detection limits of, 135
  silyl derivative of, 139
  structure of, 136
  trifluoroacetyl derivative of,
    139
Hydroxymethyltolbutamide, 293
  methyl derivative of, 293

3-Hydroxymethyltriazolo-
    phthalazine, 262, 263, 265
  silyl derivative of, 263
  structure of, 262
N-Hydroxymexiletene, 135, 136,
    138
  detection limits of, 135
  silyl derivative of, 138
  structure of, 136
p-Hydroxyphenformin, 339, 340,
    341
  detection limits of, 341
  structure of, 340
  trifluoroacetyl derivative of, 340
  structure of, 340
p-Hydroxyphenobarbital, 80, 81, 83
  glucuronide of, 80
  methoxy derivative of, 83
  silyl derivative of, 81, 83
p-Hydroxyphenylacetic acid, 178
  silyl derivative of, 178
1-(p-Hydroxyphenyl)-2-(1'-methyl-
    3'-phenylpropylamino)-1-
    propanol, see Nylidrin
5-(4-Hydroxyphenyl)-5-(2,3,4,5,6-
    pentadeuterophenyl)hydantoin,
    see p-Hydroxydiphenyl-
    hydantoin, deuterated
5-(3-Hydroxyphenyl)-5-phenyl-
    hydantoin, 95, 105
  detection limits of, 95
  methyl derivative of, 95
5-(4-Hydroxyphenyl)-5-phenylhy-
    dantoin, see p-Hydroxydi-
    phenylhydantoin
p-Hydroxyphenylpropionic acid,
    178
  silyl derivative of, 178
p-Hydroxyphenylpyruvic acid, 178
  silyl derivative of, 178
4-Hydroxypropranolol, 117, 120
  heptafluorobutyryl derivative of,
    117
  structure of, 120

SUBJECT INDEX 429

3-[α-(2-Hydroxypropyl)benzyl]-4-
    hydroxycoumarin, 186
  methyl derivative of, 186
2-Hydroxyquinidine, 41, 43, 45
  methyl derivative of, 41, 45
Hydroxyquinuclidine, 33
Hydroxysecobarbital, 80, 81, 83
  silyl derivative of, 81
Hydroxytolbutamide, 309, 310, 315,
    316, 317, 318, 319, 320, 321,
    323, 325
  methyl derivative of, 309, 310,
    315, 316, 317, 318, 319, 320,
    321, 323, 325
    deuterated, 317
  methyl/heptafluorobutyryl deriva-
    tive of, 316, 317, 318, 319,
    320, 321, 323
  methyl/pentafluoropropionyl
    derivative of, 316, 317, 318,
    319, 320, 321, 323
  methyl/trifluoroacetyl derivative
    of, 309, 310, 315, 316, 317,
    318, 319, 320, 321, 323
  trifluoroacetyl derivative of, 309,
    310, 315, 316, 317, 318, 319,
    320, 321, 323
5-Hydroxytyramine, 118
  silyl derivative of, 118
6-Hydroxywarfarin, 186
  methyl derivative of, 186
7-Hydroxywarfarin, 186
  methyl derivative of, 186
Hypoglycemic agents, 288-343
  structures of common, 289

I

ICI-45763, 117, 120
  structure of, 120
Imperatorin, 166, 174
  structure of, 174
2-Indanol, 132
  methane sulfonate derivative of,
    132

2-Indanone, 132
N-2-Indanyl-N-phenyl-1,3-
    propanediamine, 132
Indene, 132
Infusion time, 72, 279
Insulin, 332, 333
Internal standard, 6, 24, 26, 27,
    40, 41, 44, 45, 46, 47, 48,
    49, 52, 53, 56, 58, 62, 64,
    70, 74, 75, 76, 77, 83, 84,
    86, 87, 93, 94, 95, 96, 97,
    99, 102, 103, 105, 106, 107,
    109, 111, 117, 120, 122, 123,
    124, 125, 126, 128, 129, 132,
    134, 143, 144, 148, 150, 154,
    156, 157, 158, 159, 161, 163,
    164, 165, 184, 185, 189, 190,
    191, 192, 200, 206, 207, 208,
    209, 212, 214, 215, 217, 220,
    222, 223, 224, 225, 226, 227,
    231, 232, 234, 235, 256, 259,
    263, 264, 267, 268, 269, 270,
    272, 273, 274, 275, 277, 278,
    281, 283, 285, 286, 291, 292,
    293, 295, 296, 297, 298, 300,
    301, 304, 307, 310, 313, 314,
    319, 324, 328, 332, 336, 341,
    343, 345, 350, 351, 354, 370,
    377, 381, 382
Iodobutane, 231
3-Iodothyronine, 374
  silyl derivative of, 374
3-Iodotyrosine, 348, 350, 351, 352,
    360, 362, 365, 370, 371, 372,
    373, 374, 377
  detection limits of, 372, 373
  methyl derivative of, 351, 352,
    360, 362, 365
  methyl/pivalyl derivative of, 360,
    362, 365
  methyl/trifluoroacetyl derivative
    of, 351, 352
  pivalyl derivative of, 360, 362,
    365

[3-Iodotyrosine]
  silyl derivative of, 370, 371, 372, 373, 377
  structure of, 348
  trifluoroacetyl derivative of, 351, 352
Isoamyl alcohol, 234, 296, 297
Isobergapten, 166, 167, 169, 170, 172, 177
  structure of, 167
Isobutane, 197
Isoidide dinitrate, 148, 149, 150
Isomannide dinitrate, 146, 148
  detection limits of, 148
Isomannide mononitrate, 146, 148
  detection limits of, 148
Isomesuol, 175, 180, 182
  structure of, 175
Isonicotinic acid hydrazide, 67, 69, 70
  half-life of, 67, 69
Iso-octane, 224
Isopentyl alcohol, 161
Isopimpinellin, 166, 168, 169, 170, 177
  structure of, 168
Isopropanol, see 2-Propanol
4-Isopropylamino-2-phenyl-2-(2-pyridyl)butyramide, 124, 125, 126, 127, 128
  acetyl derivative of, 125
  detection limits of, 126
  half-life of, 127
  pharmacokinetics of, 126, 127
  recovery of, 126
  renal clearance of, 127
  structure of, 125
1-Isopropyl-3-p-carboxyphenyl-sulfonylurea, 296, 297, 298, 299, 300
  detection limits of, 298
  reaction product with 2,4-dinitrofluorobenzene, 297, 298, 299

[1-Isopropyl-3-p-carboxyphenyl-sulfonylurea]
  structure of, 296
Isopropyl-2-[4'-(p-chlorobenzoyl)phenoxy]-2-methylpropionate, see Procetofene
Isopropyl-2,4-dinitroaniline, 299, 300
1-Isopropyl-3-p-hydroxymethyl-sulfonylurea, 300
Isoproterenol, 32, 36, 40, 111-124, 152
  silyl derivative of, 123, 124
Isorbide dinitrate, 140, 142, 143, 144, 145, 146, 148, 149, 150, 151, 152, 153
  ^{14}C-labeled, 151, 152
  detection limits of, 143, 148, 150
  recovery of, 148, 151
  structure of, 140
2-Isorbide mononitrate, 146, 149, 150, 151, 152, 153
  recovery of, 151
5-Isorbide mononitrate, 146, 148-149, 151, 152, 153
  recovery of, 151

K

Kammogenin, 5
Ketohydroxysecobarbital, 80, 83

L

Lactic acid, 124
Lactic dehydrogenase, 331
Lactose, 124, 141
Lidocaine, 32, 34, 36, 39, 40, 49, 51, 79, 131, 134
  detection limits of, 51
  half-life of, 34
  metabolite of, 39
  plasma protein-binding of, 34
  pharmacokinetic data for, 34
  recovery of, 51

SUBJECT INDEX 431

[Lidocaine]
  renal clearance of, 34
  therapeutic concentration of, 34
  volume of distribution of, 34
Lilagenin, 30, 31
  silyl derivative of, 31
  structure of, 30
  trifluoroacetyl derivative of, 31
Limettin, 174, 177
  structure of, 174
Linoleic acid, 84
  methyl derivative of, 84
Liothyronine, see 3,3',5-
  Triiodothyronine
Liquid stationary phase (GC)
  types of
    Apiezon-series, 180, 284
    Butanediol succinate, 218
    Carbowax-series, 135, 136, 237, 291, 292, 332, 334
    DEGA (diethylene glycol adipate), 180
    Dexsil-300, 144, 145, 147, 368, 369
    E-301, 142
    EGA (ethylene glycol adipate), 224
    EGS (ethylene glycol succinate), 137, 165, 166, 167, 168, 169, 170, 171
    EGP (ethylene glycol phthalate), 165, 166, 167, 168
    EGSS-X, 223
    EGSS-Y, 33
    HIEFF-8B, 32, 33, 134, 170, 173
    JXR, 206, 212
    NPGS (neopentyl glycol succinate), 87, 92
    OV-1, 19, 21, 22, 25, 26, 27, 28, 87, 92, 105, 123, 156, 158, 177, 206, 215, 316, 317, 318, 319, 323, 337, 343, 345, 351, 366, 367, 370, 371, 374, 379, 380, 382

[Liquid stationary phase (GC)]
[types of]
    OV-3, 162
    OV-7, 41, 52, 62, 185
    OV-17, 11, 12, 14, 21, 22, 23, 25, 28, 31, 33, 34, 45, 48, 49, 51, 56, 58, 67, 70, 75, 76, 87, 92, 94, 95, 96, 99, 102, 103, 106, 107, 111, 123, 125, 126, 129, 135, 143, 154, 159, 161, 184, 189, 190, 193, 197, 198, 200, 209, 220, 230, 231, 263, 269, 272, 277, 278, 291, 293, 296, 309, 316, 317, 318, 319, 323, 327, 337, 343, 347, 351, 354, 362, 363, 364, 365, 366, 374, 377
    OV-25, 192, 322
    OV-61, 351
    OV-101, 123, 269, 355, 358
    OV-210, 286
    OV-225, 40, 102, 103, 104, 214, 215, 259, 275, 276
    Polycyclohexanedimethanoladipate, 206
    Polyethyleneglycol (PEG), see Carbowax-series
    Poly I-110, 269
    Polysulfone, 362
    PPE-20, 128, 129
    QF-1, 19, 31, 143, 146, 148, 150, 234
    SE-33, 369
    Silicone grease, 165, 166, 168, 172
    Silicone oil (DC-series), 289, 294
    Silicone rubber (SE-30), 4, 5, 7, 11, 12, 14, 17, 19, 21, 31, 32, 33, 36, 58, 81, 82, 83, 84, 140, 142, 143, 144, 145, 147, 151, 169, 170, 173, 174, 180, 182, 183, 199, 208, 212, 217, 219, 220, 222, 224, 225,

[Liquid stationary phase (GC)]
  [types of]
    [Silicone rubber (SE-30)], 227,
      232, 235, 267, 283, 340, 352,
      353, 360, 366, 367, 372, 373
    SP-series, 97, 107, 310, 311,
      315, 316, 317, 319, 323
    (3,3,3-Trifluoropropyl)methyl-
      silicone, 52
    W-98, 131, 292, 293, 308
    Versamid-900, 52
    XE-60, 32, 33, 143, 144, 146,
      148
Lithium aluminum hydride, 163
Luvangetin, 175, 180, 181, 182
  structure of, 175
Lysine, 115, 118
  silyl derivative of, 115, 118

M

Magnesium sulfate, 151, 343
Mannitol, 197, 198
Mannitol hexanitrate, 145
Manogenin, 5
Marmesin, 175, 180, 182
  structure of, 175
Marmin, 175, 180, 182
  structure of, 175
Mebaral, 94
Mebutamate, 255
Mephobarbital, 87, 91, 93
  pentafluorobenzyl derivative of,
    87, 91, 93
  detection limits of, 91
Mepivacaine, 49, 51
  recovery of, 51
Mercumallylic acid, 196
Mesantoin, 94
Mesuol, 175, 180, 182
  structure of, 175
Metformin, 289, 336, 337, 338,
    341, 343
  detection limits of, 337

[Metformin]
  reaction with monochlorodifluoro-
    acitic anhydride, 337, 338
  structure of, 289, 336
Methane, 26, 39, 76, 135, 150,
  156, 198, 200, 206, 219, 258,
  296, 301, 304, 305, 337, 353,
  368, 374
Methanol, 18, 24, 45, 67, 76, 96,
  99, 102, 106, 107, 133, 157,
  192, 200, 206, 214, 215, 218,
  220, 221, 223, 225, 227, 231,
  235, 237, 281, 284, 288, 290,
  291, 295, 302, 310, 317, 351,
  352, 359, 363, 365, 366, 370,
  380
  deuterated, 317
Methaqualone, 55
Metharbital, 94
Methetoin, 95
Methimazole, 380, 381, 382
  structure of, 382
7-Methoxycoumarin, 165, 166, 167,
    169, 176, 177, 181
  structure of, 167
6-Methoxy-7,8-dihydroxycoumarin,
    173, 176
  silyl derivative of, 176
  structure of, 173
6-Methoxy-7-hydroxycoumarin,
    see Scopoletin
3-Methoxy-4-hydroxydiphenyl-
    hydantoin, 95
  methyl derivative of, 95
1-(p-Methoxyphenethyl)-biguanide,
    343
p-Methoxyphenobarbital, 83
3-Methoxyphenylacetic acid, 226,
    227
  methyl ester of, 227
Methsuximide, 94, 97, 99
  methyl derivative of, 99
N-Methyl-p-acetylbenzenesulfona-
    mide, 332

SUBJECT INDEX

7-Methylacesculetin, see
   6-Hydroxy-7-methoxycoumarin
3-Methyl-1-butanol, 164, 165
Methyl-3-n-butylamino-5-
   dimethylsulfamyl-4-
   phenoxybenzoic acid, 209, 210
   structure of, 210
Methyl-3-(N-n-butylanilino)-5-
   dimethylsulfamyl-4-
   hydroxybenzoic acid, 209, 210
   structure of, 210
Methyl-3-(N-n-butylanilino)-5-
   dimethylsulfamyl-4-
   methoxybenzoic acid, 209, 210
   structure of, 210
N-Methyl-p-chlorobenzenesulfonamide, 322, 325
Methylclothiazide, 194, 196, 199
   structure of, 196
4-Methyldiphenylhydantoin, see
   5-(4-Methylphenyl)-5-
   phenylhydantoin
α-Methyldopa, 233
Methylene chloride, 24, 43, 48, 51,
   52, 56, 64, 65, 76, 87, 93,
   95, 111, 143, 199, 204, 205,
   208, 212, 215, 231, 234, 285,
   297, 336, 337, 341, 343, 345,
   351, 366, 367
1-(3,4-Methylenedioxybenzyl)-4-
   (2-pyrimidinyl)piperazine,
   see Piribedil
1-Methylimidazole-2-thiol, see
   Methimazole
Methyl iodide, 95, 102, 103, 204,
   205, 208, 212
Methylisobutylketone, 205
Methyl-3-methoxy-3-(3,4,5-
   trimethoxyphenyl)propionate,
   284, 285
   structure of, 285
N-Methylmexiletine, 135, 136, 138
   detection limits of, 135
   recovery of, 138

[N-Methylmexiletine]
   structure of, 136
   trifluoroacetyl derivative of, 138
Methyl myristate, 220, 222
4-Methyl-2-pentanone, 208
dl-(α-Methylphenethyl)biguanide,
   343
1-(p-Methylphenethyl)biguanide,
   343
(1-Methyl-2-phenethyl)hydrazine,
   see Pheniprazine
N-Methyl-α-phenylbutyramide,
   100, 102
5-(4-Methylphenyl)-5-phenylhy-
   dantoin, 95, 96, 97, 99, 102,
   103, 104, 107
   methyl derivative of, 95, 96, 97,
      99, 103, 104, 107
   recovery of, 97, 103
   structure of, 103
4'-Methylpropiophenone, 163
Methyl stearate, 285
Methylsuccinimide, see
   Methsuximide
6-Methyltetrazolophthalazine, 258,
   259, 262
   structure of, 258, 262
6-Methyl-2-thiouracil, see
   Methylthiouracil
Methylthiouracil, 380, 382
   structure of, 382
N-Methyltolbutamide, see
   Tolbutamide, methyl derivative of
N-Methyl-p-toluenesulfonamide,
   293, 322, 323, 332
   structure of, 293
Methyl-p-toluenesulfonylurea,
   325
3-Methyl-s-triazolo-(3,4-a)-
   phthalazine, 260, 263, 264,
   265, 266
   carboxy derivative of, 263
   deuterated, 260, 263, 264

[3-Methyl-s-triazolo-(3,4-a)-
    phthalazine]
  half-life of, 266
  hydroxyl derivative of phenyl
    ring, 263, 265
  pharmacokinetics of, 266
  recovery of, 263
  structure of, 262
Methyl-3,4,5-trimethoxybenzoate,
    284, 285
  structure of, 285
cis-Methyl-3,4,5-trimethoxycinna-
    mate, 284, 285
  structure of, 285
trans-Methyl-3,4,5-trimethoxy-
    cinnamate, 284, 285
  structure of, 285
(N-Methyl-N-trimethyl)trifluoro-
    acetamide, 40
Methylthiouracil, 380, 382
  structure of, 382
Mexiletine, 32, 131-137, 138
  butyryl derivative of, 134
  detection limits of, 134, 135
  heptafluorobutyryl derivative of,
    135
  metabolite(s) of, 135, 136
  2,4-methyl analog of, 132, 134
    butyryl derivative of, 134
  recovery of, 134, 137, 138
  structure of, 131, 136
  trifluoroacetyl derivative of, 138
Mexogenin, 5
Monochlorodifluoroacetic anhydride,
    336, 337
Monodealkylated disopyramide, see
    4-Isopropylamino-2-phenyl-2-
    (2-pyridyl)butyramide
Monohydroxyquinidine, 41
  methyl derivative of, 41
3-Monoiodothyronine, 349, 350
  structure of, 349
3'-Monoiodothyronine, 349, 350
  structure of, 349

Mononitroglycerol, 143, 148
  detection limits of, 148
  silyl derivative of, 143
Morphine, 33
Mydocalm, 162, 163, 164
  detection limits of, 164
  deuterated, 163, 164
  metabolite(s) of, 164
  ^{15}N-labeled, 162, 163, 164
    structure of, 163
  recovery of, 164
  structure of, 162
Myricetin, 179
  silyl derivative of, 179

N

Naphazoline, 277
Naphthoic acid, 232
  methyl ester of, 232
3-(α-Naphthoxy)-1,2-propanediol,
    see Propranolol glycol
Naphthylamine, 340, 341
Naringenin, 179
  silyl derivative of, 179
Neogitogenin, 30, 31
  silyl derivative of, 31
  structure of, 30
  trifluoroacetyl derivative of, 31
Neotigogenin, 30, 31
  silyl derivative of, 31
  structure of, 30
  trifluoroacetyl derivative of, 31
Nitrofurantoin, 55
Nitrogen (GC carrier gas), 7, 8,
    11, 21, 28, 40, 45, 48, 49,
    52, 58, 62, 70, 91, 92, 94,
    96, 97, 102, 103, 104, 106,
    107, 123, 124, 126, 135, 136,
    142, 143, 144, 146, 148, 154,
    159, 165, 170, 171, 180, 182,
    183, 184, 189, 190, 192, 194,
    198, 206, 208, 209, 214, 215,
    217, 223, 227, 230, 231, 232,

[Nitrogen (GC carrier gas)], 259, 267, 269, 276, 284, 286, 292, 294, 311, 317, 322, 327, 362, 366, 371, 372, 374, 377, 380, 382
Nitrogen detector (GC), 105, 106, 126, 134, 224, 225, 274, 276
Nitroglycerine, 137, 140, 141, 142, 143, 146, 148, 149
 detection limits of, 141, 148
 recovery of, 148
 structure of, 140
2-Nitroisosorbide, 148
 detection limits of, 148
5-Nitroisosorbide, 148
 detection limits of, 148
2-Nitrophenylamine, 143
N-Nitroso-N-methylurea, 234
Nitrous acid, 154, 156, 256
Nor-dalbergin, 175, 180, 182
 structure of, 175
Norepinephrine, 115, 118
 silyl derivative of, 115, 118
Normetanephrine, 115, 118
 silyl derivative of, 115, 118
Novalgin, see Dipyrone
Nylidrin, 152, 156, 157, 158
 detection limits of, 158
 recovery of, 158
 silyl derivative of, 157, 158
 structure of, 158

O

Octadecane, 230
Octopamine, 115, 118
 silyl derivative of, 115, 118
Oleic acid, 84
 methyl derivative of, 84
Ornithine, 115, 118
 silyl derivative of, 115, 118
Orphenadrine, 152
Osthol, 166, 167, 169, 176, 177
 structure of, 167

Ouabagenin, 3
 structure of, 3
Ouabain, 3, 8
 silyl derivative of, 8
 structure of, 3
Oxazepam hemisuccinate, 159, 160
Oxifedrine, 233
Oxypeucedanin, 174, 177
 structure of, 174
Oxprenolol, 120, 121, 122, 123
 detection limits of, 123
 recovery of, 123
 structure of, 121
 trifluoroacetyl derivative of, 122, 123
  structure of, 122

P

Palmitic acid, 82, 83
 methyl derivative of, 82, 83
Papaverine, 152, 164, 165
Paraformaldehyde, 163
Pargyline, 255
Pentaerythritol, 145, 146, 147
 detection limits of, 146, 147
 dinitrate/ditrifluoroacetyl derivative of, 145, 147
 mononitrate/tri-trifluoroacetyl derivative of, 145, 147
 trifluoroacetyl derivative of, 145, 147
 trinitrate/monotrifluoroacetyl derivative of, 145, 147
Pentaerythritol tetanitrate, 140, 144, 145, 146, 147
 detection limits of, 144, 146, 147
 structure of, 140
Pentafluorobenzyl bromide, 87, 189
Pentafluoropropionic anhydride, 317, 343
2,4-Pentanedione, 265, 267
 structure of, 267

Pentobarbital, 309, 381, 382
  propyl derivative of, 382
Pentyl acetate, 296, 297, 298, 301, 336
Perchloric acid, 121, 122, 123, 228
Permeability coefficient, 77
Peucedanin, 174, 177
  structure of, 174
Phellopterin, 173, 177
  structure of, 173
Phenacetin, 55
Phenanthrene, 267
2-(β-Phenethylamino)-4,6-diamino-1,3,5-triazine, 335
  structure of, 335
Pheneturide, 106, 107
  methyl derivative of, 106, 107
Phenformin, 289, 332, 334, 335, 336, 337, 338, 339, 340, 341, 342, 343
  ^{14}C-labeled, 337
  recovery of, 337
  detection limits of, 337, 341
  half-life of, 337, 341
  pharmacokinetic data for, 337, 339, 341, 342
  protein-binding of, 341
  reaction with monochlorodifluoroacetic anhydride, 337, 338
  reaction with trifluoroacetic anhydride, 340
  structure of, 340
  structure of, 289, 336
Pheniprazine, 255, 258
Phenobarbital, 80, 81, 82, 83, 86, 87, 90, 91, 92, 93, 97, 99, 100, 102, 103, 105, 106, 107, 108, 109, 110, 111, 113, 114, 309
  ^{13}C-labeled, 90, 92
  detection limits of, 90
  detection limits of, 86, 90, 97, 106

[Phenobarbital]
  methyl derivative of, 81, 82, 97, 99, 100, 102, 103, 105, 106, 107, 111
  pentafluorobenzyl derivative of, 87, 91, 93
  detection limits of, 91
  recovery of, 97, 106
Phenol, 124
Phenprocoumon, 182, 183, 184, 190, 192, 193, 194
  acetyl derivative of, 183, 184
  detection limits of, 192, 194
  methyl derivative of, 192
  recovery of, 192, 194
  silyl derivative of, 182, 183, 184
  structure of, 183
  trichloroacetyl derivative of, 183, 184
  trifluoroacetyl derivative of, 183, 184
Phensuccinimide, see Phensuximide
Phensuximide, 94, 97, 99
  methyl derivative of, 99
Phentolamine, 255
2-Phenylamino-4,6-diamino-1,3,5-triazine, 335
  structure of, 335
Phenylbiguanide, 332, 334, 335
  structure of, 334
Phenylbutazone, 185, 186, 190, 191, 192
  methyl derivative of, 186
  oxo derivative of, 190, 191, 192
    methyl derivative of, 190, 191
    recovery of, 192
    structure of, 190
  recovery of, 186
Phenylephrine, 123
  silyl derivative of, 123
Phenylethylamine, 115, 118
  silyl derivative of, 115, 118

Phenylethylmalonamide, 93, 94
  detection limits of, 93
  recovery of, 94
  silyl derivative of, 94
Phenylguanidine, 335
  structure of, 335
N-Phenyl-2-indanamine, 132
Phenyramidol, 152
Phenytoin, see Diphenylhydantoin
Phloretin, 179
  silyl derivative of, 179
Phloridzin, 179
  silyl derivative of, 179
Phosphoric acid, 231, 307
Phosphorus pentoxide, 351
Phthalazine, 260, 262, 263, 264, 265
  structure of, 262
Phthalazinone, 262, 263, 264, 265
  structure of, 262
Pilocarpine, 32, 33
Pimpinellin, 166, 167, 169, 170, 173, 177, 180, 181
  structure of, 167
Piperidine-^{15}N, 163
1-Piperidino-2,4'-dimethyl-propiophenone, see Mydocalm
3-Piperidino-2-methyl-1-(4'-carboxyphenyl)-1-propanol, 164
3-Piperidino-2-methyl-1-(4'-carboxyphenyl)-1-propanone, 164
Piribedil, 152, 154, 155
  detection limits of, 154
  mass spectrum of, 155
  recovery of, 154
  structure of, 152, 155
Pivalic anhydride, 359, 365, 367
Potassium carbonate, 135, 163, 164, 225, 235, 288
Potassium hydroxide, 133, 134, 341, 343
Potassium phosphate, 111

Practolol, 120, 121
  structure of, 121
Prenylamine, 152
O-Prenylumbelliferone, 174, 177
  structure of, 174
Primidone, 93, 94, 97, 99, 102, 103, 105, 106, 107, 108, 111, 113
  detection limits of, 93, 97, 106
  methyl derivative of, 94, 97, 99, 103, 105, 106, 107
  recovery of, 94, 97, 106
  silyl derivative of, 94
Procainamide, 32, 35, 36, 40, 47-79, 131
  comparison of GC/spectrofluorometric methods for, 51, 52, 53, 54, 56, 57
  comparison of GC/spectrofluorometric/colorimetric methods for, 54, 55
  detection limits of, 51, 52, 65
  dialysance of, 65, 66
    equation for, 65
  dialytic clearance of, 65, 66
    equation for, 65
  effect of pH on, 62, 65
  half-life of, 65
  renal clearance of, 65
  total body clearance of, 65
  ^{3}H-labeled, 74
  half-life of, 35, 59, 61, 62, 64, 67, 68, 69
  mass spectrum of, 50
  metabolic pathway of, 47
  pharmacokinetic data for, 35, 58, 59, 60, 61, 62, 63, 64, 65, 67, 68, 72, 75
  plasma protein-binding of, 35
  protein-binding of, 65
  rate of metabolite formation for, 59
    equation for, 59

[Procainamide]
  recovery of, 49, 51, 53, 54, 56, 65, 67
  renal clearance of, 59, 61, 63, 64, 68
  structure of, 47, 50
  therapeutic concentration of, 35
  total body clearance of, 61, 63, 64, 68
  two-compartment open model for, 59, 61, 63
  volume of distribution of, 35, 59, 61, 63, 64, 68
Procaine, 47, 48
Procetofene, 218, 236-238
  metabolite(s) of, 236, 237, 238
    methylation of, 237, 238
    structure(s) of, 236
  structure of, 218
2-Propanol, 82, 84, 200, 261, 263
Propoxyphene, 55
Propranolol, 32, 35, 36, 40, 111-124, 236, 255
  detection limits of, 123
  half-life of, 35
  heptafluorobutyryl derivative of, 117, 120
  metabolite(s) of, 117, 120, 121, 122, 123
  pharmacokinetic data for, 35
  plasma protein-binding of, 35
  recovery of, 123
  renal clearance of, 35
  structure of, 120, 121
  therapeutic concentration of, 35
  trifluoroacetyl derivative of, 122, 123
    structure of, 122
  volume of distribution of, 35
Propranolol glycol, 121, 122, 123
  detection limits of, 123
  recovery of, 123
  trifluoroacetyl derivative of, 122, 123

[Propranolol glycol]
  [trifluoroacetyl derivative of]
    structure of, 122
Propylbiguanide, 336, 337
  reaction with monochlorodifluoroacetic anhydride, 337
  structure of, 336
N-Propyl-p-chlorobenzenesulfonamide, 293
  structure of, 293
Propyl-2,4-dinitroaniline, 296, 299
1-Propyl-3-p-hydroxymethylsulfonylurea, 300
Propylpentanoic acid, sodium salt of, see Sodium valproate
6-n-Propyl-2-thiouracil, see Propylthiouracil
Propylthiouracil, 380, 381, 382, 383
  half-life of, 383
  pharmacokinetic data for, 383
  plasma clearance of, 383
  propyl derivative of, 382
  recovery of, 381
  structure of, 382
Prothrombin, 165
Psoralen, 166, 167, 169, 177, 181
  structure of, 167
Putrescine, 115, 118
  silyl derivative of, 115, 118
Pyridine, 6, 14, 17, 18, 21, 27, 31, 33, 220, 221, 310, 317, 373

Q

Qualitative methods of analysis, by use of
  alphabetical index, 38, 219
  base peak index, 38
  column elution temperature, 145
  digital code, 38, 219
  elution temperature, 145, 373

SUBJECT INDEX 439

[Qualitative methods of analysis, by use of]
 integrated GC-MS/GC-MS-COMP, 11, 13, 21, 33, 34, 36, 38, 39, 42, 46, 47, 49, 58, 74, 75, 76, 77, 78, 79, 80, 81, 82, 83, 84, 85, 86, 87, 88, 89, 90, 91, 92, 93, 94, 95, 96, 97, 105, 111, 115, 116, 117, 120, 129, 131, 135, 154, 156, 157, 158, 162, 163, 164, 177, 178, 179, 186, 190, 191, 192, 196, 197, 198, 199, 219, 220, 222, 237, 238, 255, 258, 261, 263, 264, 265, 269, 270, 271, 272, 273, 274, 277, 278, 280, 281, 282, 283, 286, 291, 292, 307, 309, 310, 311, 312, 313, 314, 315, 316, 317, 318, 319, 320, 321, 322, 323, 327, 328, 329, 334, 335, 337, 338, 341, 343, 344, 345, 346, 347, 350, 352, 354, 355, 356, 357, 358, 359, 361
 alphabetical index, 38, 219
 base peak index, 38
 digital code, 38, 219
 internal standard, see Internal standard
 Kovats index, 39, 40, 180, 199, 219, 255, 343, 347, 377, 381
 mass fragmentography, see Multiple/specific ion (m/e) detection
 mass spectrum (CI, EI)/specific ions (m/e), 11, 13, 14, 15, 16, 21, 30, 34, 36, 38, 39, 42, 43, 44, 46, 47, 49, 58, 75, 77, 78, 81, 84, 85, 86, 87, 88, 89, 90, 91, 92, 93, 94, 95, 96, 97, 105, 115, 116, 117, 120, 131, 135, 156, 157, 158, 162, 163, 164, 178, 179, 186, 190, 191, 192, 193,

[Qualitative methods of analysis, by use of]
 [mass spectrum (CI, EI)/specific ions (m/e)], 196, 197, 198, 199, 219, 220, 237, 238, 255, 258, 263, 264, 269, 270, 271, 273, 274, 275, 277, 278, 281, 282, 283, 292, 301, 303, 305, 309, 311, 312, 313, 314, 315, 316, 317, 318, 319, 320, 321, 322, 323, 328, 329, 334, 335, 337, 338, 341, 343, 346, 347, 353, 354, 355, 356, 357, 358, 359, 361
 methylene unit value, 11, 12, 17
 molecular ion, 29, 30, 38, 39, 42, 43, 77, 85, 86, 88, 89, 92, 93, 96, 97, 116, 131, 156, 158, 164, 177, 179, 186, 190, 191, 192, 197, 198, 219, 237, 238, 277, 281, 283, 292, 301, 303, 304, 305, 335, 347, 353
 molecular weight, 21, 23, 30, 38, 38, 39, 85, 198, 219, 258, 305, 312, 329, 334, 353
 multiple/specific ion (m/e) detection, 58, 74, 75, 77, 78, 80, 81, 84, 85, 87, 90, 91, 92, 93, 94, 95, 105, 115, 117, 120, 154, 162, 163, 164, 167, 237, 238, 263, 264, 269, 270, 273, 274, 277, 278, 281, 282, 283, 292, 303, 304, 305, 311, 313, 314, 315, 316, 341, 354, 355, 356, 357, 358, 359
 retention index, see Kovats index
 relative retention time, 4, 5, 21, 22, 23, 27, 32, 36, 38, 39, 51, 102, 107, 132, 140, 142, 146, 148, 150, 154, 166, 167, 168, 180, 182, 196, 217, 219, 255, 323, 350, 351, 362
 retention time, 5, 6, 7, 8, 14, 17, 19, 20, 21, 22, 23, 25, 26,

[Qualitative methods of analysis, by use of]
 [retention time], 27, 28, 31, 32, 41, 42, 45, 48, 49, 52, 53, 58, 62, 67, 76, 81, 82, 83, 84, 94, 96, 97, 99, 103, 107, 118, 119, 123, 124, 125, 126, 128, 129, 131, 134, 135, 137, 138, 139, 140, 141, 143, 144, 145, 146, 147, 148, 149, 150, 151, 158, 161, 162, 164, 165, 166, 169, 170, 171, 172, 174, 176, 177, 178, 179, 180, 181, 182, 183, 184, 185, 186, 189, 190, 192, 193, 198, 200, 206, 207, 208, 212, 214, 215, 217, 222, 223, 224, 226, 227, 230, 231, 232, 234, 238, 259, 260, 263, 267, 269, 270, 272, 274, 277, 278, 283, 285, 286, 290, 291, 293, 295, 299, 300, 309, 311, 313, 315, 318, 319, 322, 323, 324, 325, 332, 334, 335, 337, 340, 345, 352, 353, 354, 357, 358, 359, 360, 365, 366, 367, 368, 369, 370, 371, 372, 373, 374, 377, 378, 379, 380, 381, 382
 specific ion detection, see Multiple/specific ion (m/e) detection
Quantitative methods of analysis, by use of
 calibration curve, 10, 26, 28, 29, 49, 52, 53, 54, 56, 62, 67, 70, 75, 78, 87, 97, 104, 126, 134, 141, 148, 151, 156, 158, 189, 200, 212, 214, 269, 272, 277, 278, 291, 293, 298, 300, 303, 305, 313, 314, 324, 334, 337, 341, 364, 382
 peak area measurements, 9, 27, 28, 29, 46, 62, 67, 75, 77, 86, 104, 106, 111, 126, 148,

[Quantitative methods of analysis, by use of]
 [peak area measurements], 158, 189, 212, 269, 293, 303, 305, 341, 364
 peak height measurements, 26, 41, 46, 49, 52, 53, 56, 86, 94, 97, 99, 134, 156, 186, 200, 214, 278, 291, 298, 313, 314, 324, 334, 341, 382
Quercitin, 179
 silyl derivative of, 179
Quinic acid, 178
 silyl derivative of, 178
Quinicine, see Quinotoxine
Quinidine, 32-47, 48, 80, 124
 detection limits of, 46
 half-life of, 35
 mass spectrum of, 37
 metabolite(s) of, 33, 34, 35, 36, 41
  mass spectra of, 37
  silyl derivative of, 33, 34, 36
  structures of some, 35
 methyl derivative of, 41, 42, 43, 44, 45, 46, 47
  fragmentation patterns of, 44
 pharmacokinetic data for, 35
 plasma profiles of, 42, 43
 plasma protein-binding of, 35
 recovery of, 41, 45
 renal clearance of, 35
 silyl derivative of, 33, 34, 36, 40, 41, 42
 structure of, 33
 therapeutic concentration of, 35
 thioglycerol adduct of, 42
 volume of distribution of, 35
Quinine, 32, 33, 36, 40, 42
 silyl derivative of, 40, 42
 structure of, 33
Quininone, 40, 42
 silyl derivative of, 40, 42
2'-Quinolone, 33

SUBJECT INDEX 441

Quinotoxine, 40, 42
  silyl derivative of, 40, 42

R

Rescinnamine, 257, 284-285
  alkaline hydrolysis product of,
      284, 285
  methyl derivative of, 284, 285
  structure of, 257
Reserpine, 233, 257, 284-285
  alkaline hydrolysis product of,
      284, 285
  methyl derivative of, 284, 285
  structure of, 257
Resorcinol, 143
  silyl derivative of, 143
Rhamnose, 4

S

Sapogenins, 4, 5, 6, 29, 30, 31
  correlation between structure and
      retention time, 4-6
  Fenugreek-type, 29, 30, 31
    silyl derivative of, 31
    structure of, 30
    trifluoroacetyl derivative of, 31
Sarasapogenin, 5
Scopolamine, 33
Scopoletin, 168, 169, 171, 172, 176,
    177, 179
  acetate derivative of, 168, 172
  silyl derivative of, 171, 176, 179
  structure of, 168
Scopolin, 175, 180, 181
  structure of, 175
Secobarbital, 80, 81, 309
Serotonin, 115
  silyl derivative of, 115
Serum glutamic oxaloacetic
    transaminase, 331
Seselin, 166, 167, 169, 172, 176,
    180, 181

[Seselin]
  structure of, 167
Smilagenin, 5, 6
Sodium acetate, 221
Sodium bicarbonate, 49, 62, 157,
    205, 270, 272, 273
Sodium bisulfite, 124
Sodium carbonate, 49, 55, 129,
    277, 281
Sodium chloride, 67, 141, 336,
    345
Sodium citrate, 124
Sodium dihydrogen phosphate, 76,
    231, 288
Sodium edetate, 124
Sodium hydroxide, 27, 43, 45, 55,
    56, 67, 74, 76, 94, 122, 126,
    132, 151, 161, 186, 205, 212,
    215, 217, 223, 234, 259, 263,
    269, 272, 285, 296, 297, 336,
    343, 351
Sodium nitrite, 156, 258, 259, 261,
    263
Sodium sulfate, 126, 129, 143, 146,
    150, 157, 209, 217, 218, 224,
    263
Sodium thiosulfate, 380
Sodium valproate, 106, 107
  methyl derivative of, 106, 107
Sphondin, 166, 168, 169, 170, 172,
    173, 177
  structure of, 168
Spironolactone, 194, 196, 199,
    215-218, 233
  metabolism of, 215, 216
  structure of, 196, 216
Squalene, 370
Stearic acid, 83, 84
  methyl derivative of, 83,
      84
G-Strophanthidin, 4
2-Substituted-4-monochlorodi-
    fluoromethyl-2,6-diamino-
    1,3,5-triazines, 336

Sulfanilamide, 194, 195, 197
  structure of, 195
Sulfonylureas, 288-332
  N-methyl derivative of, 317, 320
  N-methyl/heptafluorobutyryl
    derivative of, 320
  N-methyl/pentafluoropropionyl
    derivative of, 320
  N-methylperfluoroacetyl derivative of, 317, 318, 320
  M-methyl/trifluoroacetyl derivative of, 320
  structures of common, 289
Sulfur dioxide, 313, 317
Sulfuric acid, 122, 224, 362, 381

T

Taurocholic acid, 221
  ^{14}C-labeled, 221
Temperature programming (GC), 7, 11, 12, 14, 17, 21, 23, 25, 31, 45, 46, 67, 70, 81, 82, 83, 84, 97, 99, 102, 103, 106, 123, 144, 159, 178, 179, 197, 198, 220, 222, 231, 263, 272, 315, 316, 328, 332, 360, 365, 366, 367, 370, 371, 372, 374, 380
Δ^1-Testololactone, 217
Tetrabutylammonium hydroxide, 94
3,3',5,5'-Tetrachlorothyronine, 359, 360, 361
  heptafluorobutyryl derivative of, 359, 360, 361
  methyl derivative of, 359, 360, 361
  methyl/heptafluorobutyryl derivative of, 359, 360, 361
  structure of, 360, 361
Tetracosane, 83
4-(α, α, β, β-Tetrafluorophenethyl)benzylamine, 128
  structure of, 128

[4-(α, α, β, β-Tetrafluorophenethyl)benzylamine]
  trifluoroacetyl derivative of, 128
Tetrahexylammonium hydroxide sulfate, 205, 208, 212
Tetrahydrofuran, 76, 369
Tetrahydroisoquinoline, 270, 271
  trifluoroacetyl derivative of, 270, 271
  structure of, 271
Tetraiodothyroacetic acid, 351
  methyl derivative of, 351
3,3',5,5'-Tetraiodothyronine, see Thyronine
Tetramethylammonium hydroxide, 105, 106, 200, 209, 210, 231
Tetrapropylammonium hydroxide, 382
Tetrazolo-(1,5-a)phthalazine, 256, 259, 261, 263, 264
  recovery of, 263
  structure of, 258
Thebaine, 33
Theobromine, 195
Theophylline, 152, 195, 197
Thermal conductivity detector (GC), 137, 140, 165, 174, 177
Thionyl chloride, 18, 359
Thyroid hormones, 343-383
  derivatization of, 345-380
    intermediates of, 348-349, 350, 374-379
    structures of, 348-349, 375-377
  methyl/N,O-dipivalyl derivative of, 345, 359-369
  methyl/heptafluorobutyryl derivative of, 345, 352-359, 361
  methyl/methoxy derivative of, 345-351
  methyl/trifluoroacetyl derivative of, 345, 351-352

SUBJECT INDEX 443

[Thyroid hormones]
  [derivatization of]
    silyl derivative of, 345, 369-380
Thyronine, 344, 348, 350, 365,
    370, 371, 374, 377, 380
  detection limits of, 380
  methyl derivative of, 365
  methyl/dipivalyl derivative of, 365
  pivalyl derivative of, 365
  silyl derivative of, 370, 371, 374,
    377
  structure of, 348
Thyroxine, 344, 345, 348, 350, 351,
    352, 353, 354, 357, 359, 360,
    361, 362, 363, 365, 366, 367,
    368, 369, 370, 371, 372, 373,
    374, 377, 380, 381
  detection limits of, 351, 353, 354,
    367, 372, 373, 380
  heptafluorobutyryl derivative of,
    353, 354, 359, 360, 361
  methyl derivative of, 345, 351,
    352, 353, 354, 359, 360, 361,
    362, 365, 366, 367, 368, 369
  methyl/heptafluorobutyryl derivative of, 353, 354, 359, 360,
    361
    structure of, 360
  methyl/methoxy derivative of, 345,
    351
  methyl/pivalyl derivative of, 359,
    360, 362, 365, 366, 367, 368,
    369
    structure of, 360, 362
  methyl/trifluoroacetyl derivative
    of, 351, 352, 366, 367
  pivalyl derivative of, 359, 360,
    362, 365, 366, 367, 368, 369
  recovery of, 353, 380
  silyl derivative of, 369, 370, 371,
    372, 373, 374, 377, 380, 381
  structure of, 348, 362
  trifluoroacetyl derivative of, 351,
    352, 366, 367

Tienilic acid, 213-215
  detection limits of, 214, 215
  half-life of, 215
  methyl derivative of, 214, 215
  recovery of, 214
Tigogenin, 5, 6, 30, 31
  silyl derivative of, 31
  structure of, 30
  trifluoroacetyl derivative of, 31
Tolazamide, 289, 290, 291, 292,
    309, 316, 317, 318, 319, 323
  detection limits of, 290, 291
  half-life of, 291
  methyl derivative of, 309, 316,
    317, 318, 319, 323
    deuterated, 317
  methyl/heptafluorobutyryl derivative of, 316, 317, 318, 319,
    323
  methyl/pentafluoropropionyl
    derivative of, 316, 317, 318,
    319, 323
  methyl/trifluoroacetyl derivative
    of, 316, 317, 318, 319, 323
  pharmacokinetic data for, 291
  recovery of, 290, 291, 309
  structure of, 289
  thermal degradation of, 291
Tolazoline, 277
Tolbutamide, 55, 288, 289, 290,
    292, 293, 295, 296, 297, 298,
    301, 302, 303, 304, 305, 306,
    307, 308, 309, 310, 311, 312,
    313, 314, 315, 316, 317, 318,
    319, 320, 321, 322, 323, 324,
    325, 326, 328, 330, 332
  detection limits of, 298, 301, 315,
    319
  deuterated, 301, 303, 304, 305
  evaporation profile of, 304, 305
  methyl derivative of, 301, 303,
    304, 305
  structure of, 305
  half-life of, 301, 306, 307, 308, 330

[Tolbutamide]
  metabolites of, 293, 296, 297,
    298, 299, 300, 301, 302, 303,
    309, 310, 315
  methyl derivative of, 288, 290,
    292, 293, 301, 303, 304, 305,
    308, 309, 310, 311, 312, 313,
    314, 315, 316, 317, 318, 319,
    320, 321, 322, 323, 328
    deuterated, 317
    evaporation profile of, 304, 305
    pyrolysis of, 293, 328
    structure of, 293
  methyl enol ether of, 323
  methyl/heptafluorobutyryl derivative of, 316, 317, 318, 319,
    320, 321, 323
  methyl/pentafluoropropionyl
    derivative of, 316, 317, 318,
    319, 320, 321, 323
  methyl/trifluoroacetyl derivative
    of, 309, 310, 311, 312, 313,
    314, 315, 316, 317, 318, 319,
    320, 321, 323
    structure of, 312
  pharmacokinetic data for, 301,
    302, 303, 306, 307, 308, 325,
    326, 330
  plasma clearance of, 326, 330
  protein-binding of, 325, 326, 331
  reaction product with 2,4-dinitrofluorobenzene, 296
  recovery of, 290, 293, 309, 324
  saliva/plasma concentration of
    unbound, 307
    equation for, 307
  structure of, 289
  total plasma concentration of, 307
  trifluoroacetyl derivative of, 309,
    310, 311, 312, 313, 314, 315,
    316, 317, 318, 319, 320, 321
    323
  two-compartment model for,
    307

[Tolbutamide]
  volume of distribution of, 308,
    325, 330
Toluene, 101, 231, 232, 259, 268,
  273, 307, 319, 353
p-Toluenesulfonamide, 291, 292
  structure of, 291
N-(p-Toluenesulfonyl)-N'-
  [azabicyclo(3.3.0)octyl]urea,
  327, 328, 329
  degradation pathways of, 327,
    328, 329
  products of, 327, 329
Total ion current, 311, 313, 314,
  315, 316, 356, 358
Triacetin, 143
Triamterene, 195, 197, 198, 199
  structure of, 195
s-Triazolo(3,4-a)phthalazine, 260,
  262, 263, 264, 265
  recovery of, 263
  structure of, 262
Trichloroacetic acid, 336
Trichloromethiazide, 196
Trichlorophenoxypropionic acid,
  235
  methyl ester of, 235
C-3-Trideuteromethyldiazoxide,
  see Diazoxide, deuterated
Triethylamine, 87, 343, 359, 367
Triethylene glycol dinitrate, 137,
  140, 141, 142
Trifluoroacetic anhydride, 31, 122,
  128, 135, 162, 268, 269, 309,
  310, 317, 340, 343, 351, 366
4,5,7-Trihydroxycoumarin, 172,
  173, 176
  silyl derivative of, 172, 176
  structure of, 173
3,3',5-Triiodothyronine, 348, 350,
  351, 352, 353, 354, 356, 357,
  358, 359, 360, 361, 362, 363,
  364, 365, 366, 367, 368, 369,
  370, 371, 372, 373, 374, 377,

SUBJECT INDEX

[3,3',5-Triiodothyronine], 380, 381
  detection limits of, 353, 354, 366, 367, 372, 373, 380
  heptafluorobutyryl derivative of, 353, 354, 356, 358, 359, 360, 361
  methyl derivative of, 350, 351, 352, 353, 354, 356, 358, 359, 360, 361, 362, 364, 365, 366, 367, 368, 369
  methyl/heptafluorobutyryl derivative of, 353, 354, 356, 358, 359, 360, 361
    structure of, 360
  methyl/methoxy derivative of, 350
  methyl/pivalyl derivative of, 360, 362, 364, 365, 366, 367, 368, 369
  methyl/trifluoroacetyl derivative of, 351, 352, 366, 367
  pivalyl derivative of, 360, 362, 364, 365, 366, 367, 368, 369
  recovery of, 353, 367, 380
  silyl derivative of, 369, 370, 371, 372, 373, 374, 377, 380, 381
  structure of, 348
  trifluoroacetyl derivative of, 351, 352, 366, 367
3,3',5'-Triiodothyronine, 348, 350, 353, 354, 356, 357, 358, 359, 360, 361, 369, 370, 374, 377, 380, 381
  detection limits of, 353, 354, 380
  heptafluorobutyryl derivative of, 353, 354, 356, 358, 359, 360, 361
  methyl derivative of, 353, 354, 356, 358, 359, 360, 361
  methyl/heptafluorobutyryl derivative of, 353, 354, 356, 358, 359, 360, 361
    structure of, 360
  recovery of, 353

[3,3',5'-Triiodothyronine]
  silyl derivative of, 369, 370, 374, 377, 380, 381
  structure of, 348
Triiodotyrosine, 344
Trimethadione, 94
Trimethylamine, 122, 365
Trimethylanilinium hydroxide, 41, 45, 96, 97, 99, 101, 102, 109, 111, 192, 200, 206, 209, 210, 232, 278, 308, 309
Trimethylchlorosilane, 6, 11, 14, 17, 21, 27, 33, 143, 171, 181, 221, 263, 353, 369, 370, 372, 373
Trimethylsilylimidazole, 11, 14, 123, 221
Tri-O-methyl-wedelo-lactone, 175, 180, 182
  structure of, 175
Tryptamine, 115
  silyl derivative of, 115
Tyramine, 115
  silyl derivative of, 115
Tyrosine, 344, 348, 350, 360, 369, 370, 371, 373, 374
  detection limits of, 373
  methyl derivative of, 360
  methyl/pivalyl derivative of, 360
  pivalyl derivative of, 360
  silyl derivative of, 369, 370, 371, 373, 374
  structure of, 348

U

Umbelliferone, 168, 169, 172, 176, 177, 178
  acetate derivative of, 168, 172
  silyl derivative of, 176, 178
  structure of, 168
Umbelliprenin, 166
Urea, 65, 66
  dialytic clearance of, 65

V

δ-Valerolactam-^{15}N, 163
Vanillic acid, 178
  silyl derivative of, 178
Vanillin, 178
  silyl derivative of, 178
Vitamin A, 344
Vitamin B$_6$, 230

W

Warfarin, 169, 180, 182, 183, 184, 185, 186, 189, 190
  acetyl derivative of, 183, 184
  detection limits of, 184
  metabolism of, 186
  methyl derivative of, 186
  pentafluorobenzyl derivative of, 183, 184
  protein-binding of, 186, 189
  recovery of, 186
  silyl derivative of, 182, 183, 184
  structure of, 183
  total body clearance of, 189
  trichloroacetyl derivative of, 183, 184
  trifluoroacetyl derivative of, 183, 184

X

Xanthotoxin, 168, 169, 172, 177, 180, 181
  structure of, 168
Xanthyletin, 172, 173, 176, 180, 181
  structure of, 173

Y

Yamogenin, 5, 30, 31
  silyl derivative of, 31
  structure of, 30
  trifluoroacetyl derivative of, 31
YC-93, 154, 155, 156
  ^{14}C-labeled, 156
  detection limits of, 154, 156
  mass spectrum of, 156
  nitrous acid oxidation of, 154, 156
  pyridine analog of, 154, 156
    mass spectrum of, 156
    structure of, 156
  recovery of, 156
  structure of, 155, 156
Yuccagenin, 5, 30, 31
  silyl derivative of, 31
  structure of, 30
  trifluoroacetyl derivative of, 31

DATE DUE			
AUG 0 9 2005			
AUG 0 9 2005			

DEMCO 38-297